Proteases and Their Inhibitors in Cancer Metastasis

Cancer Metastasis – Biology and Treatment

VOLUME 4

Series Editors

Richard J. Ablin, *Ph.D.*, *Innapharma, Inc., Park Ridge, NJ, U.S.A.*
Wen G. Jiang, *M.D.*, *University of Wales College of Medicine, Cardiff, U.K.*

Advisory Editorial Board

Harold F. Dvorak, *M.D.*
Phil Gold, *M.D.*, *Ph.D.*
Ian R. Hart, *Ph.D.*
Hiroshi Kobayashi, *M.D.*
Robert E. Mansel, *M.S.*, *FRCS.*
Marc Mareel, *M.D.*, *Ph.D.*

Titles published in this Series are:

Volume 1: Cancer Metastasis, Molecular and Cellular Mechanisms and
Clinical Intervention.

Editors: Wen G. Jiang and Robert E. Mansel.
ISBN 0-7923-6395-7

Volume 2: Growth Factors and Receptors in Cancer Metastasis.

Editors: Wen G. Jiang, Kunio Matsumoto and Toshikazu Nakamura.
ISBN 0-7923-7141-0

Volume 3: Cancer Metastasis-Related Genes

Editor: Danny R. Welch
ISBN 0-4020-0522-9

Proteases and Their Inhibitors in Cancer Metastasis

Edited by

Jean-Michel Foidart
Laboratoire de Biologie des Tumeurs et du Développement,
Faculté de Médecine Université de Liège, Belgium

and

Ruth J. Muschel
Department of Pathology & Laboratory Medicine,
University of Pennsylvania, U.S.A.

KLUWER ACADEMIC PUBLISHERS
DORDRECHT / BOSTON / LONDON

A C.I.P. Catalogue record for this book is available from the Library of Congress.

ISBN 1-4020-0923-2

Published by Kluwer Academic Publishers,
P.O. Box 17, 3300 AA Dordrecht, The Netherlands.

Sold and distributed in North, Central and South America
by Kluwer Academic Publishers,
101 Philip Drive, Norwell, MA 02061, U.S.A.

In all other countries, sold and distributed
by Kluwer Academic Publishers,
P.O. Box 322, 3300 AH Dordrecht, The Netherlands.

Printed on acid-free paper

TABLE OF CONTENTS

Chapter 1

MOLECULAR BIOLOGY OF THE PLASMINOGEN SYSTEM: THE DELICATE BALANCE BETWEEN TISSUE HEALING AND TISSUE DESTRUCTION

A. Luttun and P. Carmeliet
The Center for Transgene Technology and Gene Therapy, Flanders Interuniversity Institute for Biotechnology, Campus Gasthuisberg, Herestraat 49, University of Leuven, Leuven, B-3000, Belgium

Abstract
Proteinases play a central role in the complex response of tissues to injury by influencing cellular behavior and matrix remodeling. Considerable information on the biology of proteinases has been derived from gene targeting and gene transfer studies. One of the best characterised proteinase systems is the plasminogen system, belonging to the large serine proteinase family. Using mice with a targeted deficiency of plasminogen system components, it has become obvious that the plasminogen system can – directly or indirectly by activation of matrix metalloproteinases – have divergent – even opposite – roles in disease favoring healing in some cases and promoting tissue destruction in others. This Chapter discusses the mechanisms by which the plasminogen system can influence the response to injury in the vessel wall, the heart, the nervous system, the lungs and the skin.

1. INTRODUCTION

Genetic studies have provided important insights in proteinase biology. Although most of these proteinases seem dispensable during development, they have been implicated in numerous diseases often having divergent – even opposite – effects. One of the main reasons for this diversity is that proteinases can affect disease progression by different mechanisms, i.e. by influencing cellular migration, cytokine activation, extracellular matrix turnover, growth factor availability and blood vessel formation. These functions need to be carefully balanced. Consequently, the biological activity of proteinases is tightly regulated at the level of gene transcription as well as the protein level by latency of the proenzyme and by the existence of proteinase inhibitors and cellular receptors.

The group of proteinases comprises four different families based on the nature of the chemical group responsible for catalytic activity: the serine, cysteine,

1

J.-M. Foidart and R.J. Muschel (eds.), Proteases and Their Inhibitors in Cancer Metastasis, 1–22.
© 2002 *Kluwer Academic Publishers. Printed in the Netherlands.*

aspartic and metalloproteinases (Barrett, 1992). This Chapter focuses on a serine proteinase family, e.g. the plasminogen system, which plays a major role in physiologic and pathologic processes including blood coagulation, tumor growth and metastasis, cardiovascular disease and wound healing.

The plasminogen system (reviewed in Collen, 1999; Wiman, 2000) is composed of an inactive proenzyme plasminogen (Plg) that can be converted to plasmin by either of two plasminogen activators (PAs), tissue-type PA (t-PA) or urokinase-type PA (u-PA) (Collen and Lijnen, 1991; Vassalli et al, 1991). This system is controlled at the level of plasminogen activators by plasminogen activator inhibitors (PAIs), of which PAI-1 is believed to be physiologically the most important (Schneiderman et al, 1991; Wiman, 1995), and at the level of plasmin by α_2-antiplasmin (directly inhibiting plasmin) (Collen and Lijnen, 1991). Due to its fibrin-specificity, t-PA is primarily involved in clot dissolution (Collen and Lijnen, 1991; Vassalli et al, 1991). u-PA binds a cellular receptor (u-PAR) and has been implicated in cell migration and tissue remodeling (Blasi et al, 1994; Vassalli, 1994). The lipoprotein-like receptor protein (LRP) mediates rapid clearance of t-PA from plasma (Noorman and Rijken, 1997). Plasmin is able to degrade fibrin and extracellular matrix proteins directly or, indirectly, via activation of other proteinases (such as the matrix metalloproteinases or MMPs) (Carmeliet et al, 1997a; Saksela and Rifkin, 1988). Plasmin can also activate or liberate growth factors from the extracellular matrix (Saksela and Rifkin, 1988; Martin et al, 1993).

Over the last decade, mice deficient of one of the plasminogen system components have been generated (Carmeliet et al, 1993a, b, 1994; Dewerchin et al, 1996; Lijnen et al, 1999a; Ploplis et al, 1995) allowing to directly study their role in disease. Not only have these studies emphasized the complex and pleiotropic nature of this system, they also revealed that the same system can promote opposite processes like tissue healing and tissue destruction. This Chapter documents the involvement of plasminogen system components in healing and/or destruction processes in several tissues, including the vessel wall, the heart, the nervous system, the lung and the skin, as unveiled by gene targeting and gene transfer studies (Figure 1). Given the possibility that plasmin mediates some of its effects through activation of MMPs, genetic studies with MMPs will also be discussed where appropriate. The role of the plasminogen system in tumor growth and metastasis is reviewed in Chapter 2.

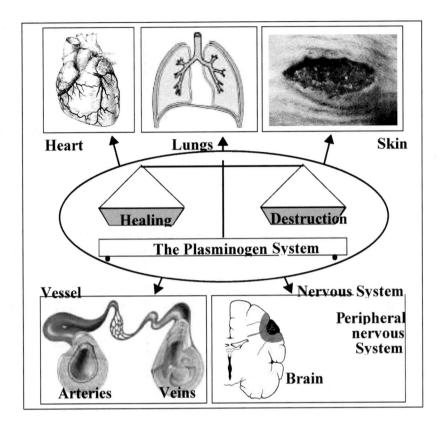

Figure 1. Role of the plasminogen system in tissue healing and destruction.

2. THE VESSEL WALL

2.1. Systemic arteries

2.1.1. *Arterial stenosis*

Vascular interventions for the treatment of atherothrombosis (balloon angio-plasty, stenting) induce restenosis of the vessel within three to six months in 30 to 50% of treated patients. Arterial stenosis may result from remodeling of the vessel wall and/or from accumulation of cells and extracellular matrix in the intimal layer. Proteinases participate in the proliferation and migration of smooth muscle cells (SMCs), and in the matrix remodeling during arterial wound healing. In a mouse model of arterial wound healing we demonstrated that u-PA but not t-PA mediates vascular wound healing and arterial neointima formation, as indicated by the significantly reduced degree and rate of arterial

3

neointima formation in u-PA-deficient mice 4 to 6 weeks after electric injury, most likely due to impairment of cellular migration. Neointima formation was not affected in u-PAR-deficient mice, indicating that, in this model, effects of u-PA were independent of u-PA binding to its receptor. Plasminogen deficiency reduced neointima formation, indicating that the effects of u-PA were mediated through plasminogen activation (for references, see Carmeliet and Collen, 2000). Consistent with the latter observations, absence of plasminogen reduced neointimal area in a recent study, although the effects on adventitial area seemed more dramatic (Busuttil et al, 2000). Surprisingly, α_2-antiplasmin, the major inhibitor of plasmin, does not play an essential role in SMC migration and neointima formation during arterial wound healing, as demonstrated by the comparable results obtained with α_2-antiplasmin-deficient and wild-type mice (Lijnen et al, 2000). Neointima formation after electric or mechanical injury in the carotid artery was accelerated in PAI-1-deficient arteries and could be inhibited by adenoviral gene transfer of human PAI-1 (Carmeliet et al, 1997b). However, using another model of injury (copper-induced injury leading to substantial fibrin deposition), Ploplis et al (2001) found that PAI-1 deficiency protected against neointima formation. Whereas in the electric or mechanical injury model neointima formation was apparently more dependent on proteolysis-mediated cell migration, the incorporation of substantial amounts of fibrin (of which removal was delayed in the presence of PAI-1) after copper-induced injury might have contributed more importantly to neointima formation. In addition, gene targeting and gene transfer studies have suggested differential roles for MMPs in arterial response to injury. Indeed, overexpression of MMP-9, achieved by seeding of stably transfected SMCs after balloon denudation enhanced SMC migration and altered post-injury vessel remodeling by thinning of the vessel wall and decreasing intimal matrix content (Mason et al, 1999). MMP-11 seemed to impair elastin degradation and cellular migration after electrical injury of the femoral artery, as derived from a study with MMP-11-deficient mice (Lijnen et al, 1999b). Genetic studies with TIMP-1 suggested a role for MMPs in promoting intimal hyperplasia, as TIMP-1 deficiency increased neointima formation after electric injury of the femoral artery (Lijnen et al, 1999c).

2.1.2. *Allograft transplant stenosis*
Accelerated coronary arteriosclerosis is an important limitation to long-term survival of patients with heart transplantation. The role of the plasminogen system in allograft transplant stenosis was studied using a mouse model of transplant arteriosclerosis that mimics in many ways the accelerated arteriosclerosis in coronary arteries of transplanted cardiac allografts in man. In this model, host-derived leukocytes adhere to and infiltrate beneath the endothelium and

form a predominantly leukocyte-rich neointima within 15 days after transplantation, whereas at later times, SMCs, derived from the donor graft, accumulate in the neointima. The role of leukocyte adhesion in the pathogenesis of transplant arteriosclerosis was recently highlighted by reduced neointimal lesions in mice deficient of intercellular adhesion molecule-1 (ICAM-1) (Dietrich et al, 2000). Since previous targeting studies had shown that migration of leukocytes and SMCs is dependent on plasmin proteolysis, carotid arteries from B.10A (2R) wild-type mice were transplanted in C57Bl/6:129 plasminogen-deficient or wild-type recipient mice. Graft arteriosclerosis was largely prevented in plasminogen-deficient recipients due to the inability of inflammatory cells to infiltrate the media and of SMCs to migrate into the intima. Fragmentation of the elastic laminae and neoadventitia formation were less severe in plasminogen-deficient than in wild-type mice, where significantly increased expression of MMPs was measured during active cell migration. Since plasmin can directly degrade some but not all matrix components in the media, it presumably activates other matrix degrading proteinases, most probably of the MMP family, that then contribute to extracellular matrix degradation (Moons et al, 1998).

2.1.3. Atherosclerosis

Atherosclerosis initiates with the formation of fatty streaks containing predominantly lipid filled macrophages and SMCs. These lesions subsequently develop to more advanced plaques consisting of a central core of lipids and necrotic material, which is covered by a fibrous cap of fibrillar collagen. Atherosclerosis often remains asymptomatic. However, complications like plaque rupture may lead to the formation of an occluding thrombus and can suddenly trigger myocardial infarction and stroke – clinical syndromes with a high morbidity and mortality. In addition, extracellular matrix breakdown in the atherosclerotic wall may lead to aneurysmal dilatation and eventually rupture of the vessel wall, causing fatal bleeding. The pathogenetic mechanisms contributing to plaque progression and complications like plaque rupture and aneurysm formation remain still incompletely defined.

Indirect evidence for a role of the plasminogen system components and MMPs was indicated by elevated levels of u-PA, t-PA, PAI-1 (Schneider et al, 1997) and several MMPs and their inhibitors in atherosclerotic lesions (reviewed in George, 1998). This is further underscored by findings that genetic polymorphisms in the promotor of several of these proteinases influence the atherosclerotic phenotype. Such genetic variants have been described for PAI-1, MMP-9 and MMP-3 (Dawson et al, 1991; Ye et al, 1996; Zhang et al, 1999). Conclusive evidence for a precipitating role of these factors in atherosclerosis *in vivo* is mostly lacking, as homozygous deficiencies for these proteinases are extremely rare in humans. However, atherosclerosis can be studied in the atherosclerosis-prone apolipoprotein E (apoE) or low density lipoprotein (LDL) receptor-deficient mice combined with a deficiency of one of the plasminogen or MMP system components.

Plaque progression. Gene targeting of plasminogen system components and MMPs in plaque growth have yielded conflicting results. In previous studies in mice with a combined deficiency of plasminogen and apoE, plaque growth was accelerated (Xiao et al, 1997), whereas in our studies, no differences in size or predilection site of early fatty streaks and more advanced plaques were observed between mice with a single deficiency of apoE and mice with a combined deficiency of apoE with t-PA or u-PA (Carmeliet et al, 1997a). Recent studies reported that combined PAI-1 and apoE deficiency did not alter plaque size in the aortic root, but significantly decreased plaque size at the carotid bifurcation (Eitzman et al, 2000; Sjoland et al, 2000). In contrast, our findings indicated a consistent increase in lesion size throughout the arterial tree in apoE$^{-/-}$:PAI-1$^{-/-}$ mice (Luttun et al, 2002). Whereas a broad-spectrum MMP inhibitor had no effect on the extent of atherosclerosis in one study (Prescott et al, 1999), another study in apoE-deficient mice reported reduction of ather-osclerotic lesions by adenoviral gene transfer of TIMP-1 (Rouis et al, 1999). These apparent contradictory findings suggest that atherosclerosis studies in knockout mice may be influenced by differences in genetic background, the type of diet or the method of analysis. For instance, PAI-1 may stimulate plaque growth by stimulating the incorporation of fibrin because it impairs fibrin breakdown. This probably occurred in the studies of Eitzman et al (2000) and Ploplis et al (2001) which both documented substantial fibrin(ogen) immunos-taining in the lesions. In contrast, PAI-1 may reduce plaque growth by inhibiting the plasmin-mediated release and activation of fibrogenic growth factors, thereby reducing extracellular matrix deposition in the plaques (Luttun et al, 2002). Collagen deposition was also reduced in the ischemic myocardium of u-PA-deficient mice, because of decreased activation of transforming growth factor-β1 (TGF-β1) (Heymans et al, 1999). The discrepant results concerning the role of PAI-1 in mouse models could reflect and extend the conflicting results that have been reported on PAI-1 as a risk factor for ischemic heart disease in humans. Indeed, elevated PAI-1 plasma levels correlated with an increased risk for ischemic heart disease in middle-aged patients with athero-sclerosis (Cortellaro et al, 1993) or a previous myocardial infarction (Hamsten et al, 1987), but not in other individuals (Cuzner et al, 1999; Jansson et al, 1991) or after correction for insulin resistance (Juhan-Vague et al, 1996).

Aneurysm formation. Significant genotypic differences were observed in the integrity of the atherosclerotic aortic wall. Indeed, destruction of the media with resultant erosion, transmedial ulceration, necrosis of medial SMCs, aneurysmal dilatation and rupture of the vessel wall were more prevalent and severe in mice lacking apoE or apoE:t-PA than in mice lacking apoE:u-PA (Carmeliet et al, 1997a). Macrophages only infiltrated the media of atherosclerotic arteries after destruction of elastin fibers. Plaque macrophages (and especially those infiltrating into the media) expressed abundant amounts of u-PA similar as in patients. Since plasmin itself is unable to degrade insoluble elastin or fibrillar collagen, it most likely activated other matrix proteinases, such as the MMPs. Wild- type and t-PA-deficient but not u-PA-deficient cultured macrophages activated secreted proMMP-3, proMMP-9, proMMP-12 and proMMP-13 but only in the presence of plasminogen, indicating that u-PA-generated plasmin was responsible for activation of these proMMPs. These plasmin-activatable metalloproteinases co-localised with u-PA in plaque macrophages. Another possible mechanism of action of plasmin is that it mediates degradation of glycoproteins in the stroma of the aortic wall, thereby exposing the highly insoluble elastin to elastases and facilitating elastolysis *in vivo*. Taken together, these results implicate an important role of u-PA in the structural integrity of the atherosclerotic vessel wall, likely via triggering activation of MMPs. A gene transfer study revealed that local overexpression of TIMP-1 in a rat aneurysm model prevents aneurysm degeneration and rupture (Allaire et al, 1998). In LDL receptor-deficient mice, aortic medial elastin degradation was reduced using a broad-spectrum MMP inhibitor (Prescott et al, 1999). However, direct proof of how and which MMPs are involved in media destruction, aneurysm formation and atherosclerotic lesion formation requires further analysis in mice that are deficient of one of these MMPs. A recent study revealed that loss of MMP-9 partially protected mice against aneurysmal dilatation of the aorta after elastase perfusion (Pyo et al, 2000). Surprisingly, single loss of MMP-12 had no effect, while combined loss of both MMP-9 and MMP-12 further protected mice. Since rupture of aneurysms in this non-atherosclerotic model does not occur, the role of these MMPs as well as of others (interstitial collagenases) remains to be defined (Carmeliet, 2000).

2.2. Pulmonary arteries

Pulmonary arteries exhibit significant structural changes in response to hypoxia (Thompson et al, 1993) or after induction of endothelial injury (Ghodsi and Will, 1981). These changes involve progressive medial thickening of the distal pulmonary arteries by accumulation of SMCs and deposition of matrix and may lead to the development of pulmonary hypertension and eventually to right heart hypertrophy and failure. The molecular mechanisms underlying these vascular changes are only partly understood. Proteinases, like the serine proteinase endogenous vascular elastase (EVE) (Cowan et al, 2000; Todorovich-Hunter et al, 1992), plasminogen activators (Bansal et al, 1997; Pinsky et al, 1998) and MMPs (Cowan et al, 1999) have been implicated in this process by their increased expression.

Several recent studies have investigated the role of these proteinases using gene targeting and gene transfer approaches. Mice with a deficiency of plasminogen, t-PA, u-PA, or its receptor u-PAR and their wild-type littermates were exposed to hypoxia for four weeks (Levi et al, 2001). Right ventricular pressure increased 2.5-fold in wild-type mice and t-PA-deficient mice, but not in mice with a deficiency of plasminogen or u-PA. Accordingly, right ventricular weight was significantly increased in wild-type and t-PA-deficient mice, whereas no such increase was seen in absence of u-PA or plasminogen. Increased medial thickness (by SMC accumulation) was measured in wild-type and t-PA-deficient mice, but not in u-PA or plasminogen-deficient mice. Interestingly, elastic lamina fragmentation, a known feature of pulmonary vascular remodeling (Rabinovitch, 1998), was evident in wild-type mice but not in u-PA or plasminogen-deficient mice, suggesting that SMC proliferation was dependent on u-PA through plasmin-mediated breakdown of elastic membranes. As plasmin is not able to degrade elastin, elastin breakdown is likely to involve plasmin-mediated activation of elastolytic MMPs. Consistent with this, wild-type mice had increased MMP-9 activity. u-PAR-deficient mice showed an intermediate response indicating that the effects of u-PA are in part dependent on its receptor. The vascular changes in wild-type mice were associated with right ventricular remodeling (as evidenced by cardiomyocyte hypertrophy and increased collagen content), but u-PA deficiency completely protected against hypoxia-induced remodeling. Together these findings implicate an essential role for u-PA (not t-PA) mediated plasmin generation in the development of the pulmonary response to hypoxia and associated pulmonary hypertension and right heart hypertrophy.

In another study (Vieillard-Baron et al, 2000), inhibition of metalloproteinases by TIMP-1 gene transfer or doxycycline was found to aggravate hypoxia-induced pulmonary hypertension in rats, suggesting that MMPs are protective. The precise reason for these different results remains unknown. Possibly, as demonstrated in systemic arteries (see above), individual MMPs may have differential roles in the response of the pulmonary vessels to injury. Conclusive evidence for a role of single MMPs in pulmonary hypertension will require studies in mice deficient of one of the MMP members. Other proteinases have also been involved in pulmonary hypertension by affecting SMC proliferation and migration. For instance, inhibition of the serine elastase EVE resulted in complete reversal of fatal monocrotaline-induced pulmonary hypertension in rats (Cowan et al, 2000).

2.3. Veins

Coronary artery bypass surgery is a frequent intervention in patients with multivessel coronary artery disease. Although arterial grafts are preferred, the saphenous vein is still used because of several advantages such as convenient harvesting and sufficient yield of graft material. However, the rate of vein graft failure is 30% to 50% within 10 years (Campeau et al, 1983), due to the combined effects of thrombosis, intimal hyperplasia and graft atherosclerosis.

The role of plasminogen in intimal hyperplasia after vein grafting was recently studied in plasminogen-deficient mice, using a model that reproduces many features of the human saphenous vein graft (Shi et al, 1999). Implantation of a vein segment on the carotid artery caused substantial intimal hyperplasia in both wild-type and plasminogen-deficient mice, but no significant differences in the extent of neointima formation were detected between both genotypes. This lack of effect is in contrast with the reduced neointima formation observed after arterial injury in plasminogen-deficient mice (Carmeliet et al, 1997c). The most likely explanation for this is the absence of well-developed elastic laminae in veins, which constitute an important barrier for SMC migration in arteries. This hypothesis is further underscored by findings that inflammatory and smooth muscle cells can only cross degraded elastic laminae in athero-sclerotic plaques or transplanted allografts (see above).

3. THE HEART

More than 1.5 million people suffer acute myocardial infarction (AMI) annually in the United States alone. About 30% of them die within the first 24 hours, due to arrhythmias or pump failure. Cardiac rupture has been reported to account for 5 to 31% of in-hospital mortality after AMI. Both plasminogen activators and MMPs have been implicated in coronary or myocardial remodeling after AMI (Carmeliet and Collen, 2000), but their precise role and their involve-ment in cardiac rupture still is unclear. A combination of gene-inactivation and gene transfer techniques in mice was applied to address these issues, using a model for AMI based on ligation of the left anterior descending coronary artery (Heymans et al, 1999).

3.1. Cardiac rupture

In male mice, cardiac rupture after AMI was observed in 30% of wild-type mice and in 30% of mice lacking t-PA, u-PAR, MMP-3 or MMP-12. In contrast, deficiency of u-PA completely protected against rupture, while lack of MMP-9 partially protected against cardiac rupture. A close correlation was observed between the number of neutrophils infiltrating the infarcts and rupture. Further, these inflammatory cells produced increased levels of u-PA and MMPs. Thus, neutrophils require proteinases to migrate into the infarct and, once arrived, contribute to myocardial destruction by generating uncontrolled proteolysis, oxidative stress and cytokine release (Heymans et al, 1999). In support of a role for MMP-9 in cardiac rupture, a recent study reported a trend to less rupture in MMP-9-deficient mice (Ducharme et al, 2000).

3.2. Cardiac healing and functional preservation

u-PA deficient mice showed impaired scar formation (as documented by impaired removal of necrotic cardiomyocytes and minimal collagen content) and infarct revascularisation, even after treatment with vascular endothelial growth factor (VEGF). In addition, they died of cardiac failure due to depressed contractility, arrhythmias and ischemia, likely because the weaker collagen-poor scar in u-PA-deficient mice imposed a larger hemodynamic load on the remote viable myocardium. This impaired wound healing and scar formation appeared to result from reduced migration of wound cells (macrophages, endothelial and smooth muscle cells, and fibroblasts), confirming the essential role of proteinases in cellular invasion. In addition, decreased activation of latent TGF-β1 in u-PA-deficient mice further contributed to the reduced collagen deposition. The recent observation that plasminogen deficiency completely abolished cardiac healing, indicates that these effects of u-PA on healing are mediated through the activation of plasminogen (Creemers et al, 2000). Formation of a collagen-rich scar after infarction was similar in MMP-9-deficient mice and in wild- type mice (on a matched mixed genetic background) implying that other MMPs (like MMP-2) might have compensated for the loss of MMP-9. However, Ducharme et al reported a decreased collagen content in MMP-9-deficient mice (on a congenic C57Bl/6 background), possibly due to compensatory up-regulation of MMP-2, MMP-3 and MMP-13, implying that in this case over-compensation resulted in more collagen breakdown in comparison with wild-type mice (Ducharme et al, 2000). Differences in genetic background or other unknown factors might have influenced the extent of the compensatory response to loss of MMP-9.

Together, these findings indicate that proteinases can promote tissue destruction (as evidenced by their involvement in cardiac rupture) as well as tissue healing (due to their effects on wound cell migration and matrix deposition). An ideal therapy would protect against rupture, without inhibiting the healing process. Temporary administration of PAI-1 or TIMP-1 by adenoviral gene transfer completely protected wild-type mice against rupture without aborting infarct healing (myocardial healing resumed beyond 14 days resulting in normal scar formation by 5 weeks after infarction), thus constituting a new medical approach to prevent cardiac rupture after AMI (Heymans et al, 1999).

4. THE NERVOUS SYSTEM

Several components of the plasminogen system, including plasminogen, t-PA and LRP are expressed in the nervous system under physiologic conditions or after neuronal stimulation (Sappino et al, 1993; Zhuo et al, 2000) and have been implicated in neuronal plasticity and learning. For instance, the late phase of long-term potentiation (L-LTP) is significantly decreased in t-PA-deficient mice (Frey et al, 1996; Huang et al, 1996) and seems to involve interactions between t-PA and LRP (Zhuo et al, 2000). Short seizures induce reorganisation of neuronal pathways, a process that was impaired in t-PA-deficient mice (Wu et al, 2000). In addition, in the context of sustained neuronal injury (Cuzner et al, 1999; Carroll et al, 1994; Dietzmann et al, 2000; Qian et al, 1993; Salles et al, 1990), plasminogen activators and their inhibitors can also be up-regulated. However, it is not clear if this altered expression has protective (healing) or deleterious (destructive) effects. The effects of plasminogen system components is discussed in different types of neuronal injury.

4.1. Ischemic stroke

Stroke is the third leading death cause and the leading cause of long-term disability in the United States (http://www.strokeassociation.org/Who_We_Are/impact.html). Approximately 80% of all strokes are ischemic in origin, the result of either thrombotic (such as formation of an occluding thrombus on top of a ruptured atherosclerotic lesion) or embolic events. Short-term ischemia for only a few minutes may cause irreversible damage to brain cells. Different mechanisms of neurotoxicity have been proposed, including excitotoxicity (mediated by the excitatory neurotransmitter glutamate) (Tsirka et al, 1997a) and endogenous zinc translocation (Choi and Koh, 1998).

Genetic studies on the role of the plasminogen system components during ischemic stroke induced by middle cerebral artery (MCA) occlusion have yielded conflicting results. Whereas t-PA deficiency reduced cerebral infarct size in some studies (Nagai et al, 1999; Wang et al, 1998), it increased infarct size in another study (Tabrizi et al, 1999). Moreover, Nagai et al (1999) indicated that t-PA and plasmin may exert opposite activities in stroke, t-PA having deleterious effects and plasmin being neuroprotective. Several reasons may underlie these apparent discrepant results. First, response to MCA occlusion in mice has been shown to differ dependent on the genetic background (Choi, 1997). Wang et al (1998) compared infarct size in pure C57Bl/6 wild-type mice to that in t-PA-deficient mice on a mixed (C57Bl/6 and 129/SvJ) genetic background, whereas Tabrizi et al (1999) compared both genotypes of a genetically matched background. Second, there were also differences in the models used in these studies. In order to study the role of t-PA independent of its fibrinolytic functions, Wang et al (1998) used a siliconised thread to induce MCA occlusion, whereas Tabrizi et al (1999) used non-siliconised threads which leads to micro-vascular thrombus formation. If fibrin deposition contributes to the disease progression, t-PA/plasmin mediated fibrinolysis would be expected to have protective effects. Alternatively, fibrin-independent activities of t-PA, such as the degradation of neuronal basal membranes, may explain the neurotoxic effects observed by Wang et al (1998). Further studies are required to explain the possible differential role of plasmin and t-PA during stroke.

Studies using models of neuro-excitotoxicity or zinc neurotoxicity have also reported opposite effects of t-PA. A number of studies has implicated t-PA-mediated plasminogen activation in the kainate-induced excitotoxicity via degradation of laminin in the basal lamina of neurons (for reference see Tsirka et al, 1997a). Recently, we demonstrated that t-PA, released by depolarized cortical neurons, could potentiate the signaling mediated by glutamatergic receptors by proteolytic cleavage of the NR1 subunit of the N-methyl-D-aspartate (NMDA) receptor, leading to increased NMDA-receptor function. These results were confirmed *in vivo* by the intrastriatal injection of recombinant t-PA, which potentiated the excitotoxic lesions induced by NMDA (Nicole et al, 2001). However, injection of t-PA into the cerebrospinal fluid after induction of kainate seizures in rats reduced zinc-associated neuronal death in the hippocampus (Kim et al, 1999). These opposite results may reflect different mechanisms of action of t-PA related to either its proteolytic or non-proteolytic properties. Indeed, whereas the neuro-excitotoxicity was dependent on the generation of plasmin, the protection against the zinc neurotoxicity appeared to be independent of its proteolytic activity as the *in vitro* protective effect of t-PA was not reversed by PAI-1 (Kim et al, 1999).

4.2. Inflammatory neuronal degeneration

t-PA has also been implicated in inflammatory neuronal degeneration in the peripheral nervous system, for instance via degradation of myelin basic protein

12

(Norton et al, 1990). However, in contrast to the neurotoxic effects after kainate injection, t-PA protected against axonal degeneration and demyelination after sciatic nerve injury (Akassoglou et al, 2000). The proposed mechanism was plasmin-mediated fibrinolysis, as fibrin may sustain nerve injury by chemoattraction of inflammatory cells, whereas kainate-induced injury was fibrin-independent (Tsirka et al, 1997b). Thus, as in ischemic stroke, the effects of t-PA and plasmin might be beneficial or deleterious, dependent on the relative contribution of fibrin in the pathogenesis of the disease.

4.3. Traumatic brain injury

Traumatic brain injury often involves disruption of the blood-brain barrier (BBB) by proteolytic breakdown of the blood vessel basement membrane. Recently, it was shown that mice deficient of u-PA had reduced extravasation of immunoglobulin three days after brain stab wounding, while PAI-1 deficiency exhibited an increased extravasation (Kataoka et al, 2000). The effects of u-PA appeared to be independent of its receptor as no differences in immunoglobin leakage were observed between u-PAR-deficient and wild-type mice. In addition, eight days after injury, PAI-1 deficiency resulted in increased vascularisation of the injured region. Thus, while u-PA might aggravate brain trauma in the acute phase by inducing BBB disruption, it might also favor post-injury healing by increasing neovascularisation in the wound.

5. THE LUNGS

Lung disease is one of the major death causes in the United States, responsible for 300,000 deaths annually (States, 1997). In most cases, acute lung injury triggers an inflammatory response, characterised by infiltration of inflammatory cells, followed by a fibrotic phase leading to excessive accumulation of fibrous connective tissue. The development of pulmonary fibrosis has been associated with changes in the activities of different proteinase families, including the plaminogen system, metalloproteinases and cathepsins (Koslowski et al, 1998; Swiderski et al, 1998). Proteinases may exert differential effects in pulmonary fibrosis both during the inflammatory and the fibrotic phase of the disease. Genetic studies in mice using a model of bleomycin-induced pulmonary fibrosis (Phan et al, 1981) have shed light on the possible mechanisms involved but the relative importance of these mechanisms remains unclear.

Increased matrix accumulation has been documented in the lungs of patients suffering inflammatory pulmonary disorders (Chapman et al, 1986). In addition, over-expression of PAI-1 or loss of plasminogen markedly increased fibrin deposition and collagen content in injured lungs, whereas PAI-1 deficiency or adenoviral gene transfer of u-PA protected against fibrin accumulation and fibrosis (Eitzman et al, 1996; Swaisgood et al, 2000; Sisson et al, 1999). These findings indicate that proteinases of the plasminogen system influence the development of pulmonary fibrosis by altering the fibrinolytic balance. Since fibrin degradation products are chemoattractive for a variety of wound cells, infiltrating fibroblasts might be responsible for the enhanced production of collagen during healing of the inflamed lung.

However, subsequent studies in fibrinogen-deficient mice indicated that fibrin deposition – while likely contributing to the disease – is not absolutely required for the development of pulmonary fibrosis (Hattori et al, 2000; Ploplis et al, 2000), implicating other – fibrin-independent – mechanisms. For instance, plasmin may promote the infiltration of inflammatory or other wound healing cells, as suggested by the reduced macrophage infiltration in inflamed lungs in mice lacking u-PA or plasminogen (Swaisgood et al, 2000). u-PA might stimulate cellular migration via interaction with u-PAR and vitronectin (Preissner et al, 1999) and/or via degradation of extracellular matrix components, either directly or indirectly via activation of MMPs (Carmeliet et al, 1997a). MMPs are likely involved in pulmonary remodeling, as suggested by the recent findings that loss of MMP-9, but not of MMP-7, protected against alveolar bronchiolisation (Betsuyaku et al, 2000), another prominent feature of pulmonary fibrosis in which clusters of cuboidal epithelial cells are formed in regions of alveolar injury (Nettesheim and Szakal, 1972). The elastolytic MMP-12 was also found to play an essential role in the development of pulmonary emphysema induced by cigarette smoking (Hautamaki et al, 1997).

It remained outstanding whether u-PA/plasmin might stimulate matrix accumulation via the release and activation of latent TGF-β1 (Rifkin et al, 1999), a potent stimulator of matrix synthesis (Lawrence, 1996). Increased expression of TGF-β1 and its receptors (Broekelmann et al, 1991; Phan and Kunkel, 1992; Zhao and Shah, 2000) as well as attenuation of lung fibrosis by administration of TGF-β1 antibodies (Giri et al, 1993) in the context of pulmonary fibrosis have indicated a role for this growth factor in the development of pulmonary fibrosis. However, recent studies indicate that plasmin is not a predominant activator of TGF-β1 in the lung (Matrat et al, 1998; Munger et al, 1999).

6. THE SKIN

Healing of skin wounds involves several sequential steps, e.g. the formation of a hemostatic fibrin-rich plug, the infiltration of inflammatory cells (neutrophils, macrophages) to remove the necrotic debris, the proliferation of keratinocytes, which cover the denuded wound from the viable wound borders, the ingrowth of new blood vessels and the formation of a collagen-rich scar by wound fibroblasts (Clark and Henson, 1988). Deficiency of plasminogen was found to delay wound healing after skin incision, presumably because the excessive fibrin deposits in the wound impaired migration of keratinocytes in the wound (Romer et al, 1996). A role for fibrin was indeed supported by subsequent findings that fibrinogen deficiency restored keratinocyte migration and healing in plasminogen- deficient mice (Bugge et al, 1996). However, the formation of a granulation tissue rich in macrophages and neovessels was comparable in all these genotypes and absence of plasminogen only delayed but did not abrogate skin healing, implicating other plasmin-independent mechanisms in the healing process. A more recent study indicated that plasminogen deficiency in combination with pharmacologic inhibition of MMPs delayed healing, suggesting that both proteinase families are involved in the healing process and have overlapping functions (Lund et al, 1999). In another study, deficiency of vitronectin slightly delayed wound healing and impaired wound angiogenesis (Jang et al, 2000).

7. CONCLUSIONS

Genetically altered mice have proven to be valuable tools to unravel the distinct functions governed by proteinases in numerous diseases. In addition, they have revealed unanticipated roles for previously characterised proteinases. The findings of these studies greatly contribute to the elucidation of the underlying molecular mechanisms in disease, but, at the same time, emphasize the complexity and diversity of the systems and processes involved. The plasminogen system is a striking example of a proteinase system that may have dual – even opposite – effects, depending on the tissue studied, the existence of other compensatory/redundant proteinase sytems, the spatio-temporal expression and the expression level of its components. Given the medical importance of the various pathologies in which the plasminogen system and other proteinases play a role, further analysis by genetic and other strategies is warranted in order to develop specific therapies based on proteinase inhibitors that prevent tissue destruction without abrogating the healing process.

ACKNOWLEDGMENTS

The authors wish to thank Mieke Derwerchin for helpful discussion and critical reading of the manuscript and Ann Vandenhoeck for artwork.

REFERENCES

Akassoglou K, Kombrinck KW, Degen JL, Strickland S. Tissue plasminogen activator-mediated fibrinolysis protects against axonal degeneration and demyelination after sciatic nerve injury. J Cell Biol 2000; 149: 1157–1166.

Allaire E, Forough R, Clowes M, Starcher B, Clowes AW. Local overexpression of TIMP-1 prevents aortic aneurysm degeneration and rupture in a rat model. J Clin Invest 1998; 102: 1413–1420.

Bansal DD, Klein RM, Hausmann EH, MacGregor RR. Secretion of cardiac plasminogen activator during hypoxia-induced right ventricular hypertrophy. J Mol Cell Cardiol 1997; 29: 3105–3114.

Barrett AJ. Cellular proteolysis. An overview. Ann NY Acad Sci 1992; 674: 1–15.

Betsuyaku T, Fukuda Y, Parks WC, Shipley JM, Senior RM. Gelatinase B is required for alveolar bronchiolization after intratracheal bleomycin. Am J Pathol 2000; 157: 525–535.

Blasi F, Conese M, Moller LB, Pedersen N, Cavallaro U, Cubellis MV, Fazioli F, Hernandez-Marrero L, Limongi P, Munoz-Canoves P, Resnati M, Rüttininen L, Sidenius N, Soravia E, Soria MR, Stoppelli MP, Talarico D, Teesalu T, Valamonica S. The urokinase receptor: structure, regulation and inhibitor-mediated internalization. Fibrinolysis 1994; 8: 182–188.

Broekelmann TJ, Limper AH, Colby TV, McDonald JA. Transforming growth factor beta 1 is present at sites of extracellular matrix gene expression in human pulmonary fibrosis. Proc Natl Acad Sci (USA) 1991; 88: 6642–6646.

Bugge TH, Kombrinck KW, Flick MJ, Daugherty CC, Danton MJ, Degen JL. Loss of fibrinogen rescues mice from the pleiotropic effects of plasminogen deficiency. Cell 1996; 87: 709–719.

Busuttil SJ, Drumm C, Ploplis VA, Plow EF. Endoluminal arterial injury in plasminogen-deficient mice. J Surg Res 2000; 91: 159–164.

Campeau L, Enjalbert M, Lesperance J, Vaislic C, Grondin CM, Bourassa MG. Atherosclerosis and late closure of aortocoronary saphenous vein grafts: sequential angiographic studies at 2 weeks, 1 year, 5 to 7 years, and 10 to 12 years after surgery. Circulation 1983; 68: II1–II7.

Carmeliet P, Kieckens L, Schoonjans L, Ream B, van Nuffelen A, Prendergast G, Cole M, Bronson R, Collen D, Mulligan RC. Plasminogen activator inhibitor-1 gene-deficient mice. I. Generation by homologous recombination and characterization. J Clin Invest 1993a; 92: 2746–2755.

Carmeliet P, Stassen JM, Schoonjans L, Ream B, van den Oord JJ, De Mol M, Mulligan RC, Collen D. Plasminogen activator inhibitor-1 gene-deficient mice. II. Effects on hemostasis, thrombosis, and thrombolysis. J Clin Invest 1993b; 92: 2756–2760.

Carmeliet P, Schoonjans L, Kieckens L, Ream B, Degen J, Bronson R, De Vos R, van den Oord JJ, Collen D, Mulligan RC. Physiological consequences of loss of plasminogen activator gene function in mice. Nature 1994; 368: 419–424.

Carmeliet P, Moons L, Lijnen R, Baes M, Lemaitre V, Tipping P, Drew A, Eeckhout Y, Shapiro S, Lupu F, Collen D. Urokinase-generated plasmin activates matrix metalloproteinases during aneurysm formation. Nat Genet 1997a; 17: 439–444.

Carmeliet P, Moons L, Lijnen R, Janssens S, Lupu F, Collen D, Gerard RD. Inhibitory role of plasminogen activator inhibitor-1 in arterial wound healing and neointima formation: a gene targeting and gene transfer study in mice. Circulation 1997b; 96: 3180–3191.

Carmeliet P, Moons L, Herbert JM, Crawley J, Lupu F, Lijnen R, Collen D. Urokinase but not tissue plasminogen activator mediates arterial neointima formation in mice. Circ Res 1997c; 81: 829–839.

Carmeliet P. Proteinases in cardiovascular aneurysms and rupture: targets for therapy? J Clin Invest 2000; 105: 1519–1520.

Carmeliet P, Collen D. Transgenic mouse models in angiogenesis and cardiovascular disease. J Pathol 2000; 190: 387–405.

Carroll PM, Tsirka SE, Richards WG, Frohman MA, Strickland S. The mouse tissue plasminogen activator gene 5′ flanking region directs appropriate expression in development and a seizure-enhanced response in the CNS. Development 1994; 120: 3173–3183.

Chapman HA Jr, Stone OL. Co-operation between plasmin and elastase in elastin degradation by intact murine macrophages. Biochem J 1984; 222: 721–728.

Chapman HA, Allen CL, Stone OL. Abnormalities in pathways of alveolar fibrin turnover among patients with interstitial lung disease. Am Rev Respir Dis 1986; 133: 437–443.

Choi DW. Background genes: out of sight, but not out of brain. Trends Neurosci 1997; 20: 499–500.

Choi DW, Koh JY. Zinc and brain injury. Annu Rev Neurosci 1998; 21: 347–375.

Clark RAF, Henson PM. The Molecular and Cellular Biology of Wound Repair. Plenum New York, 1988.

Collen D, Lijnen HR. Basic and clinical aspects of fibrinolysis and thrombolysis. Blood 1991; 78: 3114–3124.

Collen D. The plasminogen (fibrinolytic) system. Thromb Haemost 1999; 82: 259–270.

Cortellaro M, Cofrancesco E, Boschetti C, Mussoni L, Donati MB, Cardillo M, Catalano M, Gabrielli L, Lombardi B, Specchia G, et al. Increased fibrin turnover and high PAI-1 activity as predictors of ischemic events in atherosclerotic patients. A case-control study. The PLAT Group. Arterioscler Thromb 1993; 13: 1412–1417.

Cowan KN, Jones PL, Rabinovitch M. Regression of hypertrophied rat pulmonary arteries in organ culture is associated with suppression of proteolytic activity, inhibition of tenascin-C, and smooth muscle cell apoptosis. Circ Res 1999; 84: 1223–1233.

Cowan KN, Heilbut A, Humpl T, Lam C, Ito S, Rabinovitch M. Complete reversal of fatal pulmonary hypertension in rats by a serine elastase inhibitor. Nat Med 2000; 6: 698–702.

Creemers E, Cleutjens J, Smits J, Heymans S, Moons L, Collen D, Daemen M, Carmeliet P. Disruption of the plasminogen gene in mice abolishes wound healing after myocardial infarction. Am J Pathol 2000; 156: 1865–1873.

Cuzner ML, Opdenakker G. Plasminogen activators and matrix metalloproteases, mediators of extracellular proteolysis in inflammatory demyelination of the central nervous system. J Neuroimmunol 1999; 94: 1–14.

Dawson S, Hamsten A, Wiman B, Henney A, Humphries S. Genetic variation at the plasminogen activator inhibitor-1 locus is associated with altered levels of plasma plasminogen activator inhibitor-1 activity. Arterioscler Thromb 1991; 11: 183–190.

Dewerchin M, Nuffelen AV, Wallays G, Bouche A, Moons L, Carmeliet P, Mulligan RC, Collen D. Generation and characterization of urokinase receptor-deficient mice. J Clin Invest 1996; 97: 870–878.

Dietrich H, Hu Y, Zou Y, Dirnhofer S, Kleindienst R, Wick G, Xu Q. Mouse model of transplant arteriosclerosis: role of intercellular adhesion molecule-1. Arterioscler Thromb Vasc Biol 2000; 20: 343–352.

Dietzmann K, von Bossanyi P, Krause D, Wittig H, Mawrin C, Kirches E. Expression of the plasminogen activator system and the inhibitors PAI-1 and PAI-2 in posttraumatic lesions of the CNS and brain injuries following dramatic circulatory arrests: an immunohistochemical study. Pathol Res Pract 2000; 196: 15–21.

Ducharme A, Frantz S, Aikawa M, Rabkin E, Lindsey M, Rohde LE, Schoen FJ, Kelly RA, Werb Z, Libby P, Lee RT. Targeted deletion of matrix metalloproteinase-9 attenuates left ventricular enlargement and collagen accumulation after experimental myocardial infarction. J Clin Invest 2000; 106: 55–62.

17

Eitzman DT, McCoy RD, Zheng X, Fay WP, Shen T, Ginsburg D, Simon RH. Bleomycin-induced pulmonary fibrosis in transgenic mice that either lack or overexpress the murine plasminogen activator inhibitor-1 gene. J Clin Invest 1996; 97: 232–237.

Eitzman DT, Westrick RJ, Xu Z, Tyson J, Ginsburg D. Plasminogen activator inhibitor-1 deficiency protects against atherosclerosis progression in the mouse carotid artery. Blood 2000; 96: 4212–4215.

Ferrara N, Davis-Smyth T. The biology of vascular endothelial growth factor. Endocr Rev 1997; 18: 4–25.

Frey U, Muller M, Kuhl D. A different form of long-lasting potentiation revealed in tissue plasminogen activator mutant mice. J Neurosci 1996; 16: 2057–2063.

George SJ. Tissue inhibitors of metalloproteinases and metalloproteinases in atherosclerosis. Curr Opin Lipidol 1998; 9: 413–423.

Ghodsi F, Will JA. Changes in pulmonary structure and function induced by monocrotaline intoxication. Am J Physiol 1981; 240: H149–H155.

Giri SN, Hyde DM, Hollinger MA. Effect of antibody to transforming growth factor beta on bleomycin induced accumulation of lung collagen in mice. Thorax 1993; 48: 959–966.

Hamsten A, de Faire U, Walldius G, Dahlen G, Szamosi A, Landou C, Blomback M, Wiman B. Plasminogen activator inhibitor in plasma: risk factor for recurrent myocardial infarction. Lancet 1987; 2: 3–9.

Hattori N, Degen JL, Sisson TH, Liu H, Moore BB, Pandrangi RG, Simon RH, Drew AF. Bleomycin-induced pulmonary fibrosis in fibrinogen-null mice. J Clin Invest 2000; 106: 1341–1350.

Hautamaki RD, Kobayashi DK, Senior RM, Shapiro SD. Requirement for macrophage elastase for cigarette smoke-induced emphysema in mice. Science 1997; 277: 2002–2004.

Heymans S, Luttun A, Nuyens D, Theilmeier G, Creemers E, Moons L, Dyspersin GD, Cleutjens JP, Shipley M, Angellilo A, Levi M, Nube O, Baker A, Keshet E, Lupu F, Herbert JM, Smits JF, Shapiro SD, Baes M, Borgers M, Collen D, Daemen MJ, Carmeliet P. Inhibition of plasminogen activators or matrix metalloproteinases prevents cardiac rupture but impairs therapeutic angiogenesis and causes cardiac failure [see comments]. Nat Med 1999; 5: 1135–1142.

Huang YY, Bach ME, Lipp HP, Zhuo M, Wolfer DP, Hawkins RD, Schoonjans L, Kandel ER, Godfraind JM, Mulligan R, Collen D, Carmeliet P. Mice lacking the gene encoding tissue-type plasminogen activator show a selective interference with late-phase long-term potentiation in both Schaffer collateral and mossy fiber pathways. Proc Natl Acad Sci (USA) 1996; 93: 8699–8704.

Jang YC, Tsou R, Gibran NS, Isik FF. Vitronectin deficiency is associated with increased wound fibrinolysis and decreased microvascular angiogenesis in mice. Surgery 2000; 127: 696–704.

Jansson JH, Nilsson TK, Olofsson BO. Tissue plasminogen activator and other risk factors as predictors of cardiovascular events in patients with severe angina pectoris. Eur Heart J 1991; 12: 157–161.

Juhan-Vague I, Pyke SD, Alessi MC, Jespersen J, Haverkate F, Thompson SG. Fibrinolytic factors and the risk of myocardial infarction or sudden death in patients with angina pectoris. ECAT Study Group. European Concerted Action on Thrombosis and Disabilities. Circulation 1996; 94, 2057–2063.

Kataoka K, Asai T, Taneda M, Ueshima S, Matsuo O, Kuroda R, Kawabata A, Carmeliet P. Roles of urokinase type plasminogen activator in a brain stab wound. Brain Res 2000; 887: 187–190.

Keyt BA, Berleau LT, Nguyen HV, Chen H, Heinsohn H, Vandlen R, Ferrara N. The carboxyl-

18

terminal domain (111–165) of vascular endothelial growth factor is critical for its mitogenic potency. J Biol Chem 1996; 271: 7788–7795.

Kim YH, Park JH, Hong SH, Koh JY. Nonproteolytic neuroprotection by human recombinant tissue plasminogen activator. Science 1999; 284: 647–650.

Koslowski R, Knoch KP, Wenzel KW. Proteinases and proteinase inhibitors during the development of pulmonary fibrosis in rat. Clin Chim Acta 1998; 271: 45–56.

Lawrence DA. Transforming growth factor-beta: a general review. Eur Cytokine Netw 1996; 7: 363–374.

Levi M, Moons L, Bouche A, Shapiro SD, Collen D, Carmeliet P. Deficiency of urokinase-type plasminogen activator-mediated plasmin generation impairs vascular remodeling during hypoxia-induced pulmonary hypertension in mice. Circulation 2001; 103: in press.

Lijnen HR, Okada K, Matsuo O, Collen D. Dewerchin M. Alpha$_2$-antiplasmin gene deficiency in mice is associated with enhanced fibrinolytic potential without overt bleeding. Blood 1999a; 93: 2274–2281.

Lijnen HR, Van Hoef B, Vanlinthout I, Verstreken M, Rio MC, Collen D. Accelerated neointima formation after vascular injury in mice with stromelysin-3 (MMP-11) gene inactivation. Arterioscler Thromb Vasc Biol 1999b; 19: 2863–2870.

Lijnen HR, Soloway P, Collen D. Tissue inhibitor of matrix metalloproteinases-1 impairs arterial neointima formation after vascular injury in mice. Circ Res 1999c; 85: 1186–1191.

Lijnen HR, Van Hoef B, Dewerchin M, D C. a$_2$-Antiplasmin gene deficiency in mice does not affect neointima formation after vascular injury. Arterioscler Thromb Vasc Biol 2000; 20: 1488–1492.

Lund LR, Romer J, Bugge TH, Nielsen BS, Frandsen TL, Degen JL, Stephens RW, Dano K. Functional overlap between two classes of matrix-degrading proteases in wound healing. Embo J 1999; 18: 4645–4656.

Luttun A, Lupu F, Storkebaum E, Hoylaerts MF, Moons L, Crawley J, Bono F, Poole AR, Tipping P, Herbert J-M, Collen D, Carmeliet P. Lack of plasminogen activator inhibitor-1 promotes growth and abnormal matrix remodeling of advanced atherosclerotic plaques in apolipoprotein E-deficient mice. Arterioscler Thromb Vasc Biol 2002; 22: 449–505.

Martin TJ, Allan EH, Fukumoto S. The plasminogen activator and inhibitor system in bone remodelling. Growth Regul 1993; 3: 209–214.

Mason DP, Kenagy RD, Hasenstab D, Bowen-Pope DF, Seifert RA, Coats S, Hawkins SM, Clowes AW. Matrix metalloproteinase-9 overexpression enhances vascular smooth muscle cell migration and alters remodeling in the injured rat carotid artery. Circ Res 1999; 85: 1179–1185.

Matrat M, Lardot C, Huaux F, Broeckaert F, Lison D. Role of urokinase in the activation of macrophage-associated TGF-beta in silica-induced lung fibrosis. J Toxicol Environ Health A 1998; 55: 359–371.

Moons L, Shi C, Ploplis V, Plow E, Haber E, Collen D, Carmeliet P. Reduced transplant arteriosclerosis in plasminogen-deficient mice. J Clin Invest 1998; 102: 1788–1797.

Munger JS, Huang X, Kawakatsu H, Griffiths MJ, Dalton SL, Wu J, Pittet JF, Kaminski N, Garat C, Matthay MA, Rifkin DB, Sheppard D. The integrin alpha$_v$beta$_6$ binds and activates latent TGF beta 1: a mechanism for regulating pulmonary inflammation and fibrosis. Cell 1999; 96: 319–328.

Nagai N, De Mol M, Lijnen HR, Carmeliet CD. Role of plasminogen system components in focal cerebral ischemic infarction: a gene targeting and gene transfer study in mice. Circulation 1999; 99: 2440–2444.

Nettesheim P, Szakal AK. Morphogenesis of alveolar bronchiolization. Lab Invest 1972; 26: 210–219.

19

Nicole O, Docagne F, Ali C, Margaill I, Carmeliet P, MacKenzie ET, Vivien D, Buisson A. The proteolytic activity of tissue-plasminogen activator enhances NMDA receptor-mediated signaling, Nat Med 2001; 7: 59–64.

Noorman F, Rijken DC. Regulation of tissue-type plasminogen activator concentrations by clearance via the mannose receptor and other receptors. Fibrinolysis and Proteolysis 1997; 11: 173.

Norton WT, Brosnan CF, Cammer, Goldmuntz EA. Mechanisms and suppression of inflammatory demyelination. Acta Neurobiol Exp 1990; 50: 225–235.

Phan SH, Thrall RS, Williams C. Bleomycin-induced pulmonary fibrosis. Effects of steroid on lung collagen metabolism. Am Rev Respir Dis 1981; 124: 428–434.

Phan SH, Kunkel SL. Lung cytokine production in bleomycin-induced pulmonary fibrosis. Exp Lung Res 1992; 18: 29–43.

Pinsky DJ, Liao H, Lawson CA, Yan SF, Chen J, Carmeliet P, Loskutoff DJ, Stern DM. Coordinated induction of plasminogen activator inhibitor-1 (PAI-1) and inhibition of plasminogen activator gene expression by hypoxia promotes pulmonary vascular fibrin deposition. J Clin Invest 1998; 102: 919–928.

Ploplis VA, Carmeliet P, Vazirzadeh S, Van Vlaenderen I, Moons L, Plow EF, Collen D. Effects of disruption of the plasminogen gene on thrombosis, growth, and health in mice. Circulation 1995; 92: 2585–2593.

Ploplis VA, Wilberding J, McLennan L, Liang Z, Cornelissen I, DeFord ME, Rosen ED, Castellino FJ. A total fibrinogen deficiency is compatible with the development of pulmonary fibrosis in mice. Am J Pathol 2000; 157: 703–708.

Ploplis VA, Cornelissen I, Sandoval-Cooper MJ, Weeks L, Noria FA, Castellino FJ. Remodeling of the vessel wall after copper-induced injury is highly attenuated in mice with a total deficiency of plasminogen activator inhibitor-1. Am J Pathol 2001; 158: 107–117.

Preissner KT, Kanse SM, Chavakis T, May AE. The dual role of the urokinase receptor system in pericellular proteolysis and cell adhesion: implications for cardiovascular function. Basic Res Cardiol 1999; 94: 315–321.

Prescott MF, Sawyer WK, Von Linden-Reed J, Jeune M, Chou M, Caplan SL, Jeng AY. Effect of matrix metalloproteinase inhibition on progression of atherosclerosis and aneurysm in LDL receptor-deficient mice overexpressing MMP-3, MMP-12, and MMP-13 and on restenosis in rats after balloon injury. Ann NY Acad Sci 1999; 878: 179–190.

Pyo R, Lee JK, Shipley JM, Curci JA, Mao D, Ziporin SJ, Ennis TL, Shapiro SD, Senior RM, Thompson RW. Targeted gene disruption of matrix metalloproteinase-9 (gelatinase B) suppresses development of experimental abdominal aortic aneurysms. J Clin Invest 2000; 105: 1641–1649.

Qian Z, Gilbert ME, Colicos MA, Kandel ER, Kuhl D. Tissue-plasminogen activator is induced as an immediate-early gene during seizure, kindling and long-term potentiation. Nature 1993; 361: 453–457.

Rabinovitch M. Elastase and the pathobiology of unexplained pulmonary hypertension. Chest 1998; 114: 213S–224S.

Rifkin DB, Mazzieri R, Munger JS, Noguera I, Sung J. Proteolytic control of growth factor availability. Apmis 1999; 107: 80–85.

Romer J, Bugge TH, Pyke C, Lund LR, Flick MJ, Degen JL, Dano K. Impaired wound healing in mice with a disrupted plasminogen gene. Nat Med 1996; 2: 287–292.

Rouis M, Adamy C, Duverger N, Lesnik P, Horellou P, Moreau M, Emmanuel F, Caillaud JM, Laplaud PM, Dachet C, Chapman MJ. Adenovirus-mediated overexpression of tissue inhibitor of metalloproteinase-1 reduces atherosclerotic lesions in apolipoprotein E- deficient mice. Circulation 1999; 100: 533–540.

20

Saksela O, Rifkin DB. Cell-associated plasminogen activation: regulation and physiological functions. Annu Rev Cell Biol 1988; 4: 93–126.

Salles FJ, Schechter N, Strickland S. A plasminogen activator is induced during goldfish optic nerve regeneration. Embo J 1990; 9: 2471–2477.

Sappino AP, Madani R, Huarte J, Belin D, Kiss JZ, Wohlwend A, Vassalli JD. Extracellular proteolysis in the adult murine brain. J Clin Invest 1993; 92: 679–685.

Schneider DJ, Ricci MA, Taatjes DJ, Baumann PQ, Reese JC, Leavitt BJ, Absher PM, Sobel BE. Changes in arterial expression of fibrinolytic system proteins in atherogenesis. Arterioscler Thromb Vasc Biol 1997; 17: 3294–3301.

Schneiderman MH, Hofer KG, Schneiderman GS. An in vitro 125IUdR-release assay for measuring the kinetics of cell death. Int J Radiat Biol 1991; 59: 397–408.

Shi C, Patel A, Zhang D, Wang H, Carmeliet P, Reed GL, Lee ME, Haber E, Sibinga NE. Plasminogen is not required for neointima formation in a mouse model of vein graft stenosis. Circ Res 1999; 84: 883–890.

Sisson TH, Hattori N, Xu Y, Simon RH. Treatment of bleomycin-induced pulmonary fibrosis by transfer of urokinase-type plasminogen activator genes. Hum Gene Ther 1999; 10: 2315–2323.

Sjoland H, Eitzman DT, Gordon D, Westrick R, Nabel EG, Ginsburg D. Atherosclerosis progression in LDL receptor-deficient and apolipoprotein E-deficient mice is independent of genetic alterations in plasminogen activator inhibitor-1. Arterioscler Thromb Vasc Biol 2000; 20: 846–852.

States NCfHSBadU. Monthly Vital Statistics Report, Vol. 46. Atlanta, Centers for Disease Control, 1997.

Swaisgood CM, French EL, Noga C, Simon RH, Ploplis VA. The development of bleomycin-induced pulmonary fibrosis in mice deficient for components of the fibrinolytic system. Am J Pathol 2000; 157: 177–187.

Swiderski RE, Dencoff JE, Floerchinger CS, Shapiro SD, Hunninghake GW. Differential expression of extracellular matrix remodeling genes in a murine model of bleomycin-induced pulmonary fibrosis. Am J Pathol 1998; 152: 821–828.

Tabrizi P, Wang L, Seeds N, McComb JG, Yamada S, Griffin JH, Carmeliet P, Weiss MH, Zlokovic BV. Tissue plasminogen activator (tPA) deficiency exacerbates cerebrovascular fibrin deposition and brain injury in a murine stroke model: studies in tPA-deficient mice and wild-type mice on a matched genetic background. Arterioscler Thromb Vasc Biol 1999; 19: 2801–2806.

Thompson BT, Steigman DM, Spence CL, Janssens SP, Hales CA. Chronic hypoxic pulmonary hypertension in the guinea pig: effect of three levels of hypoxia. J Appl Physiol 1993; 74: 916–921.

Todorovich-Hunter L, Dodo H, Ye C, McCready L, Keeley FW, Rabinovitch M. Increased pulmonary artery elastolytic activity in adult rats with monocrotaline-induced progressive hypertensive pulmonary vascular disease compared with infant rats with nonprogressive disease. Am Rev Respir Dis 1992; 146: 213–223.

Tsirka SE, Rogove AD, Bugge TH, Degen JL, Strickland S. An extracellular proteolytic cascade promotes neuronal degeneration in the mouse hippocampus. J Neurosci 1997a; 17: 543–552.

Tsirka SE, Bugge TH, Degen JL, Strickland S.Neuronal death in the central nervous system demonstrates a non-fibrin substrate for plasmin [published erratum appears in Proc Natl Acad Sci (USA) 1997 Dec 23;94(26):14976], Proc Natl Acad Sci (USA) 1997b; 94: 9779–9781.

Vassalli JD, Sappino AP, Belin D. The plasminogen activator/plasmin system. J Clin Invest 1991; 88: 1067–1072.

Vassalli JD. The urokinase receptor. Fibrinolysis 1994; 8: 172–181.

Vieillard-Baron A, Frisdal E, Eddahibi S, Deprez I, Baker AH, Newby AC, Berger P, Levame

M, Raffestin B, Adnot S, d'Ortho MP. Inhibition of matrix metalloproteinases by lung TIMP-1 gene transfer or doxycycline aggravates pulmonary hypertension in rats. Circ Res 2000; 87: 418–425.

Wang YF, Tsirka SE, Strickland S, Stieg PE, Soriano SG, Lipton SA. Tissue plasminogen activator (tPA) increases neuronal damage after focal cerebral ischemia in wild-type and tPA-deficient mice [see comments]. Nat Med 1998; 4: 228–231.

Wiman B. The fibrinolytic enzyme system. Basic principles and links to venous and arterial thrombosis. Hematol Oncol Clin North Am 2000; 14: 325–338, vii.

Wiman B. Plasminogen activator inhibitor 1 (PAI-1) in plasma: its role in thrombotic disease. Thromb Haemost 1995; 74: 71–76.

Wu YP, Siao CJ, Lu W, Sung TC, Frohman MA, Milev P, Bugge TH, Degen JL, Levine JM, Margolis RU, Tsirka SE. The tissue plasminogen activator (tPA)/plasmin extracellular proteolytic system regulates seizure-induced hippocampal mossy fiber outgrowth through a proteoglycan substrate. J Cell Biol 2000; 148: 1295–1304.

Xiao Q, Danton MJ, Witte DP, Kowala MC, Valentine MT, Bugge TH, Degen JL. Plasminogen deficiency accelerates vessel wall disease in mice predisposed to atherosclerosis. Proc Natl Acad Sci (USA) 1997; 94: 10335–10340.

Ye S, Eriksson P, Hamsten A, Kurkinen M, Humphries SE, Henney AM. Progression of coronary atherosclerosis is associated with a common genetic variant of the human stromelysin-1 promoter which results in reduced gene expression. J Biol Chem 1996; 271: 13055–13060.

Zhang B, Ye S, Herrmann SM, Eriksson P, de Maat M, Evans A, Arveiler D, Luc G, Cambien F, Hamsten A, Watkins H, Henney AM. Functional polymorphism in the regulatory region of gelatinase B gene in relation to severity of coronary atherosclerosis. Circulation 1999; 99: 1788–1794.

Zhao Y, Shah DU. Expression of transforming growth factor-beta type I and type II receptors is altered in rat lungs undergoing bleomycin-induced pulmonary fibrosis. Exp Mol Pathol 2000; 69: 67–78.

Zhuo M, Holtzman DM, Li Y, Osaka H, DeMaro J, Jacquin M, Bu G. Role of tissue plasminogen activator receptor LRP in hippocampal long-term potentiation. J Neurosci 2000; 20: 542–549.

Chapter 2

ROLE OF SERINE PROTEASES AND THEIR INHIBITORS IN TUMOR GROWTH AND ANGIOGENESIS

A. Noël and J.-M. Foidart
Laboratory of Tumor and Development Biology, University of Liège, Tour de Pathologie (B23), Sart-Tilman, B-4000 Liège, Belgium

Abstract
Acquisition of invasive/metastatic potential through protease expression is a key event in tumor progression. The proteolytic enzyme plasmin is generated from the precursor plasminogen by the action of urokinase-type plasminogen activator (urokinase, uPA) or tissue-type plasminogen activator (tPA) under the control of plasminogen activator inhibitor-1 or PAI-1. High levels of components of this proteolytic system including uPA, its cell surface receptor (uPAR) and its inhibitor PAI-1 have been correlated with a poor prognosis for different cancers. The initial concept for the implication of serine proteases during cancer progression is that proteases degrade extracellular matrix components, a prerequisite for endothelial, inflammatory or tumor cell migration to distant sites. They have also been implicated in the activation of cytokines or other proteinases, as well as in the release of growth factors sequestered within the extracellular matrix. Recent information have underlined the importance of cell-surface proteases, their receptors/activators or their inhibitors in cell migration. This review focuses on the emerging roles of the plasminogen/plasmin system during cancer growth and angiogenesis with a special emphasis on PAI-1.

1. INTRODUCTION

The invasive process by which malignant tumors disseminate can be considered as an unregulated tissue remodeling process which progressively involves both cancer and normal cells. Recruitment and reorganization of the normal host cells lead progressively to the development of a supporting stroma infiltrated by a new blood capillary network (Noël et al, 1998). Tumor cell invasion and metastatic processes require the coordinated and temporal regulation of a series of adhesive, proteolytic and migratory events (Noël et al, 1997; Reuning et al, 1998). Extracellular proteinases, *i.e.* serine protease and matrix metallo-proteinases have been implicated in cancer metastasis.

The plasminogen system is composed of an inactive proenzyme plasminogen (Plg) that can be converted to plasmin by either of two plasminogen activators

J.-M. Foidart and R.J. Muschel (eds.), Proteases and Their Inhibitors in Cancer Metastasis, 23–38.
© *2002 Kluwer Academic Publishers. Printed in the Netherlands.*

(PA): urokinase-type (uPA) and tissue-type (tPA) plasminogen activators which are serine proteinases (Andreasen et al, 1997; Carmeliet et al, 1998; Dano et al, 1999). Their activity is controlled by plasminogen activator inhibitors, PAI-1 and PAI-2 (plasminogen activator inhibitor-type 1 and type 2), belonging to the serine proteinase inhibitor (serpin) family. Having a broad substrate specificity, plasmin is able to degrade many extracellular matrix components, to activate other proteases such as pro-metalloproteinases, and to activate or release growth factors from the extracellular matrix (Rifkin et al, 1999).

The growth factor domain of pro-uPA or uPA binds a specific, high affinity cell-surface receptor (the urokinase receptor or uPAR) increasing uPA activity and directing plasmin activity to the cell surface (Figure 1). The uPAR is a glycosylphosphatidylinositol (GPI)-linked surface receptor (Blasi, 1997, 1999). While the plasma inhibitor α_2 macroglobulin inactivates soluble uPA relatively slowly, uPA bound to uPAR appears to be protected by a steric effect (Stephens et al, 1991), thus allowing plasminogen activation to occur on the cell surface even in the presence of serum. Interaction between PAI-1 and uPA on the cell surface leads to internalization of the uPAR/uPA/PAI-1 complex and drives uPAR cycling through the endosomal compartment back to the cell surface (Andreasen et al, 1997; Blasi, 1999). The uPA activity may also be lost from the cell surface by proteolytic cleavage, leaving the so-called amino-terminal fragment (ATF) bound on the cell surface. Besides its interaction with uPA, uPAR also binds to the extracellular matrix protein vitronectin and cooperates with some integrins to modulate cell adhesion and migration (Chapman et al, 1999). Recent data suggest that uPAR is an integrin ligand rather than, or in addition to, an integrin-associated protein (Tarui et al, 2001).

2. CLINICAL RELEVANCE OF THE PLASMINOGEN/PLASMIN SYSTEM

Many studies have shown that upregulation of uPA, uPAR and PAI-1 in malignant tumors is associated with increased malignancy [for review, see (Reuning et al, 1998; Andreasen et al, 1997; Frankenne et al, 1999; Brunner et al, 1999; Schmitt et al, 2000). These proteolytic factors are very good prognostic markers, suited to identify cancer patients at risk to develop metastases (Schmitt et al, 2000). Initial studies performed on breast tumors (Duffy et al, 1988; Jaenicke et al, 1989) were extended to a variety of cancers such as ovarian, cervix, bladder, kidney, brain, lung, gastric, colon, pancreas, esophagus and liver cancers (Schmitt et al, 2000). High tumor tissue concentrations of uPA and PAI-1 were also associated to poor prognosis in early stage endometrial cancer.

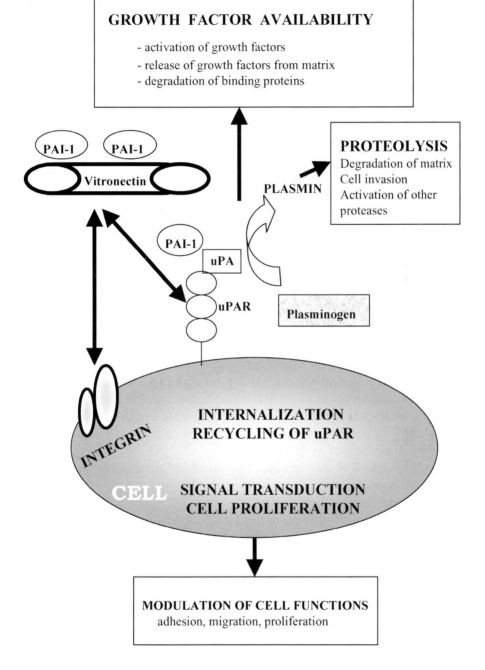

Figure 1. Interplay of components of plasminogen activator system [uPA, uPAR, PAI-1, plasmin(ogen)], integrins, and matrix vitronectin supporting tumor growth, invasion and angiogenesis.

Several publications from different laboratories have consistently reported the worse prognostic significance of high uPA in breast cancers. A recent study shows that high tumor uPA.PAI-1 complex levels were associated with a favorable prognosis (Pedersen et al, 2000). These observations are consistent with the hypothesis that regulation of uPA by PAI-1 through formation of a complex may limit tumor progression. In addition, the fact that high uPAR levels predict poor outcome for breast cancer patients (Grondahl-Hansen et al, 1995; Duggan et al, 1995) may offer an explanation of why high levels of uPA.PAI-1 complex are related to longer survival. Indeed, since uPA.PAI-1 removal could be mediated by the internalization of cell surface uPAR, high complex levels could reflect low uPAR expression. However, this does not explain why high PAI-1 levels are so strongly associated with short survival (Sugiura et al, 1999; Stephens et al, 1998; Pedersen et al, 1994). As PAI-1 is an acute-phase reactant, it remains undetermined whether the increased PAI-1 levels causally contribute to, or rather are the consequence of the malignancy. One potential explanation of this paradox could be a simultaneous enhancement in uPA and PAI-1 expression resulting in a net excess of proteolytic activity. On the opposite, the initially unexpected finding that PAI-1 is a strong negative prognostic marker in cancer may be related to a potential direct role of PAI-1 in cancer cell migration and invasion. Based on immunohistochemical data demonstrating that PAI-1 is mainly localized in endothelial cells in breast cancer, one can suggest that PAI-1 could promote tumor progression by protecting provisional pericellular matrix of neo-vessels forming through uPA-mediated proteolysis.

In contrast, high level of PAI-2 was reported associated with better prognosis in patients with breast cancers (Bouchet et al, 1994; Foekens et al, 1995) but with poor prognosis and aggressive disease in ovarian and colon cancer (Ganesh et al, 1994; Chambers et al, 1995).

The role of PAI-2, if any in cancer invasion and tumorigenesis, is unclear. The different components of the plasminogen activating system may have many different activities depending on the type of tumor.

In recent years, a soluble form of uPAR, suPAR, has been discovered in various human body fluids: in the blood of normal individuals and cancer patients, in acidic and cystic fluids, and in urine (Brunner et al, 1999). In various types of solid cancers such as non-small cell lung cancer (Pappot et al, 1997), breast (Stephens et al, 1997), colorectal (Stephens et al, 1999), prostate (Miyake et al, 1999) and ovarian cancer (Sier et al, 1998), increased levels of su-PAR have been found in plasma and serum. In acute myeloid leukemia, a high level of su-PAR at diagnosis correlates with poor response to chemotherapy (Mustjoki et al, 1999). In response to cytotoxic treatment, su-PAR levels decreased rapidly in acute myeloid leukemia, and the decreasing plasma su-PAR levels correlated highly with reducing numbers of circulating tumor cells, suggesting that the elevated plasma su-PAR was produced by circulating tumor cells (Mustjoki et al, 2000). Neither the exact mechanism(s) of su-PAR release from cells urfaces nor its biological role if any is yet clearly defined.

Altogether, these clinical data have prompted basic researchers to investigate how the plasminogen/plasmin system is involved during cancer progression, and to develop strategies to interfere with this proteolytic system in order to prevent tumor growth and metastatic dissemination.

3. IMPLICATION OF THE PLASMINOGEN/PLASMIN SYSTEM IN TUMOR PROGRESSION

3.1. The pericellular proteolysis

Data supporting the role of uPA in cellular invasion and metastases derive from *in vitro* and *in vivo* experiments demonstrating 1) a correlation between uPA expression and cell invasion and metastasis; 2) a reduction of metastatic potential by using natural or synthetic serine protease inhibitors, neutralizing antibodies to uPA, uPAR antagonists (Tressler et al, 1999) or anti-sense oligonucleotides (Ossowski et al, 1991; Yu et al, 1990); 3) an enhancement of tumor dissemination by cells overexpressing uPA [for review, see (Schmitt et al, 2000; Andreasen et al, 1997)].

UPA plays thus a key role in pericellular proteolysis. tPA, the second type of human plasminogen activator, does not promote tumour cell surface associated proteolysis since it activates plasminogen into plasmin without attaching to a specific cell surface receptor. The uPA-uPAR receptor interaction is involved in pericellular proteolysis, migration, chemotaxis and adhesion of tumoral cells.

The amino acids 13-31 of the N-terminal fragment (Amino-Terminal-Fragment ATF) of uPA binds to the uPAR. The formation of a PAI-1.uPA.uPAR complex initiates its internalization in association with another cell surface receptor, the low-density lipoprotein receptor related to protein (LRP, CD91) also termed the α_2-macroglobulin receptor. On the contrary, PAI-2 also complexes to receptor-bound uPA but does not induce the internalization of the PAI-2.uPA.uPAR complex.

It is generally believed that uPA present at the cell surface initiates a protease cascade which in turn leads to the breakdown of the extracellular matrix and thereby promotes tissue remodeling and cellular migration. In addition, proteolysis of the extracellular matrix in turn stimulate tumor growth and angiogenesis by releasing growth factors and cytokines (Figure 1). Angiogenic factors such as fibroblast growth factor (FGF) and vascular endothelial cell growth factor (VEGF) can bind to matrix in a manner that affects their availability (Rifkin et al, 1999; Bergers et al, 2000). On another hand, many growth factors circulate as latent proteins. For instances, hepatocyte growth factor (HGF), insulin-like growth factor (IGF), and transforming growth factor β (TGFβ) are all found extracellularly either in latent forms that must be activated by proteolytic cleavage, or complexed to binding proteins (such as IGF-BP) that must be removed to allow binding of the growth factor to its receptor. Latent HGF can be activated by uPA and plasmin has been implicated in the release of FGF and VEGF from the extracellular matrix and in the degradation of IGF-BP (Noël et al, 1997). In addition, plasmin can activate TGFβ which is considered as a potent inducer of PAI-1 and TIMPs gene expression and a repressor of the expression of uPA and MMPs in many cell types [for review, see (Rifkin et al, 1999)].

Thus, serine proteases in cooperation with MMPs appear to play a key role in the biological availability of growth factors, cytokines and chemokines.

3.2. Other non-proteolytic activities of the plasminogen activation system

Other uPA effects independent of its plasminogen activating function include growth factor-like function, chemotactic, adhesive and migratory properties [for review, see (Blasi, 1997; Chapman et al, 1999)]. Most of these functions are mediated by binding of uPA to its cell surface receptor.

uPA conveys a mitogenic signal, probably by several ways. Inactive forms of this enzyme or even ATF stimulate the proliferation of osteosarcoma cells (Rabbani et al, 1990) or ovarian carcinoma cells (Fischer et al, 1998). On the contrary, uPA mediated stimulation of smooth muscle cell proliferation requires its enzymatic activity. It appears therefore that several mitogenic signals can be switched on by uPA and that different parts of the uPA molecule may be involved depending upon cell type and mechanisms [for a review, see (Schmitt et al, 2000)]. The uPAR is a true chemotactic molecule whose activity lies within the protease-sensitive region linking domains 1 and 2 of uPAR, which can be cleaved by uPA. Synthetic peptides spanning this epitope promote chemotaxis and activate P56/p59 hck tyrosine kinase. Thus uPAR can be transformed through cleavage by uPA or other protease(s) into a chemokine acting on the same, or neighboring cells (Blasi, 1997; Fazioli et al, 1997).

Recent data also support the concept that plasminogen/plasmin system is an important link between pericellular proteolysis and cell adhesion to the extracellular matrix (Loskutoff et al, 1999; Chapman et al, 1999) (Figure 1). Cells transfected with uPAR bind to, adhere and spread on vitronectin in an RGD-independent way. This is due to an interaction beween uPAR and vitronectin probably *via* an induced conformational change in uPAR following uPA binding, thereby increasing its affinity to vitronectin (Wei et al, 1994; Deng et al, 1994; Kanse et al, 1996; Sidenius et al, 2000). Indeed, uPA has been demonstrated to promote the adhesion of monocyte-like U937 cells, smooth muscle cells or melanoma cells to vitronectin (Knudson et al, 1987; Stahl et al, 1997). The uPAR interacts simultaneously with vitronectin and uPA suggesting a dynamic coupling of molecular mechanisms underlaying plasminogen-dependent matrix degradation and cell adhesion and migration. PAI-1 controls cell matrix inter-action mediated through integrins or uPAR/uPA complex by regulating the accessibility of specific cell-attachment sites (Chapman, 1997; Loskutoff et al, 1999; Stefansson et al, 1996; Deng et al, 1996) (*see below*). Stable complexes between uPAR and integrins can also modulate integrin functions thereby influ-encing tumour cell adhesion and migration (Yebra et al, 1999). A specific inter-action site of a uPAR and β1 integrin was recently identified (Simon et al, 2000) that promotes spreading and migration of human vascular smooth muscle cells on fibronectin and collagen. uPAR occupancy results in an interaction between uPAR and integrins and a potentiation of integrin mediated signaling and thus in cell migration. Chapman et al (1999) have identified a peptide able to disrupt uPAR-caveolin integrin complexes. Thus, the cholesterol binding protein termed caveolin associates with β1 integrins. This association is required for src-kinases binding β1 integrins. In the presence of the peptide that disrupts the uPAR-caveolin-β1 integrin, there is a loss of focal adhesion kinase phosphorylation and no formation of focal adhesion sites (Chapman et al, 1999).

4. TARGETED GENE-INACTIVATION

Recent studies using gene-deficient mice focused on the contribution of host uPA, tPA, uPAR, plasminogen and PAI-1 in tumor growth, angiogenesis and dissemination. Plasminogen deficiency resulted in a delay, but not a complete arrest of non-neoplastic tissue remodeling processes such as wound healing and of cancer invasion and metastasis (Bugge et al, 1997). In plasminogen$^{-/-}$ mice, lung metastasis of the polyoma middle T antigen-induced mammary cancer was substantially delayed, but did eventually occur (Bugge et al, 1998). Primary Lewis lung carcinomas developed both in wild-type and plasminogen$^{-/-}$ mice (Bugge et al, 1997). However, dissemination of such tumors to regional lymph node was delayed in plasminogen$^{-/-}$ mice. Nevertheless, sufficient proteolytic activity is generated in plasminogen$^{-/-}$ mice for efficient tumor development and metastasis. Consistently, tumor vascularization was delayed but not completely impaired in plasminogen$^{-/-}$ mice transplanted with transformed keratinocytes (Bajou et al, 2001). Altogether, these data suggest that plasmin-mediated proteolysis is essential, but not sufficient for tumor growth and angiogenesis. This could be due to a functional overlap between plasmin and certain MMPs in matrix degradation (Dano et al, 1999).

Evidence for a role of uPA in malignant progression was provided by Shapiro et al (1996), in carcinogen-induced melanocytic neoplasms. However, more than 95% of cellular blue nevi invaded the underlying tissues in wild-type and uPA-deficient mice. While lack of uPA reduced primary tumor growth, it did have a substantial effect on tumor angiogenesis (Gutierrez et al, 2000). This is consistent with the fact that similar vascularization was observed in malignant keratinocyte transplants in wild-type and uPA$^{-/-}$ mice (Bajou et al, 2001).

Based on its ability to block uPA proteolysis, PAI-1 would be anticipated to impair tumorigenesis. Accordingly, Lewis lung carcinoma cells injected into mice over-expressing human PAI-1 showed a reduction of lung metastasis (Donati, 1995). However, deficiency of host PAI-1 or elevation of systemic levels in transgenic mice did not influence neither the primary tumor growth, nor the metastatic potential of B16 melanoma cells (Eitzman et al, 1996). Such a discrepancy may reflect tumor-specific differences in the relative importance of the plasminogen system. Human ocular melanoma cells implanted ortho-topically in the eyes of nude mice are reduced in their metastatic potential by both local gene transfer of PAI-1 into the tumor and systemic enhancement of PAI-1 levels using liver gene transfer (Ma et al, 1997). PAI-1 inhibited meta-stasis of HT1080 cells when expressed by tumor cells, suggesting autocrine or paracrine effects. However, PAI-1 was not efficient when over-expressed in the circulation (Praus et al, 1999). The reason for these controversial data remains to be elucidated, but may be due to differences in the level of uPA produced by tumor cells. Indeed, the 10 times higher uPA level produced by HT1080 cells as compared to melanoma cells may explain why PAI-1 liver gene transfer reduced metastasis and prolonged survival in the melanoma model, but not in the HT1080 one (Praus et al, 1999).

The balance between plasminogen activators and PAI-1 could also affect metastasis by modulating angiogenesis and, thereby the access of tumor cells to the vascular system. The overexpression of PAI-1 in PC-3 human prostate carcinoma cells reduced tumor growth, vascularization and metastasis to lung and liver (Soff et al, 1995). In order to investigate the role played by host PAI-1 in tumor invasion and angiogenesis, more recently, murine malignant keratinocytes plated on a collagen gel were implanted into PAI-1-deficient mice (Bajou et al, 1998). These cancer cells invaded the tissues of wild-type host, but not those of PAI-1$^{-/-}$ mice. Moreover, endothelial cells from PAI-1-deficient hosts failed to migrate and to vascularize the implanted. As malig-nant PDVA cells produced uPA, tPA and PAI-1, the genotypic effect on tumor invasion and vascularization was attributable to PAI-1 produced by host mesenchymal cells and/or sprouting endothelial cells. Obviously, PAI-1 produced by the cancer cells was not sufficient to overcome the host cell deficiency. This conclusion was further strengthened by the finding that the tumor invasion and vascularisation in PAI-1$^{-/-}$ mice were both restored by systemic adenoviral PAI-1 gene transfer (Bajou et al, 1998).

Although the exact mechanism of PAI-1 action remains to be elucidated, different hypothesis could be formulated. PAI-1 may be implicated in the stabilization of the extracellular matrix surrounding sprouting neovessels. Migration of endothelial cells requires proteolytic remodeling of the extracellular matrix (Schnaper et al, 1995). Plasmin activity is not an absolute requirement for physiological angiogenesis, as mice deficient in plasminogen, tPA or uPA develop relatively normally [for a review see (Carmeliet and Collen, 1998; Carmeliet et al, 1997). In accordance, vascularization of malignant keratinocyte transplants was not affected in mice deficient in tPA, uPA, both uPA and tPA, or uPAR (Bajou et al, 2001). Lack of one plasminogen activator could be compensated by the other. Interestingly, plasmin activity was still detected in double uPA and tPA-deficient mice. The reduced tumor invasion and vascularization in plasminogen$^{-/-}$ mice further emphasizes the requirement of plasmin for optimal tumor progression (Bajou et al, 2001). Altogether, the data obtained with the transplantation model of keratinocytes (Bajou et al, 2001) suggest that optimal tumor vascularization requires a tightly controlled plasmin-mediated proteolysis. It is well known that endothelial cell invasion is enhanced *in vitro* in the presence of plasminogen, as a result of cell-mediated plasmin formation. However, excessive proteolysis prevents the coordinated assembly of endothelial cells into capillaries, suggesting that proteolytic activity needs to be tightly controlled (Montesano et al, 1990). The sequestration of PAI-1 in the extracellular matrix is consistent with this role in the maintenance of a certain degree of matrix integrity for capillary morphogenesis (Loskutoff et al, 1999). A precise balance between proteolytic enzyme and their inhibitors may be essential for endothelial cell migration and differentiation into functional vessels. This appears also to be the case for tumor cell migration and invasion. Indeed, Tsuboi and Rifkin (1990) have previously demonstrated that production of high levels of either tPA or uPA blocks cell invasion, whereas synthesis of moderate to low levels of uPA promotes cell invasion.

A second mechanism of PAI-1 action is that PAI-1 promotes tumor angiogenesis by inhibiting angiostation generation. Angiostatin, a kringle containing peptide from plasminogen, is a potent inhibitor of angiogenesis (O'Reilly et al, 1997) which can be generated by limited proteolysis of plasminogen by plasmin, uPA, tPA or matrix metalloproteinases (Stack et al, 1999; Gately et al, 1997). Although angiostatin has been shown to inhibit both endothelial cell migration and proliferation, recent data demonstrate that it might regulate tPA activity. Indeed, it binds tPA and blocks its association to matrix components and hence the matrix-enhanced plasminogen activation by tPA (Stack et al, 1999). Nevertheless, the lack of plasminogen in mice was associated with a decreased rather than an increased formation of blood vessels (Bajou et al, 2001), suggesting that, in the transplantation system, angiostatin formation is not a critical event.

Alternatively, PAI-1 may potentiate cell migration by regulating cell adhesion and migration. There is an accumulating evidence that both the uPAR and PAI-1 are multifunctional proteins involved not only in extracellular matrix proteolysis, but also in cellular adhesion and migration *via* their binding sites for vitronectin (Chapman, 1997). PAI-1 may potentiate tumor cell migration by promoting uPA turnover from its receptor, with subsequent attachment of uPAR to vitronectin. PAI-1 could also be considered as the molecular switch that governs uPAR- and/or integrin-mediated cell adhesion and release. Vitronectin contains a RGD sequence recognized by integrins and located C-terminally and to the vicinity of its somatomedin B domain. Although plasma vitronectin is in a 'closed conformation' that does not interact with integrins, PAI-1 converts this latent form to the open integrin binding conformation of vitronectin (Deng et al, 1996). Paradoxically, PAI-1 inhibits the binding of the integrin $\alpha_v\beta_3$ to vitronectin and in this way blocks smooth muscle cell migration (Stefansson and Lawrence, 1996). The $\alpha_v\beta_3$ attachment site on vitronectin was found to overlap with the binding for PAI-1. Therefore, the binding of PAI-1 to the somatomedin B domain of vitronectin not only directly blocks uPAR-mediated adhesion, but also sterically inhibits $\alpha_v\beta_3$ binding to vitronectin RGD sequence. PAI-1 competes with the binding of vitronectin to different integrins such $\alpha_v\beta_1$, $\alpha_v\beta_3$, $\alpha_v\beta_5$, $\alpha_{IIb}\beta_3$ and $\alpha_8\beta_1$ (Sugiura et al, 1999). Accordingly, PAI-1 was reported to inhibit integrin-dependent migration of human amnion WISH cells and human carcinoma Hep-2 cells on vitronectin (Kjoller et al, 1997). Altogether, these observations suggest that although the interactions between PAI-1 and vitronectin induce the cell binding conformation of vitronectin, it simultaneously blocks the cell binding site via both integrins and uPAR.

Cellular migration has been considered as resulting from a succession of attachment and detachment events. Thus, the capability of PAI-1 in inhibiting vitronectin/ uPAR and vitronectin/integrin binding would make PAI-1 anti-migratory at the leading edge. On the other hand, the PAI-1-stimulated endo-cytosis of uPAR/uPA complex would remove adhesive cell-surface molecules and eliminate PAI-1 through internalization. Since the uPAR is recycled at the cell surface and preferentially at the leading edge, it would facilitate new rounds of adhesion as the cells moves along the substrates. However, when malignant keratinocytes were transplanted into PAI-1$^{-/-}$ mice, neither tumor vascularization, nor invasion was restored by injection of an adenovirus expressing a mutant of PAI-1 that binds normally to vitronectin, but that is inactive as protease inhibitor (Bajou et al, 2001). Furthermore, deficiency of vitronectin in mice did not affect the invasive and angiogenic phenotype of malignant keratinocytes. On the opposite, restoration of tumor invasion and vascularization in PAI-1$^{-/-}$ mice was observed after adenovirus-mediated transfer of a mutant PAI-1 defective in binding to vitronectin, but able to inhibit proteolytic activity. This further supports the importance of a precise balance between protease and inhibitors for optimal angiogenesis.

5. CONCLUSIONS

Therapeutic strategies that counteract tumour invasion, metastasis and tumoral angiogenesis are being developed. Such combined treatments with radiotherapy, chemotherapy, surgery, hormone therapy might reveal useful approaches. They are indeed targeting key gene products of tumour associated host cells such as inflammatory cells, endothelial cells, fibroblasts . . . These cells are indeed responsible for the bulk production of proteases in many tumors. Since tumor invasion, growth and angiogenesis result from a coordinated interaction between tumoral cells and host cells, it is anticipated that the selective inhibition of host cells activation in tumor might block cancer progression. Protease inhibitors of the MMPs and of the plasminogen activation system and antiangiogenic agents might therefore be excellent candidates to cancer treatments targeting normal host cells. In contrast, to tumoral cells, they are indeed genetically stable and do not regularly develop mutational resistance to anti-cancerous agents. Naturally occurring and synthetic inhibitors of uPA, antibodies to uPAR and uPA, antisense oligodeoxynucleotides, recombinant and synthetic ATF or soluble uPAR are being evaluated (Schmitt et al, 2000) in various tumor models in animals.

Finally, the overproduction of proteases and particularly plasmin may be exploited by the use of pro-drugs consisting of chemotherapeutic agents linked to a blocking peptide. The selective activation of such pro-drugs is then achieved preferentially in tumors during tumor-associated protease plasmin expression that removes the inactivating peptide (de Groot et al, 2000).

ACKNOWLEDGMENTS

This work was supported by grants from the Communauté Française de Belgique (Actions de Recherches Concertées), the Commission of European Communities, the Fonds de la Recherche Scientifique Médicale, the Fonds National de la Recherche Scientifique (FNRS, Belgium), the Fédération Belge Contre le Cancer, the Fonds spéciaux de la Recherche (University of Liège), the Centre Anticancéreux près l'Université de Liège, the CGER-FORTIS-Assurances, the Fondation Léon Frédéricq (University of Liège), the D.G.T.R.E. from the 'Région Wallonne', and the Fonds d'Investisse-ments de la Recherche Scientifique (CHU, Liège, Belgium). A.N. is a Senior Research Associate from the FNRS.

REFERENCES

Andreasen PA, Kjoller L, Christensen L, Duffy MJ. The urokinase-type plasminogen activator system in cancer metastasis: a review. Int J Cancer 1997; 72: 1–22.

Bajou K, Masson V, Gerard RD, Schmitt P, Albert V, Praus M, Lund LR, Frandsen TL, Brunner N, Dano K, Fusenig NE, Weidle UH, Carmeliet G, Loskutoff DJ, Collen D, Carmeliet P, Foidart JM, Noël A. The plasminogen activator inhibitor PAI-1 controls in vivo tumor vascularization by interaction with proteases, not vitronectin: implications for antiangiogenic strategies. J Cell Biol 2001; 152: 777–784.

Bajou K, Noël A, Gerard RD, Masson V, Brunner N, Holst-Hansen C, Skobe M, Fusenig NE, Carmeliet P, Collen D, Foidart JM. Absence of host plasminogen activator inhibitor 1 prevents cancer invasion and vascularization. Nat Med 1998; 4: 923–928.

Bergers G, Brekken R, McMahon GA, Vu TH, Itoh T, Tamaki K, Tanzawa K, Thorpe P, Werb Z, Hanahan D. Matrix metalloproteinase-9 triggers the angiogenic switch during carcinogenesis. Nat Cell Biol 2000; 2: 737–744.

Blasi F. uPA, uPAR, PAI-1: key intersection of proteolytic, adhesive and chemotactic highways? Immunol Today 1997; 18: 415–417.

Blasi F. The urokinase receptor. A cell surface, regulated chemokine. APMIS 1999; 107: 96–101.

Bouchet C, Spyratos F, Martin PM, Hacene K, Gentile A, Oglobine J. Prognostic value of urokinase-type plasminogen activator and 2 inhibitors PAI-1 and PAI-2 in breast cancer. Bull Cancer 1994; 81: 770–779.

Brunner N, Nielsen HJ, Hamers M, Christensen IJ, Thorlacius-Ussing O, Stephens RW. The urokinase plasminogen activator receptor in blood from healthy individuals and patients with cancer. APMIS 1999; 107: 160–167.

Bugge TH, Kombrinck KW, Xiao Q, Holmback K, Daugherty CC, Witte DP, Degen JL. Growth and dissemination of Lewis lung carcinoma in plasminogen-deficient mice. Blood 1997; 90: 4522–4531.

Bugge TH, Lund LR, Kombrinck KK, Nielsen BS, Holmback K, Drew AF, Flick MJ, Witte DP, Dano K, Degen JL. Reduced metastasis of Polyoma virus middle T antigen-induced mammary cancer in plasminogen-deficient mice. Oncogene 1998; 16: 3097–3104.

Carmeliet P, Collen D. Development and disease in proteinase-deficient mice: role of the plasminogen, matrix metalloproteinase and coagulation system. Thromb Res 1998; 91: 255–285.

Carmeliet P, Moons L, Lijnen R, Baes M, Lemaitre V, Tipping P, Drew A, Eeckhout Y, Shapiro S, Lupu F, Collen D. Urokinase-generated plasmin activates matrix metalloproteinases during aneurysm formation. Nat Genet 1997; 17: 439–444.

Chambers SK, Gertz RE, Ivins CM, Kacinski BM. The significance of urokinase-type plasminogen activator, its inhibitors and its receptor in ascites of patients with epithelial ovarian cancer. Cancer 1995; 75: 1627–1633.

Chapman HA. Plasminogen activators, integrins and the coordinated regulation of cell adhesion and migration. Curr Opin Cell Biol 1997; 9: 714–724.

Chapman HA, Wei Y, Simon DI, Waltz DA. Role of urokinase receptor and caveolin in regulation of integrin signaling. Thromb Haemost 1999; **82**: 291–297.

Dano K, Romer J, Nielsen BS, Bjorn S, Pyke C, Rygaard J, Lund LR. Cancer invasion and tissue remodeling-cooperation of protease systems and cell types. APMIS 1999; 107: 120–127.

de Groot FMH, van Berkom LWA, Scheeren HW. Synthesis and biological evaluation of 2'-carbamate-linked and 2'-carbonate-linked prodrugs of paclitaxel: Selective activation by the tumor-associated protease plasmin. J Med Chem 2000; 43: 3093–3102.

Deng G, Curriden SA, Wang S, Rosenberg S, Loskutoff DJ. Is plasminogen activator inhibitor-1 the molecular switch that governs urokinase receptor-mediated cell adhesion and release? J Cell Biol 1996; 134: 1–9.

Deng G, Waltz DA, Navaneetha R, Drummond RJ, Rosenberg S, Chapman HA. Identification of the urokinase receptor as an adhesion receptor for vitronectin. J Biol Chem 1994; 269: 32380–32388.

Donati MD. Cancer and thrombosis: from phlegmasia alba dolens to transgenic mice. Thromb Haemost 1995; 74: 278–281.

Duffy MJ, O'Grady PDDOLFJLHJ. Urokinase-plasminogen activator, a marker for aggressive breast carcinomas. Preliminary report. Cancer 1988; 62: 351–353.

Duggan C, Maguire T, McDermott E, O'Higgins N, Fennelly JJ, Duffy MJ. Urokinase plasminogen activator and urokinase plasminogen activator receptor in breast cancer. Int J Cancer 1995; 61: 597–600.

Eitzman DT, Krauss JC, Shen T, Cui J, Ginsburg. Lack of plasminogen activator inhibitor-1 effect in a transgenic mouse model of metastatic melanoma. Blood 1996; 87: 4718–4722.

Fazioli F, Resnati M, Sidenius N, Higashimoto Y, Appella E, Blasi F. A urokinase-sensitive region of the human urokinase receptor is responsible for its chemotactic activity. EMBO J 1997; 16: 7279–7286.

Fischer K, Lutz V, Wilhelm O, et al. Urokinase induces proliferation of human ovarian cancer cells: characterization of structural elements required for growth factor function. FEBS Lett 1998; 438: 101–105.

Foekens JA, Buessecker F, Peters HA, et al. Plasminogen activator inhibitor-2: prognostic relevance in 1012 patients with primary breast cancer. Cancer Res 1995; 55: 1423–1427.

Frankenne F, Noël A, Bajou K, Sounni NE, Goffin F, Masson V, Munaut C, Remacle A, Foidart JM. Molecular interactions involving urokinase plasminogen activator (uPA), its receptor (uPAR) and its inhibitor, plasminogen activator inhibitor-1 (PAI-1), as new targets for tumour therapy. Emerging Therapeutic Targets 1999; 3: 469–481.

Ganesh S, Sier CF, Griffioen G, et al. Prognostic relevance of plasminogen activators and their inhibitors in colorectal cancer. Cancer Res 1994; 54: 4065–4071.

Gately S, Twardowski P, Stack MS, Cundiff DL, Grella D, Castellino FJ, Enghild J, Kwaan HC, Lee F, Kramer RA, Volpert O, Bouck N, Soff GA. The mechanism of cancer-mediated conversion of plasminogen to the angiogenesis inhibitor angiostatin. Proc Natl Acad Sci (USA) 1997; 94: 10868–10872.

Grondahl-Hansen J, Peters HA, van Putten WL, Look MP, Pappot H, Ronne E, Dano K, Klijn JG, Brunner N, Foekens JA. Prognostic significance of the receptor for urokinase plasminogen activator in breast cancer. Clin Cancer Res 1995; 1: 1079–1087.

Gutierrez LS, Schulman A, Brito-Robinson T, Noria F, Ploplis VA, Castellino FJ. Tumor development is retarded in mice lacking the gene for urokinase-type plasminogen activator or its inhibitor, plasminogen activator inhibitor-1. Cancer Res 2000; 60: 5839–5847.

Jaenicke F, Schmitt M, Graeff H. Urokinase-type plasminogen activator antigen and early relapse in breast cancer [letter]. Lancet 1989; 2: 1049.

Kanse S, Kost C, Wilhelm O andreasen PA, Preissner KT. The urokinase receptor is a major vitronectin-binding protein on endothelial cells. Exp Cell Res 1996; 224: 344–353.

Kjoller L, Kanse SM, Kirkegaard T, Rodenburg KW, Ronne E, Goodman SL, Preissner KT, Ossowski L, Andreasen PA. Plasminogen activator inhibitor-1 represses integrin- and vitronectin-mediated cell migration independently of its function as an inhibitor of plasminogen activation. Exp Cell Res 1997; 232: 420–429.

Knudson BS, Hapel PC, Nachman RL. Plasminogen activator inhibitor is associated with the extracellular matrix of cultured bovine smooth muscle cells. J Clin Invest 1987; 80: 1082–1089.

Loskutoff DJ, Curriden SA, Hu G, Deng G. Regulation of cell adhesion by PAI-1. APMIS 1999; 107: 54–61.

Ma D, Gerard RD, Li XY, Alizadeh H, Niederkorn JY. Inhibition of metastasis of intraocular melanomas by adenovirus-mediated gene transfer of plasminogen activator inhibitor type 1 (PAI-1) in an athymic mouse model. Blood 1997; 90: 2738–2746.

Miyake H, Hara I, Yamanaka K, Gohji K, Arakawa S, Kamidono S. Elevation of serum levels of urokinase-type plasminogen activator and its receptor is associated with disease progression and prognosis in patients with prostate cancer. Prostate 1999; 39: 123–129.

Montesano R, Pepper MS, Mohle-Steinlein U, Risau W, Wagner EF, Orci L. Increased proteolytic activity is responsible for the aberrant morphogenetic behavior of endothelial cells expressing the middle T oncogene. Cell 1990; 62: 435–445.

Mustjoki S, Alitalo R, Stephens RW, Vaheri A. Blast cell-surface and plasma soluble urokinase receptor in acute leukemia patients: relationship to classification and response to therapy. Thromb Haemost 1999; 81: 705–710.

Mustjoki S, Sidenius N, Sier CF, Blasi F, Elonen E, Alitalo R, Vaheri A. Soluble urokinase receptor levels correlate with number of circulating tumor cells in acute myeloid leukemia and decrease rapidly during chemotherapy. Cancer Res 2000; 60: 7126–7132.

Noël A, Foidart JM. The role of extra-cellular matrix and fibroblasts in breast carcinoma growth in vivo. J Mammary Gland Biol Neoplasia 1998; 3: 215–225.

Noël A, Gilles C, Bajou K, Devy L, Kebers F, Lewalle JM, Maquoi E, Munaut C, Remacle A, Foidart JM. Emerging roles for proteinases in cancer. Invasion Metastasis 1997; 17: 221–239.

O'Reilly MS, Boehm T, Shing Y, Fukai N, Vasios G, Lane WS, Flynn E, Birkhead JR, Olsen BR, Folkman J. Endostatin: an endogenous inhibitor of angiogenesis and tumor growth. Cell 1997; 88: 277–285.

Ossowski L, Russo-Payne H, Wilson EL. Inhibition of urokinase-type plasminogen activator by antibodies: the effects on dissemination of a human tumor in the nude mouse. Cancer Res 1991; 51: 274–281.

Pappot H, Hoyer-Hansen G, Ronne E, Hoi-Hansen H, Brunner N, Dano K, Grondahl-Hansen J. Elevated levels of receptor for urokinase plasminogen activator in patients with non-small cell lung cancer. Eur J Cancer 1997; 33: 867–872.

Pedersen AN, Christensen IJ, Stephens RW, Briand P, Mouridsen H, Dano K.The complex between urokinase and its type-1 inhibitor in primary breast cancer: relation to survival. Cancer Res 2000; 60: 6927–6934.

Pedersen H, Brunner N, Francis D, Osterlind K, Ronne E, Hansen HH, Dano K, Grondahl-Hansen J. Prognostic impact of urokinase, urokinase receptor and type 1 plasminogen activator inhibitor in squamous and large cell lung cancer tissue. Cancer Res 1994; 54: 4671–4675.

Praus M, Wauterickx K, Collen D, Gerard RD. Reduction of tumor cell migration and metastasis by adenoviral gene transfer of plasminogen activator inhibitors. Gene Therapy 1999; 6: 236.

Rabbani SA, Desjardins J, Bell AW, et al. An aminotemial fragment of urokinase isolated from a prostate cancer cell line (PC-3) is mitogenic for osteoblast-like cells. Biochem Biophys Res Commun 1990; 173: 1058–1064.

Reuning U, Magdolen V, Wilhelm O, Fischer K, Lutz V, Graeff H, Schmitt M. Multifunctional potential of the plasminogen activation system in tumor invasion and metastasis (review). Int J Oncol 1998; 13: 893–906.

Rifkin DB, Mazzieri R, Munger JS, Noguera I, Sung J. Proteolytic control of growth factor availability. APMIS 1999; 107: 80–85.

Schmitt M, Wilhelm O, Reuning U, Kruger A, Harbeck. The urokinase plasminogen activator system as a novel target for tumour therapy. Fibrinolysis & Proteolysis 2000; 14: 114–132.

Schnaper HW, Barnathan ES, Mazar A, Maheshwari S, Ellis S, Cortez SL, Baricos WH, Kleinman HK. Plasminogen activators augment endothelial cell organization in vitro by two distinct pathways. J Cell Physiol 1995; 165: 107–118.

Shapiro RL, Duquette JG, Roses DF, Nunes I, Harris MN, Kamino H, Wilson EL, Rifkin DB. Induction of primary cutaneous melanocytic neoplasms in urokinase-type plasminogen activator (uPA)-deficient and wild-type mice: cellular blue nevi invade but do not progress to malignant melanoma in uPA-deficient animals. Cancer Res 1996; 56: 3597–3604.

Sidenius N, Blasi F. Domain 1 of the urokinase receptor (uPAR) is required for uPAR-mediated cell binding to vitronectin. FEBS Lett 2000; 470: 40–46.

Sier CF, Stephens RW, Bizik J, Mariani A, Bassan M, Pedersen N, Frigerio L, Ferrari A, Dano K, Brunner N, Blasi F. The level of urokinase type plasminogen activator receptor is increased in serum of ovarian cancer patients. Cancer Res 1998; 58: 1843–1849.

Simon DI, Wei Y, Zhang L, Rao NK, Xu H, Chen Z, Liu Q, Rosenberg S, Chapman HA. Identification of a urokinase receptor-integrin interaction site. Promiscuous regulator of integrin function. J Biol Chem 2000; 275: 10228–10234.

Soff GA, Sanderowitz J, Gately S, Verrusio E, Weiss I, Brem S, Kwaan HC. Expression of plasminogen activator inhibitor type 1 by human prostate carcinoma cells inhibits primary tumor growth, tumor-associated angiogenesis and metastasis to lung and liver in an athymic mouse model. J Clin Invest 1995; 96, 2593–2600.

Stack MS, Gately S, Bafetti LM, Enghild J, Soff GA. Angiostatin inhibitits endothelial and melanoma cellular invasion by blocking matrix-enhanced plasminogen activation. Biochem J 1999; 340: 77–84.

Stahl A, Mueller BM. Melanoma cell migration on vitronectin: regulation by components of the plasminogen activation system. Int J Cancer 1997; 71: 116–122.

Stefansson S, Lawrence DA. The serpin PAI-1 inhibits cell migration by blocking integrin alpha V beta 3 binding to vitronectin [see comments]. Nature 1996; 383: 441–443.

Stephens R, Pedersen AN, Nielsen HJ, Hamers M, Hoyer-Hansen G, Ronne E, Dybkjaer E, Dano K, Brunner N. ELISA determination of soluble urokinase receptor in blood from healthy donors and cancer patients. Clin Chem 1997; 43: 1868–1876.

Stephens RW, Brunner N, Janicke F, Schmitt M. The urokinase plasminogen activator system as a target for prognostic studies in breast cancer. Breast Cancer Res Treat 1998; 52: 99–111.

Stephens RW, Nielsen HJ, Christensen IJ, Thorlacius-Ussing O, Sorensen S, Dano K, Brunner N. Plasma urokinase receptor levels in patients with colorectal cancer: relationship to prognosis. J Natl Cancer Inst 1999; 91: 869–874.

Stephens RW, Tapiovaara HRTBJVA. Alpha$_2$-macroglobulin restricts plasminogen activation to the surface of RC2A leukemia cells. Cell Regul 1991; 2: 1057–1065.

Sugiura Y, Ma L, Sun B, Shimada H, Laug WE, Seeger RC, Declerck YA. The plasminogen-

plasminogen activator (PA) system in neuroblastoma: role of PA inhibitor-1 in metastasis. Cancer Res 1999; 59: 1327–1336.

Tarui T, Mazar AP, Cines DB, Takada Y. Urokinase receptor (uPAR/CD87) is a ligand for integrins and mediates cell-cell interaction. J Biol Chem 2001; 276: 3983–3990.

Tsuboi R, Rifkin DB. Bimodal relationship between invasion of the amniotic membrane and plasminogen activator activity. Int J Cancer 1990; 46: 56–60.

Tressler RJ, Pitot PA, Stratton-Thomas JR, Forrest LD, Zhuo S, Drummond RJ, Fong S, Doyle MV, Doyle LV, Min HY, Rosenberg S. Urokinase receptor antagonists: discovery and application to in vivo models of tumor growth. APMIS 1999; 107: 168–173.

Wei Y, Waltz DA, Rao NK, Drummond RJ, Rosenberg S, Chapman HA. Identification of the urokinase receptor as an adhesion receptor for vitronectin. J Biol Chem 1994; 269: 32380–32388.

Yebra M, Goretzki L, Pfeifer M, Mueller BM. Urokinase-type plasminogen activator binding to its receptor stimulates tumor cell migration by enhancing integrin-mediated signal transduction. Exp Cell Res 1999; 250: 231–240.

Yu HR, Schultz RM. Relationship between secreted urokinase plasminogen activator activity and metastatic potential in murine B16 cells transfected with human urokinase sense and antisense genes. Cancer Res 1990; 50: 7623–7633.

38

Chapter 3

THE GELATINASES, MMP-2 AND MMP-9-IMPLICATIONS FOR INVASION AND METASTASIS

Ruth J. Muschel and Jiang Yong
Department of Pathology and Laboratory Medicine, Rm 269 John Morgan Bld., University of Pennsylvania, Philadelphia, PA 19104, USA

1. INTRODUCTION

The gelatinase subgroup of matrix metalloproteinases consists of two highly homologous members, a larger 92 kDa enzyme MMP-9 and a smaller 72 kDa, MMP-2. These enzymes have been shown to be frequently overexpressed in carcinomas and there is considerable evidence pointing to the involvement of these enzymes, MMP-2 and 9, that have also been termed gelatinase A and B or the 72 and 92 kDa Type IV collagenase in malignant progression of tumors and in invasion and metastasis. Their expression is frequently elevated in carcinomas compared to comparable normal tissues [for review see Curran and Murray (Curran and Murray, 2000)]. In some cases the overexpression of MMP-9, or of activation of MMP-2 can be shown to correlate with a worse prognosis. Interestingly, sometimes the elevation in expression is in the tumor cells themselves, but it can also be in the host stroma. In this review we will consider the structure of these two homologous enzymes, the evidence for their biological functions *in vivo* and for their involvement in invasion and metastasis.

2. THE GELATINASES-STRUCTURE AND FUNCTION

These two enzymes are highly homologous and have overlapping, but distinctive substrate specificity. However, their expression patterns and transcriptional control vary considerably. Both have been hypothesized to play major roles in tumor progression, tumor cell invasion and angiogenesis. As more has been learned, it has become apparent that the actual situation is much more complex than the original idea that tumor cells secreting these proteases could use that

J.-M. Foidart and R.J. Muschel (eds.), Proteases and Their Inhibitors in Cancer Metastasis, 39–52.
© 2002 *Kluwer Academic Publishers. Printed in the Netherlands.*

activity to digest the underlying basement membrane and hence gain access to the mesenchymal tissue as part of the invasive phenotype distinguishing benign from malignant cancers.

The matrix metalloproteinase family has many members and is subdivided into four families. Two members of this family have marked activity against gelatin and hence are termed the gelatinase members of the family. One member of 72 kDa has variously been called MMP-2 or gelatinase A or the 72 kDa Type IV collagenase and the other, a 92 kDa protein is MMP-9 or gelatinase B or the 92 kDa Type IV collagenase. Comparison of their gene structure have shown them to be highly homologous (Collier et al, 1988; Huhtala et al, 1990; Huhtala et al, 1991; Wilhelm et al, 1989). Each gene has the same number of exons and introns with a high degree of homology in exons 2, 3, 4 and 75% in exons 5, 6 and 7. Exon 9, the most distal or 3′ exon that is translated has little homology and differences in this exon account for the size difference between the two with an additional 48 amino acids in the MMP-9. The murine MMP-9 additionally has an insert of 24 amino acids making it larger than that of other species (Tanaka et al, 1993).

The domain structure of these proteins is also homologous. Both are secreted proteins and both have a typical signal peptide at the N terminal end. The propeptide domain is responsible for inhibition of the active site and maintains both proteins in a latent state until cleavage of the propeptide at a conserved amino acid sequence PRCGVPPV. This sequence is conserved not only within the gelatinases, but also throughout the MMP family. The rest of the propeptide diverges between MMP-9 and 2. The catalytic domains of both enzymes contain a zinc binding domain including 3 histidines that can complex a zinc ion that is a critical component of the active site. In this region the gelatinases MMP-2 and MMP-9 are homologous to each other and to other members of the family. Within the catalytic region however MMP-2 and 9 also contain a region capable of binding gelatin. This is unique to the gelatinases and accounts for their high affinity and activity against gelatin. Further distal is a domain with structure reminiscent of the tandem repeat of hemopexins. This domain is divergent between the two gelatinases and some of their distinctive biochemical properties can be attributed to this region (Bode et al, 1999; Cockett et al, 1998; Massova et al, 1998; Nagase and Woessner, 1999). In particular binding to the natural inhibitors TIMPS is facilitated by binding in this region. This binding in turn is responsible for the localization of MMP-2 to the cellular surface and more recently it has become apparent that substrate specificity is also conferred by this region (Bode et al, 1999; Brew et al, 2000; Massova et al, 1998; Overall et al, 1999). A specific substrate of MMP-2, monocyte chemoattractant protein-3 was identified using a two hybrid screen with the hemopexin domain of MMP-2 as the bait (McQuibban et al, 2000).

The C terminal end of the gelatinases binds to the C terminal region of TIMPS, MMP-2 to TIMP-2 and MMP-9 to TIMP-1. Inhibition of enzyme activity is mediated by the N terminal regions of the TIMPs that bind to the active site of the MMPs. This binding can occur to MMPs in either the latent or the activated forms (Brew et al, 2000). In the case of MMP-2, the binding of TIMP-2 to the membrane bound MT1 MMP leads to the formation of a complex that essentially can act as a receptor for MMP-2 and may also be critical for the cleavage of the proform leading to the activation of MMP-2 (see Itoh and Seiki, Chapter 6). MMP-9 binds TIMP-1 through interactions in this domain. While MMP-9 is capable of binding both TIMP-1 and 2, the binding of TIMP-1 is preferential due to higher affinity in this region and similarly the binding of MMP-2 to TIMP-2 is mediated through higher affinity in this region (Olson et al, 1997). The interactions of MMP-2 or 9 with TIMP-3 a TIMP localized to the extracellular matrix is also mediated through interactions with the C terminal region of these MMPs (Butler et al, 1999).

The interactions of MMP-2 with TIMP-2 lead to the cell surface and interestingly association of MMP-2. MMP-2 is enriched in the regions of pseudopod extension during invasion in outcroppings of membrane termed invadapodia by Chen's group (Nakahara et al, 1997). MMP-2 also binds to the integrin alpha$_v$ beta$_3$ and this binding may be of significance not only in tumor cell association of MMP-2, but also in MMP-2 localization in tumor cell blood vessels since these endothelia characteristically express that integrin in contrast to established vessels in normal tissue (Brooks et al, 1996).

In some instances it appears that MMP-2 is synthesized by the host tissue yet may then bind to the tumor cell surface. Thus expression of MMP-2 may be necessary for its actions in tumor progression but additionally tumor cell expression of a MT MMP would then be necessary for invasion.

The evidence for membrane association for MMP-9 is less concrete. Yu and Stamenkovic have shown that MMP-9 can bind to CD44 and have postulated that this is necessary for its biological roles in cancer (Yu and Stamenkovic, 1999; Yu and Stamenkovic, 2000). In addition Fridman has shown that MMP-9 can bind to the alpha$_2$ (IV) chain of Type IV collagen a potential receptor, but also a potential substrate of MMP-9 (Olson et al, 1998; Toth et al, 1999).

3. ACTIVATION

The activation of both gelatinases can readily be detected due to the loss in molecular weight after cleavage of the N termnal end. MMP-2 is cleaved from a 72 kDa molecule to one of 62 kDa while MMP-9 at 92 kDa can be cleaved to a still latent form at 87 kDa into an active forms at 84 kDa. Smaller active forms of MMP-9 at 68 kDa are also sometimes seen (Murphy et al, 1999; Ogata et al, 1995). The activation of MMP-2 can clearly be mediated *in vivo* and *in vitro* by MT MMPs. In MT1 MMP deficient mice, MMP-2 activation in skin and lung is strongly diminished, but not absent while MMP-9 activation is unaffected (Holmbeck et al, 1999; Zhou et al, 2000). In addition to the MT1 MMP activation of MMP-2, protein C a component of the anticoagulant system has also been reported to be able to activate MMP-2 (Nguyen et al, 2000). The activation of MMP-9 can proceed enzymatically mediated by plasmin, matrilysin stromeylsin, but the *in vivo* activators have not been firmly established (Hahn-Dantona et al, 1999; Ramos-DeSimone et al, 1999; von Bredow et al, 1998). Stromelysin deficient mice still can activate MMP-9 in a model system based upon endothelial injury (Lijnen et al, 1999). The activation of MMP-2 has been correlated with tumor progression and is required for invasion suggesting that expression MT1-MMP expression may be a controlling event (Nagase, 1998). The activation and significance of the activation of MMP-9 is less carefully documented.

4. SUBSTRATES

Initially the MMPs were defined by their ability to degrade extracellular matrix and both MMP-2 and 9 fit that pattern with activity against denatured collagens of many types including collagens Type IV and V, elastin, gelatin, and fibronectin. More recently however a variety of additional non-matrix physiological targets have been identified including basic fibroblast growth factor, the cell surface protein galectin and a variety of proteins affecting inflammation. Specificity can be discerned. MMP-2 can cleave monocyte chemotactic factor, while it is resistant to MMP-9 and MMP-9 can cleave interleukin-8, or the alpha-1-proteinase inhibitor that are resistant to MMP-2.

5. EXPRESSION PATTERNS

In general MMP-9 is rarely expressed in adult tissues whereas in embryonic development, it is frequently observed in a complex spacial and temporal pattern. While many workers have stressed its high expression in the osteoclasts in the developing embryo, it is also expressed in the neuroblasts, liver and lung especially at the time when these organs are undergoing vasculogenesis (Canete-Soler et al, 1995; Canete-Soler et al, 1994; Okada et al, 1995; Reponen et al, 1994). And indeed activated MMP-9 can be detected using gelatin substrate gels in some, but not all of these organs. In spite of the abundance of MMP-9, its absence in knockout mice has little effect upon the development and subsequent maturation of these animals. One phenotype observed so far is that of smaller mice which seems to be triggered by shorter long bones (Vu et al, 1998). The change in size of the bones is coincident with a transient delay in vascularization of the growth plate resulting in a widened growth plate without timely ossification. This pathology can be seen 3 weeks after birth, but resolves quickly into histologically normal bone. This work led to the suggestion that MMP-9 contributes to angiogenesis. Additionally Dubois et al (1999) has reported a decrease in viable offspring in MMP-9 deficient mice, a result perhaps reflective of the high levels of MMP-9 seen in invasive trophoblastic cells of the placenta (Alexander et al, 1996; Canete-Soler et al, 1995).

The absence of gelatinases in knockout mice while not altering the phenotype of healthy mice has been shown to alter the course of disease in several murine models. Absence of MMP-9 in genetically altered mice leads to significant changes in pathological responses to injury. That secretion of MMP-9 can contribute in general to the remodeling of extracellular matrix is apparent from these experiments implicating MMP-9 in pathological processes. MMP-9 is overexpressed after myocardial infarction. When infarction is induced in MMP-9 deficient mice, the mice are less prone to go on to develop myocardial rupture and show more collagen deposition at the site of the infarct (Ducharme et al, 2000). Similarly MMP-9 deficiency can stave off the rupture of abdominal aneurysms. In a model of abdominal aneurysm in which elastase is instilled into the aorta leading to aneurysm formation, MMP-9 expression was found to be associated with the inflammatory response accompanying the destruction of the aortic wall elastin (Pyo et al, 2000). Mice deficient in MMP-9 had substantially reduced aneurismal dilatation in this model raising the possibility that MMP-9 inhibition might be beneficial for patients with abdominal aneurysms.

The use of MMP-9 deficient mice has also led to identification of its involvement in a murine model for multiple sclerosis, experimental autoimmune encephalomyelitis and additionally in a model for bullous pemphigoid in which mice are given an intradermal injection of anti-murine immunoglobulin (IgG) (Dubois et al, 1999; Liu et al, 1998). In both cases induction of the disease is accompanied by infiltration of MMP-9 positive cells. Absence of MMP-9 in mice recently born – up to 3–4 weeks post natal – resulted in reduced manifestations of the disease compared to heterozygote or wild type litter mates. However older mice showed no differences. Interestingly this is the time period over which bone development can be shown to be altered, in neonatal mice but not in adult mice. These observations lead to the suggestion that compensatory mechanisms can develop with age although these have not yet been identified. The disease related target for MMP-9 in bullous pemphigoid has been identified as a serpin alpha$_1$-proteinase inhibitor, a protease inhibitor that acts to inhibit neutrophil elastase (Liu et al, 2000b). Induction of MMP-9 leads to destruction of the inhibitor thus unleashing the elastase that cleaves the epithelial-dermal contacts leading to the skin blistering characteristic of bullous pemphigoid. MMP-9 can also affect the inflammatory response in other ways since it has enzymatic activity allowing the degradation of some inflammatory cytokines and activates interleukin-8 by cleaving it to a smaller more active form (Van Den Steen et al, 2000).

6. MMP-9 AND TUMOR PROGRESSION

Evidence of the effects of these gelatinases on tumor progression and metastasis comes both from studies *in vitro*, in tumor models and in knock out mice. Both gelatinases have been shown to be involved in invasion in cell culture based assays. This data while interesting must always be considered in the light of the differences between invasion and migration in actual tissue as compared to invasion in cell culture through an artificial barrier composed of components of the extracellular matrix. While much has been learned about cellular behavior using these assays and in many cases the extent of invasion correlates with metastatic capacity, there are a wide range of examples of a lack of correlation with these assays and activity *in vivo* (Simon et al, 1992). Nonetheless there are a number of intriguing correlations between apparent physiological inducers of metastasis triggering MMP-9 expression and affecting invasion in these tissue culture assays. For example, E cadherin has been shown to inhibit invasion and metastasis. Downregulation of E cadherin in skin carcinoma cells leads to MMP-9 expression and coincides with invasion (Llorens et al, 1998). Conversely upregulation of N-cadherin leads to increased invasion and enhanced expression of MMP-9 (Hazan et al, 2000). Other stimulators of MMP-9 that are known to be overexpressed in carcinomas such as EGF1 also stimulate invasion. EGFR signalling in carcinoma cells of the head and neck also leads to MMP-9 dependent invasion (Charvat et al, 1998; Chen et al, 1993; Hazan et al, 2000; Kondapaka et al, 1997; McCawley et al, 1998). Expresion of several integrins can be shown to be associated with carcinoma and signalling through these integins leads to gelatinase expression. We have cited here only a few of many such examples so that the principle that signalling through various characteristic autocrine factor involved in carcinoma leads to MMP-9 expression and to invasion in culture. Additionally MMP-9 activation through a plasmin mediated pathway also enhances invasion *in vivo* further making the case of MMP-9 involvment in invasion in cell culture (Ramos-DeSimone et al, 1999). Expression and activation of MMP-2 similarly can affect invasion in cell culture although the interaction with MT1-MMP complicates

44

this analysis (see review by Itoh and Seiki in Chapter 6). These data then lead to the question of the roles that expression of gelatinases might affect the biological behavior of tumors *in vivo*.

The timing of MMP-9 induction during tumor progression is in accord with data showing that the MMP-9 promoter is activated in breast carcinoma progression induced by the MMTV- polyoma middle T transgene at the time when lesions become invasion, but is not active while the carcinoma remains non-invasion or is a carcinoma *in situ* (Kupferman et al, in press). Furthermore in a variety of systems MMP-2 and 9 expression can be seen coincident with tumor progression, invasion or metastasis in naturally occurring carcinomas (Ara et al, 2000; Arenas-Huertero et al, 1999; Arii et al, 1996; Cox et al, 2000; Davidson et al, 1999; Etoh et al, 2000; Rao et al, 1996; Talvensaari-Mattila et al, 1999). These data further implicate these gelatinases in the development of aggressive malignancy.

Various data implicates both of these MMPs in the processes of metastasis and angiogenesis. MMP-2 but not MMP-9 has also been suggested to affect tumor growth.

Manipulation of MMP-9 can also be seen to affect metastasis. In a sarcoma model system in which MMP-9 expression correlated with the ability to metastasize, over-expression of MMP-9 those cell lines lacking MMP-9 expression induced metastatic potential. Tumor growth was unaffected (Bernhard et al, 1994). Similar experiments in melanoma cells also demonstrated the ability of MMP-9 to augment metastasis (MacDougall et al, 1999). In complementary experiments, downregulation of MMP-9 using a ribozyme, curtailed metastasis in a sarcoma model system or a prostatic carcinoma model, while this down regulation did not alter tumor growth rate (Hua and Muschel, 1996; Sehgal et al, 1998).

Thus strong evidence exists demonstrating the importance of MMP-9 expression in tumor cells contributing to metastasis. This data has been confirmed and extended using mice with genetic elimination of MMP-9. In these mice experimental lung metastasis was reduced between 45 and 59% compared to wild type mice. The potential contribution of MMP-9 from the tumor was not addressed by these studies (Itoh et al, 1999). In this case absence of MMP-9 production by the host, impaired metastatic potential even though the tumor had at least a theoretical capacity of MMP-9 expression. It still remains to be determined whether host derived MMP-9 can substitute for tumor derived MMP-9.

Overexpression of MMP-2 accelerated the metastatic phenotype in a bladder carcinoma cell line, but that effect may be attributable to enhanced tumor growth (Kawamata et al, 1995). Additional evidence favoring an effect of MMP-2 on tumor growth comes from experiments in knockout mice. Tumor cells implanted

45

in MMP-2 deficient mice exhibited a slightly decreased tumor growth and a more significant lag in lung colonization after intravenous injection. These tumor cells were still capable of synthesizing MMP-2 (Itoh et al, 1998). Conversely downregulation of MMP-2 in chrondrosarcoma cells resulted in growth suppression in mice with wild type MMP-2 (Fang et al, 2000). Whether MMP-2 contributes to different aspects of tumor growth invasion or metastasis when made by the tumor or by the host is not yet established. This effect of MMP-2 may be due to its functions in angiogenesis.

Chambers has suggested that the production of MMPs in general affect angiogenesis during the early colony formation in metastasis. Her group found that microscropic liver metastases were not inhibited by a pharmacological MMP inhibitor- one that blocks all MMP activity-but that macroscopic metastases were impaired leading to the suggestion that angiogenesis was the key component being regulated by the MMPs (Wylie et al, 1999). Certainly MMPs in general are likely to play a role in angiogenesis since non specific MMP inhibitors block angiogenesis in a variety of assays of angiogenesis.

Itoh et al as noted above found that tumor growth both subcutaneously and as lung colonies after intravenous injection was impaired in MMP-2 knockout mice and that the density of blood vessels appeared to be reduced. Furthermore these tumor cells generated fewer vessels in a dorsal air sac assay leading to the conclusion that MMP-2 deficiency in the host led to impaired angiogenesis (Itoh et al, 1998). Manipulation of MMP-2 in tumor cells by antisense oligonucleotides decreased angiogenesis using the chrondrosarcoma cells noted above as stimulators of angiogenesis in a chorioallonaotic membrane assay for angiogenesis (Fang et al, 2000). In a different system however Hanahan observed that tumor growth, but not angiogenesis was impaired during islet cell tumor progression *in vivo* when the Sv-T Ag transgene was activated in MMP-2 deficient mice (Bergers et al, 2000). There are also potential anti angiogenic effects of MMP-2 since O'Reilly et al has reported that MMP-2 can cleave plasminogen into the anitangiogenic fragments known as angiostatin (O'Reilly et al, 1999). Additionally a fragment of MMP-2 consisting mainly of the hemopexin domain called PEX can bind to the MMP-2 alpha$_v$beta$_3$ integrin complex on endothlial cells and in doing so disrupts angiogenesis (Brooks et al, 1998). Both MMP-2 and MMP-9 bind to thrombospondin 1 and 2, inhibitors of angiogenesis and this binding inhibits enzyme activity *in vitro* (Bein and Simons, 2000). The potential effects of MMP-2 on angiogenesis involve both stimulation and inhibition.

While both gelatinases A and B or MMP-2 and MMP-9 are produced in model systems during angiogenesis whether the cells were grown on collagen or on fibrin, the importance of that production is still unclear. In spite of the production of these proteases during formation of endothelial channels *in vitro* on fibrin, inhibition of MT1-MMP blocked angiogenesis, but blockade of either of the gelatinases did not (Hotary et al, 2000). Zhu et al had shown that regression of vessels may also be influenced by MMPs (Zhu et al, 2000). Some of the effects of MMP-2 on angiogenesis may also be due to the activity of MMP-2 on bFGFR 1. MMP-2 has enzymatic activity that is capable of resulting in the release of the ectodomain of FGFR, a domain that is able to bind to bFGF and hence might modulate the activity of FGF (Levi et al, 1996).

In experiments that point to MMP-9 as playing an important role in angiogenesis in tumor progression Bergers et al (2000) observed that angiogenesis was impaired during tumor formation in mice bearing a ? SV-40 T antigen transgene, mice that first develop hyperplastic islet cell nodules followed by *in situ* and invasive carcinoma formation. MMP-9 knockout mice had decreased angiogenesis and reduced tumor progression. In contrast MMP-2 mice has slower tumor growth but unaltered induction of malignancy (Bergers et al, 2000).

7. SECRETION

While there is an extensive literature on the regulation of gelatinases through transcription, headway has only recently been made regarding potential regulation of secretion. Takahashi et al found after cloning a gene based upon its ability to reverting transformation that this gene RECK a membrane bound protein suppresed secretion of MMP-9 from cells containing MMP-9 mRNA (Takahashi et al, 1998). MMP-2 secretion may also be regulated through signalling through src (Liu et al, 2000a).

Thus, there is a large body of literature implicating the gelatinase family in metastasis, but much remains to be learned. Both MMP-2 and 9 are overexpressed in cancers. However the mechanisms leading to that overexpression are not known and are clearly different for each. Both MMP-2 and 9 are frequently found in metastatic carcinomas and in specific instances blocking their expression can decrease invasion and metastasis. However in many settings their actions appear to be distinct. Both may be synthesized by either tumor cells or host cells. Whether the site of synthesis matters is unknown. The actual substrates of each *in vivo* involved in tumor progression have not yet been identified. The steps in tumor progression that each affect are also not clearly delineated. And finally whether either would be a useful therapeutic target is largely in question.

REFERENCES

Alexander CM, Hansell EJ, Behrendtsen O, Flannery ML, Kishnani NS, Hawkes SP, Werb Z. Expression and function of matrix metalloproteinases and their inhibitors at the maternal-embryonic boundary during mouse embryo implantation. Development 1996; 122: 1723–1736.

Ara T, Kusafuka T, Inoue M, Kuroda S, Fukuzawa M, Okada A. Determination of imbalance between MMP-2 and TIMP-2 in human neuroblastoma by reverse-transcription polymerase chain reaction and its correlation with tumor progression. J Pediatr Surg 2000; 35: 432–437.

Arenas-Huertero FJ, Herrera-Goepfert R, Delgado-Chavez R, Zinser-Sierra JW, De la Garza-Salazar JG, Herrera-Gomez A, Perez-Cardenas E. Matrix metalloproteinases expressed in squamous cell carcinoma of the oral cavity: correlation with clinicopathologic features and neo-adjuvant chemotherapy response. J Exp Clin Cancer Res 1999; 18: 279–284.

Arii S, Mise M, Harada T, Furutani M, Ishigami S, Niwano M, Mizumoto M, Fukumoto M, Imamura M. Overexpression of matrix metalloproteinase 9 gene in hepatocellular carcinoma with invasive potential. Hepatology 1996; 24: 316–322.

Bein K, Simons M. Thrombospondin type 1 repeats interact with matrix metalloproteinase 2. Regulation of metalloproteinase activity. J Biol Chem 2000; 275: 32167–32173.

Bergers G, Brekken R, McMahon G, Vu TH, Itoh T, Tamaki K, Tanzawa K, Thorpe P, Itohara S, Werb Z, Hanahan D. Matrix metalloproteinase-9 triggers the angiogenic switch during carcinogenesis. Nat Cell Biol 2000; 2: 737–744.

Bernhard EJ, Gruber SB, Muschel RJ. Direct evidence linking expression of matrix metallopro-teinase 9 (92-kDa gelatinase/collagenase) to the metastatic phenotype in transformed rat embryo cells. Proc Natl Acad Sci (USA) 1994; 91: 4293–4297.

Bode W, Fernandez-Catalan C, Tschesche H, Grams F, Nagase H, Maskos K. Structural prop-erties of matrix metalloproteinases. Cell Mol Life Sci 1999; 55: 639–652.

Brew K, Dinakarpandian D, Nagase H. Tissue inhibitors of metalloproteinases: evolution, struc-ture and function. Biochim Biophys Acta 2000; 1477: 267–283.

Brooks PC, Silletti S, von Schalscha TL, Friedlander M, Cheresh DA. Disruption of angiogen-esis by PEX, a noncatalytic metalloproteinase fragment with integrin binding activity. Cell 1998; 92: 391–400.

Brooks PC, Stromblad S, Sanders LC, von Schalscha TL, Aimes RT, Stetler-Stevenson WG, Quigley JP, Cheresh DA. Localization of matrix metalloproteinase MMP-2 to the surface of invasive cells by interaction with integrin alpha,beta$_3$. Cell 1996; 85: 683–693.

Butler GS, Apte SS, Willenbrock F, Murphy G. Human tissue inhibitor of metallo-proteinases 3 interacts with both the N- and C-terminal domains of gelatinases A and B. Regulation by polyanions. J Biol Chem 1999; 274: 10846–10851.

Canete-Soler R, Gui YH, Linask KK, Muschel RJ. Developmental expression of MMP-9 (gelati-nase B) mRNA in mouse embryos. Dev Dyn 1995; 204: 30–40.

Canete-Soler R, Litzky L, Lubensky I, Muschel RJ. Localization of the 92 kd gelatinase mRNA in squamous cell and adenocarcinomas of the lung using in situ hybridization. Am J Pathol 1994; 144: 518–527.

Charvat S, Chignol MC, Souchier C, Le Griel C, Schmitt D, Serres M. Cell migration and MMP-9 secretion are increased by epidermal growth factor in HaCaT-ras transfected cells. Exp Dermatol 1998; 7: 184–190.

Chen LL, Narayanan R, Hibbs MS, Benn PA, Clawson ML, Lu G, Rhim JS, Greenberg B, Mendelsohn J. Altered epidermal growth factor signal transduction in activated Ha-ras-trans-formed human keratinocytes. Biochem Biophys Res Commun 1993; 193: 167–174.

Cockett MI, Murphy G, Birch ML, O'Connell JP, Crabbe T, Millican AT, Hart IR, Docherty AJ. Matrix metalloproteinases and metastatic cancer. Biochem Soc Symp 1998; 63: 295–313.

Collier IE, Wilhelm SM, Eisen AZ, Marmer BL, Grant GA, Seltzer JL, Kronberger A, He CS, Bauer EA, Goldberg GI. H-ras oncogene-transformed human bronchial epithelial cells (TBE-1) secrete a single metalloprotease capable of degrading basement membrane collagen. J Biol Chem 1988; 263: 6579–6587.

Cox G, Jones JL, O'Byrne KJ. Matrix metalloproteinase 9 and the epidermal growth factor signal pathway in operable non-small cell lung cancer. Clin Cancer Res 2000; 6: 2349–2355.

Curran S, Murray GI. Matrix metalloproteinases. molecular aspects of their roles in tumour invasion and metastasis. Eur J Cancer 2000; 36: 1621–1630.

Davidson B, Goldberg I, Kopolovic J, Lerner-Geva L, Gotlieb WH, Ben-Baruch G, Reich R. MMP-2 and TIMP-2 expression correlates with poor prognosis in cervical carcinoma-a clinicopathologic study using immunohistochemistry and mRNA in situ hybridization. Gynecol Oncol 1999; 73: 372–382.

Dubois B, Masure S, Hurtenbach U, Paemen L, Heremans H, van den Oord J, Sciot R, Meinhardt T, Hammerling G, Opdenakker G, Arnold B. Resistance of young gelatinase B-deficient mice to experimental autoimmune encephalomyelitis and necrotizing tail lesions. J Clin Invest 1999; 104: 1507–1515.

Ducharme A, Frantz S, Aikawa M, Rabkin E, Lindsey M, Rohde LE, Schoen FJ, Kelly RA, Werb Z, Libby P, Lee RT. Targeted deletion of matrix metalloproteinase-9 attenuates left ventricular enlargement and collagen accumulation after experimental myocardial infarction. J Clin Invest 2000; 106: 55–62.

Etoh T, Inoue H, Yoshikawa Y, Barnard GF, Kitano S, Mori M. Increased expression of colla-genase-3 (MMP-13) and MT1-MMP in oesophageal cancer is related to cancer aggressive-ness. Gut 2000; 47: 50–56.

Fang J, Shing Y, Wiederschain D, Yan L, Butterfield C, Jackson G, Harper J, Tamvakopoulos G, Moses MA. Matrix metalloproteinase-2 is required for the switch to the angiogenic phenotype in a tumor model. Proc Natl Acad Sci (USA) 2000; 97: 3884–3889.

Hahn-Dantona E, Ramos-DeSimone N, Sipley J, Nagase H, French DL, Quigley JP. Activation of proMMP-9 by a plasmin/MMP-3 cascade in a tumor cell model. Regulation by tissue inhibitors of metalloproteinases. Ann N Y Acad Sci 1999; 878: 372–387.

Hazan RB, Phillips GR, Qiao RF, Norton L, Aaronson SA. Exogenous expression of N-cadherin in breast cancer cells induces cell migration, invasion, and metastasis [published erratum appears in J Cell Biol 2000; 149: following 236]. J Cell Biol 2000; 148: 779–790.

Holmbeck K, Bianco P, Caterina J, Yamada S, Kromer M, Kuznetsov SA, Mankani M, Robey PG, Poole AR, Pidoux I, Ward JM, Birkedal-Hansen H. MT1-MMP-deficient mice develop dwarfism, osteopenia, arthritis, and connective tissue disease due to inadequate collagen turnover. Cell 1999; 99: 81–92.

Hotary K, Allen E, Punturieri A, Yana I, Weiss SJ. Regulation of cell invasion and morphogen-esis in a three-dimensional type I collagen matrix by membrane-type matrix metalloproteinases 1, 2, and 3. J Cell Biol 2000; 149: 1309–1323.

Hua J, Muschel RJ. Inhibition of matrix metalloproteinase 9 expression by a ribozyme blocks metastasis in a rat sarcoma model system. Cancer Res 1996; 56: 5279–5284.

Huhtala P, Chow LT, Tryggvason K. Structure of the human type IV collagenase gene. J Biol Chem 1990; 265: 11077–11082.

Huhtala P, Tuuttila A, Chow LT, Lohi J, Keski-Oja J, Tryggvason K. Complete structure of the human gene for 92-kDa type IV collagenase. Divergent regulation of expression for the 92- and 72-kilodalton enzyme genes in HT-1080 cells. J Biol Chem 1991; 266: 16485–16490.

Itoh T, Tanioka M, Matsuda H, Nishimoto H, Yoshioka T, Suzuki R, Uehira M. Experimental metastasis is suppressed in MMP-9-deficient mice. Clin Exp Metastasis 1999; 17: 177–181.

Itoh T, Tanioka M, Yoshida H, Yoshioka T, Nishimoto H, Itohara S. Reduced angiogenesis and tumor progression in gelatinase A-deficient mice. Cancer Res 1998; 58: 1048–1051.

Kawamata H, Kameyama S, Kawai K, Tanaka Y, Nan L, Barch DH, Stetler-Stevenson WG, Oyasu R. Marked acceleration of the metastatic phenotype of a rat bladder carcinoma cell line by the expression of human gelatinase A. Int J Cancer 1995; 63: 568–575.

Kondapaka SB, Fridman R, Reddy KB. Epidermal growth factor and amphiregulin up-regulate matrix metalloproteinase-9 (MMP-9) in human breast cancer cells. Int J Cancer 1997; 70: 722–726.

Levi E, Fridman R, Miao HQ, Ma YS, Yayon A, Vlodavsky I. Matrix metalloproteinase 2 releases active soluble ectodomain of fibroblast growth factor receptor 1. Proc Natl Acad Sci (USA) 1996; 93: 7069–7074.

Lijnen HR, Lupu F, Moons L, Carmeliet P, Goulding D, Collen D. Temporal and topographic matrix metalloproteinase expression after vascular injury in mice. Thromb Haemost 1999; 81: 799–807.

Liu E, Thant AA, Kikkawa F, Kurata H, Tanaka S, Nawa A, Mizutani S, Matsuda S, Hanafusa H, Hamaguchi M. The Ras-mitogen-activated protein kinase pathway is critical for the activation of matrix metalloproteinase secretion and the invasiveness in v-crk-transformed 3Y1. Cancer Res 2000a; 60: 2361–2364.

Liu Z, Shipley JM, Vu TH, Zhou X, Diaz LA, Werb Z, Senior RM. Gelatinase B-deficient mice are resistant to experimental bullous pemphigoid. J Exp Med 1998; 188: 475–482.

Liu Z, Zhou X, Shapiro SD, Shipley JM, Twining SS, Diaz LA, Senior RM, Werb Z. The serpin alpha1-proteinase inhibitor is a critical substrate for gelatinase B/MMP-9 in vivo. Cell 2000b; 102: 647–655.

Llorens A, Rodrigo I, Lopez-Barcons L, Gonzalez-Garrigues M, Lozano E, Vinyals A, Quintanilla M, Cano A, Fabra A. Down-regulation of E-cadherin in mouse skin carcinoma cells enhances a migratory and invasive phenotype linked to matrix metalloproteinase-9 gelatinase expression. Lab Invest 1998; 78: 1131–1142.

MacDougall JR, Bani MR, Lin Y, Muschel RJ, Kerbel RS. 'Proteolytic switching': opposite patterns of regulation of gelatinase B and its inhibitor TIMP-1 during human melanoma progression and consequences of gelatinase B overexpression. Br J Cancer 1999; 80: 504–512.

Massova I, Kotra LP, Fridman R, Mobashery S. Matrix metalloproteinases: structures, evolution, and diversification. Faseb J 1998; 12: 1075–1095.

McCawley LJ, O'Brien P, Hudson LG. Epidermal growth factor (EGF)- and scatter factor/hepatocyte growth factor (SF/HGF)- mediated keratinocyte migration is coincident with induction of matrix metalloproteinase (MMP)-9. J Cell Physiol 1998; 176: 255–265.

McQuibban GA, Gong JH, Tam EM, McCulloch CA, Clark-Lewis I, Overall CM. Inflammation dampened by gelatinase A cleavage of monocyte chemoattractant protein-3. Science 2000; 289: 1202–1206.

Murphy G, Stanton H, Cowell S, Butler G, Knauper V, Atkinson S, Gavrilovic J. Mechanisms for pro matrix metalloproteinase activation. Apmis 1999; 107: 38–44.

Nagase H. Cell surface activation of progelatinase A (proMMP-2) and cell migration. Cell Res 1998; 8: 179–186.

Nagase H, Woessner JF Jr. Matrix metalloproteinases. J Biol Chem 1999; 274: 21491–21494.

Nakahara H, Howard L, Thompson EW, Sato H, Seiki M, Yeh Y, Chen WT. Transmembrane/cytoplasmic domain-mediated membrane type 1-matrix metalloprotease docking to invadopodia is required for cell invasion. Proc Natl Acad Sci (USA) 1997; 94: 7959–7964.

Nguyen M, Arkell J, Jackson CJ. Activated protein C directly activates human endothelial gelatinase A. J Biol Chem 2000; 275: 9095–9098.

O'Reilly MS, Wiederschain D, Stetler-Stevenson WG, Folkman J, Moses MA. Regulation of angiostatin production by matrix metalloproteinase-2 in a model of concomitant resistance. J Biol Chem 1999; 274: 29568–29571.

Ogata Y, Itoh Y, Nagase H. Steps involved in activation of the pro-matrix metalloproteinase 9 (progelatinase B)-tissue inhibitor of metalloproteinases-1 complex by 4-aminophenylmercuric acetate and proteinases. J Biol Chem 1995; 270: 18506–18511.

Okada Y, Naka K, Kawamura K, Matsumoto T, Nakanishi I, Fujimoto N, Sato H, Seiki M. Localization of matrix metalloproteinase 9 (92-kilodalton gelatinase/type IV collagenase = gelatinase B) in osteoclasts: implications for bone resorption. Lab Invest 1995; 72: 311–322.

Olson MW, Gervasi DC, Mobashery S, Fridman R. Kinetic analysis of the binding of human matrix metalloproteinase-2 and -9 to tissue inhibitor of metalloproteinase (TIMP)-1 and TIMP-2. J Biol Chem 1997; 272: 29975–29983.

Olson MW, Toth M, Gervasi DC, Sado Y, Ninomiya Y, Fridman R. High affinity binding of latent matrix metalloproteinase-9 to the alpha$_2$(IV) chain of collagen IV. J Biol Chem 1998; 273: 10672–10681.

Overall CM, King AE, Sam DK, Ong AD, Lau TT, Wallon UM, DeClerck YA, Atherstone J. Identification of the tissue inhibitor of metalloproteinases-2 (TIMP-2) binding site on the hemopexin carboxyl domain of human gelatinase A by site-directed mutagenesis. The hierarchical role in binding TIMP-2 of the unique cationic clusters of hemopexin modules III and IV. J Biol Chem 1999; 274: 4421–4429.

Pyo R, Lee JK, Shipley JM, Curci JA, Mao D, Ziporin SJ, Ennis TL, Shapiro SD, Senior RM, Thompson RW. Targeted gene disruption of matrix metalloproteinase-9 (gelatinase B) suppresses development of experimental abdominal aortic aneurysms [see comments]. J Clin Invest 2000; 105: 1641–1649.

Ramos-DeSimone N, Hahn-Dantona E, Sipley J, Nagase H, French DL, Quigley JP. Activation of matrix metalloproteinase-9 (MMP-9) via a converging plasmin/stromelysin-1 cascade enhances tumor cell invasion. J Biol Chem 1999; 274: 13066–13076.

Rao JS, Yamamoto M, Mohaman S, Gokaslan ZL, Fuller GN, Stetler-Stevenson WG, Rao VH, Liotta LA, Nicolson GL, Sawaya RE. Expression and localization of 92 kDa type IV collagenase/gelatinase B (MMP-9) in human gliomas. Clin Exp Metastasis 1996; 14: 12–18.

Reponen P, Sahlberg C, Munaut C, Thesleff I, Tryggvason K. High expression of 92-kD type IV collagenase (gelatinase B) in the osteoclast lineage during mouse development. J Cell Biol 1994; 124: 1091–1102.

Sehgal G, Hua J, Bernhard EJ, Sehgal I, Thompson TC, Muschel RJ. Requirement for matrix metalloproteinase-9 (gelatinase B) expression in metastasis by murine prostate carcinoma. Am J Pathol 1998; 152: 591–596.

Simon N, Noel A, Foidart JM. Evaluation of in vitro reconstituted basement membrane assay to assess the invasiveness of tumor cells. Invasion Metastasis 1992; 12: 156–167.

Takahashi C, Sheng Z, Horan TP, Kitayama H, Maki M, Hitomi K, Kitaura Y, Takai S, Sasahara RM, Horimoto A, Ikawa Y, Ratzkin BJ, Arakawa T, Noda M. Regulation of matrix metalloproteinase-9 and inhibition of tumor invasion by the membrane-anchored glycoprotein RECK. Proc Natl Acad Sci (USA) 1998; 95: 13221–13226.

Talvensaari-Mattila A, Paakko P, Turpeenniemi-Hujanen T. MMP-2 positivity and age less than 40 years increases the risk for recurrence in premenopausal patients with node-positive breast carcinoma. Breast Cancer Res Treat 1999; 58: 287–293.

Tanaka H, Hojo K, Yoshida H, Yoshioka T, Sugita K. Molecular cloning and expression of the mouse 105-kDa gelatinase cDNA. Biochem Biophys Res Commun 1993; 190: 732–740.

Toth M, Sado Y, Ninomiya Y, Fridman R. Biosynthesis of alpha$_2$(IV) and alpha$_1$(IV) chains of collagen IV and interactions with matrix metalloproteinase-9. J Cell Physiol 1999; 180: 131–139.

Van Den Steen PE, Proost P, Wuyts A, Van Damme J, Opdenakker G. Neutrophil gelatinase B potentiates interleukin-8 tenfold by aminoterminal processing, whereas it degrades CTAP-III, PF-4, and GRO-alpha and leaves RANTES and MCP-2 intact. Blood 2000; 96: 2673–2681.

von Bredow DC, Cress AE, Howard EW, Bowden GT, Nagle RB. Activation of gelatinase-tissue-inhibitors-of-metalloproteinase complexes by matrilysin. Biochem J 1998; 331: 965–972.

Vu TH, Shipley JM, Bergers G, Berger JE, Helms JA, Hanahan D, Shapiro SD, Senior RM, Werb Z. MMP-9/gelatinase B is a key regulator of growth plate angiogenesis and apoptosis of hypertrophic chondrocytes. Cell 1998; 93: 411–422.

Wilhelm SM, Collier IE, Marmer BL, Eisen AZ, Grant GA, Goldberg GI. SV40-transformed human lung fibroblasts secrete a 92-kDa type IV collagenase which is identical to that secreted by normal human macrophages [published erratum appears in J Biol Chem 1990; 265: 22570]. J Biol Chem 1989; 264: 17213–17221.

Wylie S, MacDonald IC, Varghese HJ, Schmidt EE, Morris VL, Groom AC, Chambers AF. The matrix metalloproteinase inhibitor batimastat inhibits angiogenesis in liver metastases of B16F1 melanoma cells. Clin Exp Metastasis 1999; 17: 111–117.

Yu Q, Stamenkovic I. Localization of matrix metalloproteinase 9 to the cell surface provides a mechanism for CD44-mediated tumor invasion. Genes Dev 1999; 13: 35–48.

Yu Q, Stamenkovic I. Cell surface-localized matrix metalloproteinase-9 proteolytically activates TGF-beta and promotes tumor invasion and angiogenesis. Genes Dev 2000; 14: 163–176.

Zhou Z, Apte SS, Soininen R, Cao R, Baaklini GY, Rauser RW, Wang J, Cao Y, Tryggvason K. Impaired endochondral ossification and angiogenesis in mice deficient in membrane-type matrix metalloproteinase I. Proc Natl Acad Sci (USA) 2000; 97: 4052–4057.

Zhu WH, Guo X, Villaschi S, Francesco Nicosia R. Regulation of vascular growth and regression by matrix metalloproteinases in the rat aorta model of angiogenesis. Lab Invest 2000; 80: 545–555.

Chapter 4

THE COLLAGENASES: NOVEL ROLES FOR MATRIX METALLOPROTEINASES (MMPS) IN INVASION AND METASTASIS

Constance E. Brinckerhoff, Ulrike Benbow and Grant B. Tower
Dartmouth Medical School, Hanover, NH 03755, USA

1. INTRODUCTION

Malignant tumors have the ability to invade normal tissue and spread to distant sites, giving rise to metastases, which are major factors in the morbidity and mortality of cancer. Invasion and metastasis involve attachment of tumor cells to the basement membrane, degradation of the local connective tissue, and penetration and migration through proteolyzed stroma (Basset et al, 1997; Chambers and Matrisian, 1997; Parsons et al, 1997; Curran and Murray, 1999; Westermarck and Kahari, 1999; Koblinski et al, 2000; Nelson et al, 2000). An integral component of these events is the capacity of tumor cells to enter (intravasate) and exit (extravasate) the blood stream or lymphatic system before they can become established at a distant site. All these steps require destruction of the extracellular matrix, a process that is mediated by the concerted action of several proteinases, including members of the serine, cysteine, aspartate, and matrix metalloproteinase (MMP) families.

Despite the contributions of these various proteinases, matrix degradation is carried out primarily by the MMPs, a family of zinc dependent enzymes that collectively degrades all components of connective tissues (Ohuchi et al, 1997; Nagase and Woessner, 1999; Pei, 1999; Westermarck and Kahari, 1999; Hotary et al, 2000; Nelson et al, 2000; Velesco et al, 2000). Currently, 26 human MMPs have been identified, and they can be classified into four main sub-groups, according to their substrate specificity and structural similarities (1) interstitial collagenases, (2) gelatinases, (3) stromelysins, and (4) membrane-type MMPs (MT-MMPs) (Ohuchi et al, 1997; Nagase and Woessner, 1999; Pet, 1999; Hotary et al, 2000; Velesco et al, 2000) (Table 1 and Figure 1). The interstitial collagenases degrade the structural collagens types I, II and III, while the gelatinases are effective mainly against type IV collagen. The MT-MMPs represent membrane bound forms of the enzymes, and at least some members of this

J.-M. Foidart and R.J. Muschel (eds.), Proteases and Their Inhibitors in Cancer Metastasis, 53–79.
© 2002 *Kluwer Academic Publishers. Printed in the Netherlands.*

Table 1. Matrix metalloproteinases (MMPs).

Enzyme	MMP No.	Matrix substrates
Collagenases		
Interstitial collagenase-1	MMP-1	Collagens I, II, III, VII, X, gelatins, aggrecan, entactin
Neutrophil collagenase-1	MMP-8	Collagens I, II, III, aggrecan, link protein
Collagenase-3	MMP-13	Collagens I, II, III
MT1-MMP	MMP-14	Collagens I, II, III, fibronectin
Gelatinases		
Gelatinases A	MMP-2	Gelatins, collagens I, IV, V, VII, X, XI, bibronectin, laminin, elastin, aggrecan, vitronectin
Gelatinases B	MMP-9	Gelatins, collagens IV, V, XIV, elastin, aggrecan, vitronectin
Stromelysins		
Stromelysins-1	MMP-3	Collagens III, IV, IX, gelatins, aggrecan, fibronectin, laminin
Stromelysins-2	MMP-10	Aggrecan, fibronectin, collagen IV
Membrane-type MMPs		
MT2-MMP	MMP-15	Collagens I, II, III, fibronectin
MT3-MMP	MMP-16	Collagens III, gelatins, fibronectin
MT4-MMP	MMP-17	Not known
MT5-MMP	MMP-24	Gelatins
MT6-MMP	MMP-25	Gelatins
Others		
Matrilysin	MMP-7	Collagen IV, gelatins, aggrecan, fibronectin, elastin, laminin
Stromelysin-3	MMP-11	Collagen IV, gelatins, aggrecan, fibronectin, elastin, laminin
Metalloelastase	MMP-12	Elastin

sub-group can degrade collagen, thus qualifying them as collagenases (Ohuchi et al, 1997; Hotary et al, 2000). The stromelysins have a broad substrate specificity, degrading non-collagen matrix molecules, such as proteoglycans, laminin, fibronectin and importantly, also contributing to the activation of other latent MMP family members (Nagase and Woessner, 1999). Most MMPs are secreted as proenzymes, which are then activated extracellularly by serine proteinases such as plasmin or urokinase, or by other members of the MMP family (Nagase and Woessner, 1999; Westermarck and Kahari, 1999). In contrast, the membrane-bound MMPs are activated intracellularly and are inserted into the membrane in an active form (Nagase and Woessner, 1999; Westermarck and Kahari, 1999 – see below).

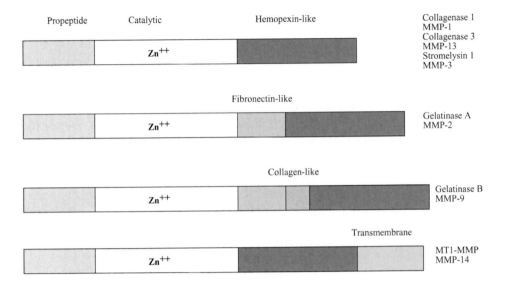

Figure 1. Domain structure of MMPs. The functional structure of MMPs consists of a propeptide domain, catalytic domain, which contains Zn++, and the hemopexin-like domain. Additional structural features of the gelatinases and the membrane type MMPs are indicated.

The importance of MMPs in tumor invasion and metastasis has been well-documented (Basset et al, 1997; Chambers and Matrisian, 1997; Parsons et al, 1997; Curran and Murray, 1999; Westermarck and Kahari, 1999; Koblinski et al, 2000; Nelson et al, 2000) Because the gelatinases (MMP-2 and MMP-9) cleave type IV collagen, the main component of the basement membrane, these enzymes have a major role in mediating invasion and facilitating metastasis. However, the basement membrane is not the only barrier that needs to be crossed. The interstitial collagens, type I and III, are the body's most abundant proteins and comprise stromal tissue that must also be destroyed for tumor invasion to occur. This destruction is accomplished principally by collagenases, i.e. collagenase-1 (MMP-1), neutrophil collagenase-2 (MMP-8), collagenase-3 (MMP-13) and some MT-MMPs. MMP-8 is expressed by neutrophils, and is thought to contribute more to the connective tissue degradation seen in inflammatory arthritic disease, rather than to cancer (Vincenti et al, 1996). Thus, this chapter will consider the contributions of MMP-2, MMP-9, MMP-1, MMP-13 and the MT-MMPs. Since the classical roles of these enzymes in connective tissue degradation and in tumor invasion/metastasis have been amply discussed (Basset et al, 1997; Chambers and Matrisian, 1997; Parsons et al, 1997; Curran and Murray, 1999; Westermarck and Kahari, 1999; Koblinski et al, 2000; Nelson et al, 2000), we will summarize these and then focus on some of the more novel aspects of collagenase behavior in tumor biology.

2. COLLAGENASE GENE EXPRESSION

2.1. Host/tumor cell interactions

As tumors progress, an increasing number of MMP family members are expressed, either by the tumor cells, and/or by the adjacent stromal cells. Ultimately, production of the collagenases correlates with the metastatic potential of the tumor (Basset et al, 1997; Chambers and Matrisian, 1997; Parsons et al, 1997, Curran and Murray, 1999; Westermarck and Kahari, 1999; Brinckerhoff et al, 2000; Koblinski et al, 2000; McCawley and Matrisian, 2000; Nelson et al, 2000). However, the contribution of each enzyme probably varies considerably through-out the stages of malignancy, which include (a) the initial and early stages of local tumor invasion, (b) the processes of metastasis to distant sites and eventually, (c) growth of the tumor at this metastatic site.

In vitro studies with cell lines have provided insight into the nature of the interactions that may occur between tumor cells and host cells (Heppner et al, 1996; Guo et al, 1997; Sato et al, 1999). The tumor cells may secrete factors that induce MMPs in the adjacent stromal cell, such as EMMPRIN (extracellular matrix metalloproteinase inducer), a 58 kDa protein that belongs to the immunoglobulin superfamily and induces MMP-1 and MMP-2 in fibroblasts (Guo et al, 1997). Alternatively, however, the stromal cells may induce expression of MMPs in the tumor cells. For example, collagenolytic MMPs can be induced in several different types of tumor cells, including lung, renal, colon squamous cell carcinoma (reviewed in Brinckerhoff et al, 2000), perhaps in response to cytokines and growth factors secreted by infiltrating stromal cells or macrophages (Borden et al, 1996; Heppner et al, 1996; Guo et al, 1997; Sato et al, 1999; Westermarck and Kahari, 1999). In some instances, however, the need for direct cell-cell contact has been documented, as in the induction of collagenase in bone cells in contact with breast cancer cells (Ohishi et al, 1995), an important event in mediating the ability of breast cancer cells to metastasize to bone. Finally, there may be simultaneous expression of the collagenases by stromal cells and tumor cells, and when both cell types express heightened levels of the collagenases, the invasive and metastatic potential of the tumor is enhanced (Heppner et al, 1996; Guo et al, 1997; Sato et al, 1999; Westermarck and Kahari, 1999; Brinckerhoff et al, 2000).

2.2. Regulation of gene expression

Host/tumor cell interactions culminate in increased expression of collagenase genes, which usually occurs at the level of transcription. In non-malignant cells, i.e. stromal, epithelial and endothelial cells, that may be adjacent to the tumor, basal transcription of MMP-1, MMP-13 and MMP-9 is normally low, but is readily induced by growth factors and cytokines (Vincenti et al, 1996; Borden et al, 1996; Benbow and Brinckerhoff, 1997; Borden and Heller, 1997). In contrast, MMP-2 and MT1-MMP are constitutively expressed at moderate to high levels, although they, too, may be further induced under certain conditions. (see below). Some additional regulation of gene expression may be conferred by mRNA stability. The 3' untranslated region (3'-UTR) of several collagenases contains the AUUUA motif, which may mediate an increase in the stability of mRNA, particularly if the inducer is an inflammatory cytokine, such as tumor necrosis factor or interleukin-1 (Vincenti et al, 1996).

Maximal transcriptional activation of the collagenase genes involves cooperation among a variety of cis-acting sequences in their promoters (Figure 2) (Borden et al, 1996; Vincenti et al, 1996; Benbow and Brinckerhoff, 1997; Borden and Heller, 1997). With the exception of MMP-2 and MT1-MMP, these promoters contain a TATA box and one or more Activator Protein-1 (AP-1) sites, which play critical roles in controlling both basal and induced transcription. The AP-1 sites are located in the proximal region of the promoters as well as in upstream regions of MMP-1 and MMP-9 (Figure 2), and they generally bind heterodimers composed of members of the Fos and Jun families of transcription factors. Different family members, e.g. c-Jun, Jun B, c-Fos and Fra-2, bind differentially to the various AP-1 sites (White and Brinckerhoff, 1995; Vincenti et al, 1996; Westermarck and Kahari, 1999), and this differential binding may govern the subtle differences in the contribution of various AP-1 elements to the expression of these genes. In addition, although knock out studies of c-Fos in mice reveal that it has an essential role in the progression of skin papillomas (Saez et al, 1995), Fos homodimers can not transactivate AP-1 sites, while Jun homodimers can (Vincenti et al, 1996; Benbow and Brinckerhoff, 1997; Borden and Heller, 1997; Westermarck and Kahari, 1999). Despite the essential role of AP-1, it must cooperate with other elements in order to maximally active transcription. ETS (E26 transformation specific) sites are scattered throughout the promoters of the collagenases and AP-1/ETS interactions represent a prominent mechanism for controlling transcription of these genes (Wasylyk et al, 1993; Buttice et al, 1996; Vincenti et al, 1996; Basuyaux et al, 1997; Benbow and Brinckerhoff, 1997; Borden and Heller, 1997; Westermarck and Kahari, 1999). However, other cis-acting sequences, such as NFkB or CBFA1 may also contribute (Vincenti et al, 1998; Jimenez et al, 1999; Westermarck and Kahari, 1999).

As tumors progress and become more invasive, production of the collagenases is increasingly linked to the tumor cells, and this production often becomes constitutively high (Durko et al, 1997; Benbow et al, 1999; Benbow et al, 1999;

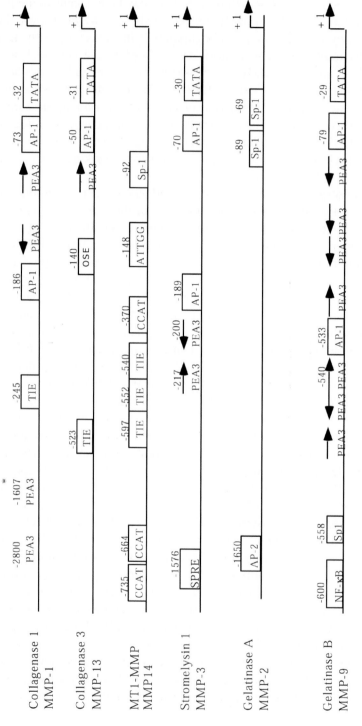

Figure 2. Regulatory elements of the MMP promoters showing location of major cis-acting elements known to contribute to transcription. AP-1, Activator Protein-1 site; PEA3, Polyomavirus EnhancerA-binding Protein-3 site, also known as ETS, E26 transformation specific; TIE, TGF-β Inhibitory Element. * = location of the single nucleotide polymorphism in the MMP-1 promoter.

58

Schoenermarck et al, 1999; Westermarck and Kahari, 1999; Brinckerhoff et al, 2000). This suggests that the mechanisms controlling MMP transcription have become dysregulated, perhaps as a function of aberrations in the signal/transduction pathways that control MMP gene expression (Figure 3) (Rowinsky et al, 1999; Westermarck and Kahari, 1999; Mengshol et al, 2000). In particular, the mitogen activated protein kinases (MAPK)and extracellular regulated kinase (ERK) pathways that involve growth receptors and/or stress activated signaling pathways such as MEKK 1,3, JNK, p38, and MEK 1,2 represent major signaling cascades, which culminate in the phosphorylation and transactivation of various transcription factors. Indeed, the AP-1 and ETS families are common downstream targets of these signal/transduction pathways, which in turn, stem from the upstream activation of the Ras oncoprotein. Dysregulation of these signaling pathways, therefore, with subsequent constitutively high expression of MMPs, implies continuous transactivation through these sites. Since Ras is constitutively active in many tumors, ETS/AP-1 proteins that are Ras responsive may be overly activated in those instances (Rowinsky et al, 1999; Westermarck and Kahari, 1999). This may contribute to the inappropriate overexpression of the proteins/enzymes that play a critical role in metastasis, such as the MMPs.

2.3. The proteolytic cascade

The conversion of proMMPs to enzymatically active forms is absolutely essential to invasion. This conversion is a function of an activation cascade that depends not only on MMPs but also on serine proteinases (Durko and Brodt, 1998; Aguirre Ghiso et al, 1999; Benbow et al, 1999; Benbow et al, 1999; Kim et al, 1999; Ramos-deSimone et al, 1999). Sometimes, the cascade is 'self-contained' within the tumor cells, so that they can invade the extracellular matrix by themselves, without the 'help' of stromal cells. Under these conditions, the tumor cells must have an inherent mechanism for activating latent MMPs, thereby mediating their own invasion, as has been described for MIM human melanoma cells and for MDA231 breast cancer cells (Durko et al, 1997; Benbow et al, 1999). The critical role of serine proteinases is apparent from the fact that the serine proteinase inhibitor, aprotinin, can block invasion (Benbow et al, 1999).

On the other hand, the cascade may not always function solely with proteinases produced by the tumor cells, and enzymes from the stromal cells may be required. For example, another human melanoma cell line (A2058 cells) secretes copious amounts of MMP-1, but can not invade a matrix of type I collagen unless the cells are cultured in the presence of conditioned medium derived from stromal cells (Benbow et al, 1999). Apparently, the A2058 cells

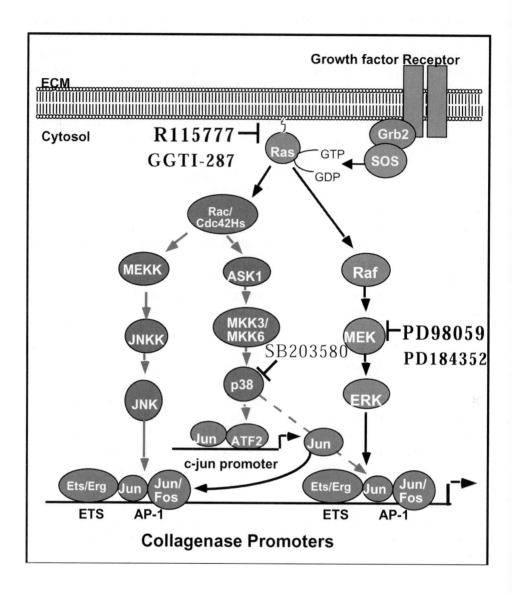

Figure 3. Signaling pathways involved in MMP gene expression. MAP kinase signaling pathways contribute to the activation of ETS and AP-1 transcription factor families, which are important for the expression of the collagenase genes. Induction and constitutive expression of the collagenase genes can be blocked by pharmacological agents that inhibit the activation of MAP kinase signaling proteins. R115777 and GGTI-287 are inhibitors of Ras farnesylation and geranylgeranylation, respectively. PD98059 and PD184352 are MEK inhibitors, while SB203580 inhibits p38 (Buolamwini, 1999; Heimbrook and Oliff, 1999; Westermarck and Kahari, 1999; Mengshol et al, 2000).

are unable to activate the proMMP-1 they have secreted, while a factor(s) produced by the stromal cells can, thus allowing invasion to proceed. Here, too, a serine proteinase is required, but it is not sufficient to fully activate latent MMP-1 (Benbow et al, 1999). The addition of active stromelysin-1 (MMP-3) completes the enzymatic cascade and then the tumor cells can invade the collagen (Benbow et al, 1999; Nagase and Woessner, 1999). MMP-3 is a constitutive product of stromal cells, where basal levels of expression are very low (Buttice et al, 1996; Benbow and Brinckerhoff, 1997; Borden and Heller, 1997; Benbow et al, 1999). Nonetheless, these low levels are sufficient since serum-free medium from resting stromal cells can mediate the activation process (Benbow et al, 1999). Thus, even though MMP-3 (stromelysin-1) is not a collagenase, it is an essential, player in the cascade leading to collagenolysis.

Several other reports also describe serine/MMP proteolytic cascades needed for the activation of proMMPs (Durko and Brodt, 1998; Aguirre Ghiso et al, 1999; Kim et al, 1999; Ramos-deSimone et al, 1999). Expression of MMP-2 or MMP-9 was not sufficient to permit intravasation of tumor cells, with subsequent invasion of a chick embryo chorioallantoic membrane. Urokinase plasminogen activator (uPA) and its receptor (uPAR) were also needed, and only tumor cells that expressed this serine protease could intravasate and invade (Kim et al, 1999; Ramos-deSimone et al, 1999). Another study supports the important role of uPA/uPA receptor in MMP-mediated invasion, and the interconnected regulation of these two classes of proteinases (Durko and Brodt, 1998). Suppression of MMP-1 resulted in a decrease in uPA receptors, suggesting that coordinated expression was necessary for MMP-1 activity. Thus, even though the collagenases are the direct mediators of matrix degradation, the serine proteinases represent a critical component of the invasive process (Aguirre Ghiso et al, 1999). We can, therefore, develop a model of (1) secretion of proMMPs by either tumor cells and/or stromal cells (2) partial activation of latent MMPs by a serine proteinase, such as uPA, which may be produced by either the tumor cells or stromal cells, and (3) full activation by MMP-3 (Durko and Brodt, 1998; Aguirre Ghiso et al, 1999; Ramos-deSimone et al, 1999; Kim et al, 1999).

3. GELATINASE-A (MMP-2) AND GELATINASE-B (MMP-9)

Because of their specificity for cleaving type IV collagen and thus breaching the basement membrane, MMP-2 and MMP-9 have a major role in initiating tumor invasion. As a result, they have received considerable attention and their presence has been described in many tumors (Basset et al, 1997, Chambers and Matrisian, 1997; Parsons et al, 1997, Curran and Murray, 1999;

Westermarck and Kahari, 1999; Koblinski et al, 2000; Nelson et al, 2000). Although there have been numerous attempts to link expression of these MMPs with patient outcome, no consistent pattern of prognosis has emerged (Allgayer et al, 1998; Remacle et al, 1998; Talvensaari-Mattila et al, 1998; Vaisanen et al, 1998; Kuniyasu et al, 1999; Moser et al, 1999; Vaisanen et al, 1999; O-Charoenrat et al, 2000; Oberg et al, 2000), even within similar types of cancers (Remacle et al, 1998; Talvensaari-Mattila et al, 1998; Vaisanen et al, 1998; Vaisanen et al, 2000). Recently, however, a new role for these MMPs as potential markers of tumor aggression has been demonstrated in a variety of tumor cell lines and in ovarian cancer. Vesicles are shed from tumors and these vesicles contain MMP-2 and MMP-9 (Dolo et al, 1998; Ginestra et al, 1998; Ginestra et al, 1999). A positive correlation has been noted between tumor malignancy, the number of vesicles, and the amount of enzyme they contain. Along with MMP-2 and MMP-9, they also contain uPA, leading to the speculation that the vesicle contents promote the proteolytic cascade required for localized destruction of the extracellular matrix.

In contrast to MMP-9, the MMP-2 gene lacks a TATA box and proximal AP-1 site, and it is expressed constitutively in many cells (Benbow and Brinckerhoff, 1997; Borden and Heller, 1997; Westermarck and Kahari, 1999). Therefore, MMP-2 is seen in many tumors and at several stages of tumor progression (Basset et al, 1997; Chambers and Matrisian, 1997; Parsons et al, 1997; Curran and Murray, 1999; Westermarck and Kahari, 1999; Koblinski et al, 2000; Nelson et al, 2000). Since expression is constitutive and does not need to be induced, MMP-2 produced by the stromal cells may actually facilitate the local invasion of tumor cells, particularly since it is readily activated by MT1-MMP, which is also constitutively expressed (Li et al, 1998; Nagase and Woessner, 1999; Seiki, 1999; Westermarck and Kahari, 1999). Since these two MMPs are common products of stromal cells, it may well be that the early stages of tumor invasion are mediated primarily by the host stroma immediately adjacent to the tumor cells, rather than by the malignant tumor cells. However, MMP-2 can also be expressed by tumor cells, and as tumors progress and metastases occur, MMP-2 production by tumor cells may increase, perhaps due to an increase in transcriptional activators or, alternatively, to mutations in a tumor suppressor gene(s).

Indeed, a recent report links mutations in a tumor suppressor gene, Von-Hippel Lindau (VHL), to an increase in MMP-2 and MMP-9 mRNAs and to angiogenesis (Koochekpour et al, 1999). VHL syndrome is an inherited cancer, characterized by extensive vascularization and increased angiogenesis. Compared to wild-type cells, VHL null renal cell carcinoma cells exhibited an increase in invasive behavior through Matrigel® and type IV collagen. Furthermore, when the tumor cells with the VHL null gene were treated with hepatocyte growth factor/scatter factor (HGF/SF), there was an increase in branching morphogenesis and a decrease in tissue inhibitor of metalloproteinase 1 and 2 (TIMP 1 and TIMP 2), endogenous inhibitors of MMP activity. Treating the cells with recombinant TIMPs abolished this branching, confirming that it was mediated by the action of MMPs. Although the mechanisms connecting VHL, angiogenesis and MMPs remain unclear, one possible link in these cells is the vascular endothelial growth factor (VEGF) receptor (Wang and Keiser, 1998). This receptor is a tyrosine kinase that responds to HGF/SF and thus, may act as an angiogenic trigger as well as an inducer of MMPs (Unemori et al, 1992; Wang and Keiser, 1998). Two high affinity VEGF receptors are Flt-1 and kinase insert domain-containing receptor (KDR), and their tissue specific expression may explain the ability of endothelial cells and smooth muscle cells to respond to VEGF with an increase in MMP expression, while fibroblasts do not (Unemori et al, 1992).

The emerging role of MMP-2 and MMP-9 in angiogenesis represents one of the most important developments in MMP research (Hanahan and Folkman, 1996; Vu et al, 1998; Fang et al, 2000). By digesting the matrix and allowing migration of new endothelial cells with subsequent formation of new vessels, MMP-2 may participate in one of the earliest and most important stages of tumorigenesis, i.e., helping to activate the angiogenesis and the 'switch to the angiogenic phenotype' (Hanahan and Folkman, 1996; Vu et al, 1998; Fang et al, 2000). Thus, even though the ability of MMP-2 and MMP-9 to degrade type IV collagen may be responsible for their reputation as major mediators of tumor invasion, recent studies indicate that these enzymes have novel roles.

4. COLLAGENASE-1 (MMP-1) AND COLLAGENASE-3 (MMP-13)

MMP-1 is the most ubiquitously expressed of the interstitial collagenases (Vincenti et al, 1996; Nagase and Woessner, 1999; Brinckerhoff et al, 2000; McCawley and Matrisian, 2000). Many normal cells, including fibroblasts, keratinocytes, macrophages, smooth muscle cells and endothelial cells, produce low basel levels of this enzyme. Although it is readily induced by growth factors and cytokines (Borden et al, 1996; Vincenti et al, 1996; Benbow and Brinckerhoff, 1997; Borden and Heller, 1997), several tumor cell lines display high constitutive expression, probably resulting from dysregulated signal/transduction pathways (Rowinsky et al, 1999; Westermarck and Kahari, 1999; Mengshol et al, 2000). This high expression often occurs along with the transition to a more mesenchymal phenotype (Gilles et al, 1997), a transition characterized by expression of vimentin and loss of keratin and E-cadherin. These changes are associated with more aggressive tumor behavior, and they suggest that a cohort of genes, including MMP-1, is involved in the progression of tumors (Murrey et al, 1996; Murray et al, 1998; Airola et al, 1999; Inoue et al, 1999; Ito et al, 1999; Kanamori et al, 1999; Nakopoulou et al, 1999; Pickett et al, 1999; Brinckerhoff et al, 2000; Nishioka et al, 2000).

Recent studies by Rutter et al. (1998) describe how an increase in MMP-1 expression may be mediated. They report the presence of a single nucleotide polymorphism (SNP) in the human MMP-1 promoter, which is an insertion/deletion polymorphism of a guanine base (G) at position -1607 bp. The additional G creates a binding site, 5'-GGA(A/T)-3', for the ETS family of transcription factors (Wasylyk et al, 1993; Buttice et al, 1996; Basuyaux et al, 1997), and transient transfection of promoter constructs containing either 1G or 2Gs reveals that DNA with 2Gs is transcribed at a higher level than is DNA containing only 1G. The increase in transcription is seen in both normal stromal cells and in tumor cells, suggesting that increased MMP-1 expression by either cell type could enhance the invasive behavior of tumors.

The SNP is a true polymorphism and not a rare mutation found only in a few tumor cells (Rutter et al, 1998). The distribution of this SNP in the normal population is approximately 30% = 1G homozygous; 30% = 2G homozygous; 40% = 1G/2G heterozygous. Interestingly, the presence of the 2G allele increases to 62% in tumor cell lines cultured *in vitro* ($P < 0.001$), supporting the hypothesis that it correlates with aggressive tumors. Further, two separate studies provide important clinical evidence for a functional role of the SNP in cancer biology. Patients with ovarian (Kanamori et al, 1999) or endometrial (Nishioka et al, 2000) cancers had a significantly higher incidence of the 2G allele, compared to non-cancer controls, and the 2G allele correlated with the expression of higher levels of MMP-1 protein.

Compared to MMP-1, MMP-13 (collagenase-3) has a more restricted pattern of expression but broader substrate specificity (Freije et al, 1994; Balbin et al, 1999; Nagase and Woessner, 1999; Pendas et al, 2000). MMP-13 was originally identified in breast carcinoma, and it was thought that the enzyme was produced by the tumor cells and was specifically associated with malignancy (Freije et al, 1994). Indeed, expression of MMP-13 has been documented in certain cancers, particularly squamous cell carcinomas of the head and neck, which are noted for their aggressive behavior and for propensity for rapid progression (Kahari et al, 1998; Johansson et al, 1999; Tsukifuji et al, 1999). Only malignant squamous cell tumors, not premalignant or benign lesions, express MMP-13. However, MMP-13 is not uniquely associated with tumor cells. Its expression has been demonstrated in non-malignant conditions, such as chronic ulcers (Vaalamo et al, 1997; Uitto et al, 1998) and osteoarthritis (Mitchell et al, 1996; Rebous et al, 1996; Mengshol et al, 2000). It has also been found in the stromal cells immediately adjacent to some tumors (Kahari et al, 1998;

Balbin et al, 1999; Johansson et al, 1999; Tsukifuji et al, 1999), and since MMP-13 gene expression is rare in stromal cells, production may be occurring in response to stimuli produced by the tumors.

Despite similarities in gene structure with MMP-1, our understanding of the mechanisms controlling MMP-13 gene expression is limited. The MMP-13 gene resides on chromosome 11q22, distal to the MMP-1 gene (Pendas et al, 1997; Tardiff et al, 1997). It contains a traditional TATA box, and the transcription start site(s) is located about 22 nucleotides upstream of the ATG translation start codon. As with other MMPs, the proximal AP-1 site has been identified as an important regulator of this gene, and Cbfa1/Runx-2 and NFkB have also been implicated as playing a role in the transcriptional control of this gene (Jimenez et al, 1999; Mengshol et al, 2000). However, expression of MMP-13 appears to be confined to a few normal tissues and perhaps to particular types of tumors, leading to the speculation that a negative regulator may contribute to the stringent control of this gene (Pendas et al, 1997; Tardiff et al, 1997).

5. MT-MMPS

To date, six membrane-bound MMPs (MT-MMPs) have been identified (Ohuchi et al, 1997; Polette and Birembaut, 1998; Nagase and Woessner, 1999; Pei, 1999; Westermarck and Kahari, 1999; Hotary et al, 2000; Velesco et al, 2000). Like other MMPs, the MT-MMPs are synthesized in a latent form. In contrast to the secreted MMPs, they contain an RXXR motif, which renders them susceptible to activation intracellularly by furin. In addition, MT-MMPs contain a short carboxy-terminal transmembrane domain, which results in their becoming embedded in the plasma membrane. This surface localization suggests that they may modulate a number of important cell-matrix interactions. The transmembrane/cytoplasmic domain may mediate the spatial organization of MT1-MMP to the invadopodia, with subsequent localized degradation of the extracellular matrix (Ohuchi et al, 1997; Polette and Birembaut, 1998; Nagase and Woessner, 1999; Pei, 1999; Westermarck and Kahari, 1999; Hotary et al, 2000; Velesco et al, 2000). Another function of the MT-MMPs is activating latent MMPs, i.e. MMP-2 and MMP-13, indicating that they can participate indirectly in collagen degradation. Since MMP-2 has been immunolocalized to the cell membrane of the tumor cells, the model is that MT-MMPs may function as receptor molecules to capture proMMP-2 on the cell surface before activating it. However, MT1-MMP is not a universal activator of all MMPs since it fails to activate MMP-7 (matrilysin) and MMP-3 (stromelysin-1) (Li et al, 1998; Nagase and Woessner, 1999).

The potential of several MT-MMPs to contribute to tumor invasion is illustrated in a recent study that describes the ability of MT1-MMP-1, 2 and 3 to regulate cell invasion and branching morphogenesis in three-dimensional collagen matrices (Hotary et al, 2000). In this study, the epithelial line of MDCK cells was stably transfected to express each of ten different MMPs. The cells were then stimulated with HGF/SF as an inducer of invasion and branching morphogenesis. None of the secreted interstitial collagenases (MMP-1, MMP-13) or the gelatinases (MMP-2, MMP-9) was able to mediate invasion in response to HGF/SF, perhaps because the necessary components for a proteolytic cascade that could activate these latent MMPs were not present. In contrast, two of the three membrane-bound MMPs, MT1-MMP and MT2-MMP, which are activated intracellularly, enabled the MDCK cells to penetrate matrices containing type I collagen and to initiate tubulogenesis. Of particular importance is the finding that soluble forms of these enzymes were ineffective, suggesting that they must be confined to the pericellular space/compartment. Here they can be concentrated at the cell-matrix interface and be protected from circulating proteinase inhibitors.

MT-MMPs have been detected in the stromal cells adjacent to the invading tumor, again suggesting that host cells may be mediating matrix degradation and tumor invasion (Gilles et al, 1996; Bando et al, 1998; Imamura et al, 1998; Kitagawa et al, 1998; Polette and Birembaut, 1998; Tanney et al, 1998; Ishigake et al, 1999; Kitagawa et al, 1999; Kjellman et al, 1999; Kurahara et al, 1999; Ellenrieder et al, 2000). However, as the tumors progress, expression of MT-MMP is increasingly associated with the tumor cells in a wide variety of carcinomas, where they are thought to contribute substantially to the metastatic phenotype (Gilles et al, 1996; Bando et al, 1998; Li et al, 1998; Imamura et al, 1998; Kitagawa et al, 1998; Polette and Birembaut, 1998; Ishigake et al, 1999; Kitagawa et al, 1999; Kjellman et al, 1999; Kurahara et al, 1999; Ellenrieder et al, 2000). Enhanced expression of MT-MMP has also been described in a number of advanced genito-urinary cancers (Gilles et al, 1996; Kitagawa et al, 1998; Kitagawa et al, 1999). Since these tissues express MT-MMPs during normal development (Bjorn et al, 1997; Lui et al, 1998; Tanney et al, 1998), it is interesting to speculate that there is a link between the expression of MT-MMPs during the highly regulated processes of normal development and their re-expression during the dysregulation seen in carcinogenesis. Given their constitutively active state in the membrane and their potential to carry out a multiplicity of functions, the MT-MMPs appear to have a number of important roles in tumor invasion.

6. COLLAGENASES AS THERAPEUTIC TARGETS

6.1. Natural inhibitors

Metastasis, not the primary tumor, usually causes death from cancer, and metastasis depends on MMP expression (Basset et al, 1997; Chambers and Matrisian, 1997; Parsons et al, 1997; Curran and Murray, 1999; Westermarck and Kahari, 1999; Koblinski et al, 2000; Nelson et al, 2000). There is, therefore, tremendous appeal in targeting these enzymes for therapeutic strategies that block either enzyme *activity* or enzyme *synthesis*. The key for success with this strategy may lie in specificity, i.e., the ability of certain compounds to specifically block the particular collagenases that are mediating the invasive behavior of a tumor at a particular time.

Originally, there was some interest in utilizing naturally occurring inhibitors of enzyme activity to halt invasion. One natural inhibitor is alpha$_2$-macroglobulin, a 725 kDa plasma protein, that complexes with all active proteinases and inactivates them (Barrett and Starkey, 1973; Nagase et al, 1994). Although this broad activity could be considered a bonus in an environment filled with many different classes of proteinases, its large size generally precludes access to localized tissues where it could inhibit enzymes, and thus retard tumor invasion. Other natural inhibitors are the TIMPs, which, in constrast to alpha$_2$-macroglobulin, are specific for MMPs. TIMPs are small (~25 kDa) proteins that are produced by stromal cells and that complex with active MMPs in a 1:1 molar ratio (Cawston et al, 1994; Gomez et al, 1997). Presently, four TIMPs have been identified. TIMP-1 is the most abundant, and its expression can be increased by compounds such as transforming growth factor-β and the vitamin A analogs, the retinoids, thereby leading to the suggestion that up-regulation of TIMP-1 might be therapeutically effective (Cawston et al, 1994; Gomez et al, 1997). However, despite the attractiveness of this concept, their therapeutic efficacy has not been demonstrated. Although endogenous and non-toxic, TIMPs are probably not suitable therapeutic agents for several reasons (Greenwald et al, 1999). First, they bind to nearly all MMPs and thus, they lack specificity. Second, in contrast to TIMP-2, TIMP-1 does not effectively inhibit the MT-MMPs, enzymes known to have critical roles in invasion. Third, and perhaps most important, the levels of MMPs usually exceed TIMP levels, and increases in TIMP expression caused by inducers are generally not as great as increases in the expression of MMPs.

6.2. Synthetic inhibitors

Because of the limitations associated with naturally occurring inhibitors, attention has turned to synthetic compounds. Although inhibiting enzyme activity with synthetic compounds is an attractive concept there are the difficulties of enzyme specificity, drug delivery, drug stability, rates of clearance, and achievement of clinically effective concentrations (Vincenti et al, 1994; Greenwald et al, 1999). Some of these difficulties may be circumvented with the introduction of new 'second generation' inhibitors, which are directed against a specific MMP.

One group of second generation inhibitors are the chemically modified tetracyclines (CMTs). These have received considerable attention, especially in the treatment of arthritic disease where the collagenases are overexpressed and connective tissue destruction is rampant (Vincenti et al, 1996; Greenwald et al, 1999; Mengshol et al, 2000). The CMTs chelate the di-valent Ca^{++} required for MMP function, and thus inhibit their activity. *In vitro* experiments suggest that the CMTs are more effective against collagenase-3 than against collagenase-1 (Greenwald et al, 1998; Greenwald et al, 1999), thereby demonstrating the selectivity that may be important for therapeutic efficacy.

The hydroxamate compounds are another class of MMP inhibitors. These small peptides compete with the natural substrate for the active site of the enzyme (Rasmussen and McCann, 1997; Wojtowicz-Praga et al, 1998; Wojtowicz-Praga et al, 1998; Greenwald et al, 1999). One compound, Batimastat®, is effective against most MMPs *in vitro*, with an IC_{50} ranging from 0.5 to 10 ng/ml. It has been used in both animal and human studies, with some clinical success and without systemic toxicities. However, the principal difficulty with this drug is its extreme insolubility, although it may be effective and appropriate in the treatment of certain tumors (Haq et al, 2000). In contrast, Marimastat® is a more soluble hydroxamate compound, with an inhibitory profile similar to Batimastat® (Rasmussen and McCann, 1997; Wojtowicz-Praga et al, 1998; Wojtowicz-Praga et al, 1998; Greenwald et al, 1999). It has been tested in phase I/II trials in patients with several types of advanced-stage solid tumors, and substantial clinical improvement has been noted. The major side effects are musculoskeletal pain, which are dose and time dependent in their appearance. These side effects might be related to the inhibition of the low basal expression of MMPs that is part of normal physiology.

Nonetheless, newer drugs, which make use of our knowledge of the crystal structures of the different MMPs (Greenwald et al, 1999; Lovejoy et al, 1999) and are thus directed against a specific enzyme, are being developed. There are several promising specific MMP inhibitors, and perhaps they will circumvent the problem of debilitating side effects (Rasmussen and McCann, 1997; Greenwald et al, 1999). Another intriguing therapeutic approach is the use of two or more drugs with totally different targets (Shalinsky et al, 1999; Haq et al, 2000). The efficacy of this strategy has been tested with two MMP inhibitors, AG3340 (Shalinsky et al, 1999) and Batimastat® (Haq et al, 2000). When used in combination with standard chemotherapeutic agents, the resulting therapies were successful by being both anti-proliferative and anti-invasive.

Inhibiting the *synthesis* of the collagenases, mediated at the level of gene expression, is another therapeutic possibility (Vincenti et al, 1996; Borden and Heller, 1997; Durko et al, 1997; Benbow et al, 1999; Benbow et al, 1999; Greenwald et al, 1999; Schoenermark et al, 1999; Westermarck and Kahari, 1999;). MMP synthesis can be inhibited by only a few compounds, transforming growth factor-β, which has pleotrophic affects on many cells (Zimmerman and Padgett, 2000), the glucocorticoid hormones, which are commonly used to suppress the excessive MMP production seen in rheumatoid arthritis (Vincenti et al, 1994), and the vitamin A analogues, retinoids (Sporn et al, 1994; Schroen and Brinckerhoff, 1997), which have a history as effective suppressors of malignancy (Sporn et al, 1994; Issing and Wustrow, 1996; Lotan, 1996; Zhang et al, 1996; Tallman et al, 1997). In addition, a synthetic triterpenoid compound, a plant derivative, has been described for its inhibitory effect on MMP synthesis (Mix et al, 2000). At nanomolar concentrations, this triterpenoid, 2-cyano-3,-12-dioxoolean-1,9, dien-28-oic acid (CDDO) selectively inhibits the transcriptional induction of MMP-1 and MMP-13 by inflammatory cytokines in a cell line. Additionally, CDDO prevents invasion of the cells through a matrix of type I collagen. Although still in the preliminary stages of investigation, this novel compound may hold promise as a therapeutic agent.

The retinoids exert their therapeutic effects through several mechanisms, including inhibition of cell proliferation, induction of apoptosis, enhanced cell differentiation, repression of cell motility, and inhibition of MMP synthesis (Sporn et al, 1994; Schroen and Brinckerhoff, 1997; Spanjaard et al, 1997). Retinoids act through two classes of nuclear hormone receptors, the retinoic acid receptors (RARs) and retinoid X receptors (RXRs), both of which belong to the steroid hormone receptor super-family (Sporn et al, 1994; Schroen and Brinckerhoff, 1997). In the presence of ligand, RAR/RXR heterodimers or RXR homodimers act through a variety of retinoic acid response element (RARE) motifs that resemble the sequence AG[G/T]TCA. However, with the exception of MMP-3 (stromelysin 1), the MMP promoters do not contain a classical RARE (Schroen and Brinckerhoff, 1997; Westermarck and Kahari, 1999), and retinoid-mediated repression occurs by a number of mechanisms that include (a) upregulation of RAR mRNAs, (b) down-regulation of Fos and Jun mRNAs, (c) sequestration of Fos and Jun proteins, and (d) indirect association of RAR/RXR heterodimers with the AP-1 sites in the promoter (Sporn et al, 1994; Schroen and Brinckerhoff, 1997).

Retinoids have been particularly successful in the treatment of head and neck cancers and acute promyelocytic leukemia, and their application to the treatment of breast cancer is now emerging (Zhang et al, 1996; Tallman et al, 1997). Retinoids have had only limited success with other tumors. However, recent reports suggest that RAR/RXR specific ligands, i.e. 'designer retinoids' are effective against certain tumors (Schadendorf et al, 1996; Spanjaard et al, 1997) and perhaps against specific MMPs (Schoenermarck et al; 1999), thus renewing interest in their use as therapeutic agents.

Finally, our increasing knowledge of the signal/transduction pathways involved in MMP gene expression has lead to the development of a novel therapeutic strategy designed to block specific pathways, with subsequent inhibition of MMP synthesis (Rowinsky et al, 1999; Westermarck and Kahari, 1999; Mengshol et al, 2000) (Figure 3). Some of these therapies are in various stages of clinical trials where, in addition to inhibiting cell growth, they may be blocking MMP gene expression (Heimbrook and Oliff, 1998; Buolamwini, 1999; Rowinsky et al, 1999). For example, Ras and MAPK signaling are important for MMP expression (Rowinsky et al, 1999; Westermarck and Kahari, 1999; Mengshol et al, 2000). Ras function depends on post-translational modifications such as farnesylation and geranylgeranylation for plasma membrane localization. Farnesylation inhibitors or geranylgeranytransferase inhibitors can block ras localization, hence blocking the ability of Ras to transduce signals through the various pathways involved in the transcriptional regulation of oncogenes and MMPs (Heimbrook and Oliff, 1998; Buolamwini, 1999; Rowinsky et al, 1999). Furthermore, the downstream pathways, by MEK/ERK, can be targeted by compounds such as PD98059 (Rowinsky et al, 1999; Westermarck and Kahari, 1999; Mengshol et al, 2000) and its orally available counterpart, PD-184352, thereby potentially increasing the specificity of targets and decreasing more generalized toxicities. These drugs are an attractive alternative for blocking MMP gene expression and subsequent metastases since they may block both tumor invasion and tumor growth.

7. CONCLUSION AND FUTURE DIRECTIONS

Our traditional views on the functions of MMPs are being challenged as we re-evaluate the matrix substrates that each enzyme can degrade, assign new functions to 'old' MMPs, and discover new members of this increasingly diverse family (Ohuchi et al, 1997; Nagase and Woessner, 1999; Pei, 1999; Hotary et al, 2000; Velesco et al, 2000). For example, some MMPs degrade components of the extracellular matrix that have not been considered their 'natural' substrates (Durko et al, 1997). Experiments with MMP-1 anti-sense constructs have shown that this enzyme can mediate cellular invasion through Matrigel®, implying that MMP-1, traditionally an interstitial collagenase, also degrades type IV collagen. In addition, the ability of several MT-MMPs to degrade interstitial collagen (Ohuchi et al, 1997; Hotary et al, 2000) indicates that these MMPs may be directly involved in the invasive behavior of tumors, rather than functioning primarily as activators of proMMP-2.

Several papers raise questions about possible additional roles for MMPs in tumor biology. First, the ability of aggressive and invasive melanoma cells to form their own blood vessels, without recruiting host endothelial cells has been described (Maniotis et al, 1999). Might MMPs produced by the tumor cells contribute to this 'auto-angiogesis'? Second, the intravascular origin of metastases has been demonstrated (Al-Mehdi et al, 2000). This new model proposes that tumor cells attach to the endothelium, where they proliferate and give rise to metastatic foci without the need to extravasate. Eventually, the colonies outgrow the vascular walls, destroy them and migrate into tissues. What is the role of MMPs in this process? Third, and equally intriguing, however, is the fact that MMPs can also have anti-angiogenic activity, when for example, they are involved in the generation of endostatin (Hanahan and Folkman, 1996;; Stetler-Stevenson, 1999; Wen et al, 1999 Fang et al, 2000). Can we utilize the anti-angiogenic properties of MMPs in a therapeutic manner? Lastly, Loss of Heterozygosity (LOH) at the MMP-1 locus of chromosome 11q.22 has been described and linked to metastatic melanomas (Driouch et al, 1998; Noll et al, 2000). LOH is usually associated with the loss of a tumor suppressor gene, and several putative tumor suppressors have been assigned to this locus (Driouch et al, 1998). However, LOH in these metastatic tumors is significantly associated with retention of the 2G allele, i.e. the allele expressing higher levels of MMP-1. Although LOH is a random event with an equal probability of losing either allele, the hypothesis is that heterozygotic tumors retaining the 2G allele have a selective aggressive and invasive advantage, which is manifested in an increased number of metastases. How will knowledge of the MMP-1 SNP increase our understanding of tumor invasion? Will this SNP be a useful prognostic marker?

Thus, the role of MMPs in cancer is complex, and tumor cells are a complex and heterogeneous population. They are constantly changing their genotype and their phenotype, in response to genetic, physiologic and pharmacologic pressures (Bae et al, 1997; Baldini, 1997; Wosikowski et al, 1997; Yoon et al, 1997; Hanahan and Weisberg, 2000). Errors in gene regulation continue to accrue as tumors metastasize, and as cancers progress. Furthermore, as cells in different metastatic sites respond to local environments, subpopulations of tumor cells may arise. Quite possibly, these subpopulations express different levels of the collagenolytic MMPs, and these different levels of expression may influence the invasive behavior of tumors. Once thought to only degrade the collagens that comprise the extracellular matrix, it is now clear that the collagenases have numerous functions. As our knowledge of the diverse roles of MMPs in tumor invasion and metastasis continues to increase, we may be successful in developing therapies directed against specific enzymes at particular stages of tumor progression.

NOTE ADDED IN PROOF

Since this chapter was submitted, several additional papers have documented the role of the 2G SNP in the MMP-1 promoter in cancer. These are: Noll et al, 2001; Ye et al, 2001; Zhu et al, 2001; Gilhardi et al, 2001.

REFERENCES

Aguirre Ghiso JA, Alonso DF, Farias EF, Gomez DE, Bal de Kier Joffe E. Deregulation of the signaling pathways controlling urokinase production. Eur J Biochem 1999; 263: 295–304.

Airola K, Karonen T, Vaalamo M, Lehti K, Lohi J, Kariniemi AL, Keski-Oja J, Saarialho-Kee U. Expression of collagenases-1 and -3 and their inhibitors TIMP-1 and -3 correlates with the level of invasion in malignant melanomas. Br J Cancer 1999; 80: 733–743.

Allgayer H, Babic R, Beyer BC, Grutzner KU, Tarabichi A, Schildberg FW, Heiss MM. Prognostic relevance of MMP-2 (72-kD collagenase IV) in gastric cancer. Oncology 1998; 55: 152–160.

Al-Mehdi AB, Tozawa K, Fisher AB, Shientag L, Lee A, Muschel RJ. Intravascular origin of metastasis from the proliferation of endothelium-attached tumor cells a new model for metastasis. Nature Med 2000; 6: 100–102.

Bae RC, Jurchott K, Wagener C, Bergmann S, Metzner S, Bommert K, Mapara MY, Winzer K-J, Dietel M, Dorken B, Royer HD. Nuclear localization and increased levels of transcription factor YB-1 in primary human breast cancers are associated with intrinsic MDR1 gene expression. Nature Med 1997; 3: 447–450.

Balbin M, Pendas AM, Uria JA, Jimenez MG, Freije JP, Lopez-Otin C. Expression and regulation of collagenase-3 (MMP-13) in human malignant tumors. APMIS 1999; 107: 45–53.

Baldini N. Multidrug resistance – a muliplex phenomenon. Nature Med 1997; 3: 378–380.

Bando E, Yonemura Y, Endou Y, Sasaki T, Taniguchi K, Fujita H, Fushida S, Fujimura T, Nishimura G, Miwa K, Seiki M. Immunohistochemical study of MT-MMP tissue status in gastric carcinoma and correlation with survival analyzed by univariate and multivariate analysis. Oncol Rep 1998; 5: 1483–1488.

Barrett AJ, Starkey PM. The interaction of alpha-2-macroglobulin with proteases. Biochem J 1973; 133: 709–724.

Basset P, Okada A, Chenard M-P, Kannan R, Stoll I, Anglard P, Bellocq J-P, Rio M-C. Matrix metalloproteinases as stromal effectors of human carcinoma progression therapeutic implications. Matrix Biol 1997; 15: 535–541.

Basuyaux JP, Ferreira E, Stehlin D, Buttice G. The Ets transcription factors interact with each other and with the c-Fos/c-Jun complex via distinct protein domains in a DNA-dependent and independent manner. J Biol Chem 1997; 272: 26188–26195.

Benbow U, Brinckerhoff CE. The AP-1 site and MMP gene regulation what is all the fuss about? Matrix Biology 1997; 15: 519–526.

Benbow U, Schoenermark MP, Mitchell TI, Rutter JL, Shimokawa K, Nagase H, Brinckerhoff CE. A novel host/tumor cell interaction activates matrix metalloproteinase 1 and mediates invasion through type I collagen. J Biol Chem 1999; 274: 25371–25378.

Benbow U, Schoenermark MP, Orndorff KA, Given AL, Brinckerhoff CE. Human breast cancer cells activate procollagenase-1 and invade type I collagen invasion is inhibited by all-trans retinoic acid. Clin Exp Metastasis 1999; 17: 213–238.

Bjorn SF, Hastrup N, Lund LR, Dano K, Larsen JF, Pyke C. Co-ordinated expression of MMP-2 and its putative activator MT1-MMP in human placentation. Mol Hum Reprod 1997; 8: 713–723.

Borden P, Solymjar D, Swcharczuk A, Lindman B, Cannon P, Heller RA. Cytokine control of interstitial collagenase and collagenase-3 gene expression in human chondrocytes. J Biol Chem 1996; 271: 23577–23581.

Borden P, Heller RA. Transcriptional control of matrix metalloproteinases and the tissue inhibitors of matrix metalloproteinases. Critical Reviews in Eukaryotic Gene Expression 1997; 7: 159–178.

Buolamwini JK. Novel anticancer drug discovery. Current Opin Chem Biol 1999; 3: 500–509.

Buttice G, Duterque-Coquillaud M, Basuyaux JP, Carrere S, Kurkinen M, Stehlin D. Erg an Ets-family member differentially regulates human collagenase-1 (MMP-1) and stromelysin-1 (MMP-3) expression by physically interacting with the Fos/Jun complex. Oncogene 1996; 9: 2241–2246.

Cawston T, Plumpton T, Curry V, Ellis A, Powell L. Role of TIMP and MMP inhibition in preventing connective tissue breakdown. Ann NY Acad Sci 1994; 732: 75–83.

Chambers AF, Matrisian LA. Changing views on the role of matrix metalloproteinases in metastasis. J Natl Cancer Inst 1997; 89: 1260–1270.

Curran S, Murray GI. Matrix metallo-proteinases in tumor invasion and metastasis. J Pathol 1999; 189: 300–308.

Dolo V, Ginestra A, Cassara D, Violini S, Lucania G, Torrisi MR, Nagase H, Canevari S, Pavan A, Vitorelli ML. Selective localization of matrix metalloproteinase 9 beta1 integrins and human lymphocyte antigen class I molecules on membrane vesicles shed by 8701-BC breast cancer cells. Cancer Res 1998; 58: 4468–4474.

Driouch K, Briffod M, Bieche I, Champeme M-H, Lidereau R. Location of several putative genes possibly involved in human breast cancer progression. Cancer Res 1998; 58: 2081–2086.

Durko M, Navab R, Shibata HR, Brodt P. Suppression of basement membrane type IV collagen degradation and cell invasion in human melanoma cells expressing an antisense RNA for MMP-1. Biochem Biophys Acta 1997; 1356: 271–280.

Durko M, Brodt N. Suppression of type I collagenase expression by antisense RNA in melanoma cells results in reduced synthesis of the urokinase-type plasminogen activator receptor. Biochem Biophys Res Communications 1998; 247: 342–348.

Ellenrieder V, Alber B, Lacher U, Hendler SF, Menke A, Boeck W, Wagner M, Wilda M, Friess H, Buchler M, Adler G, Gress TM. Role of MT-MMPs and MMP-2 in pancreatic cancer progression. Int J Cancer 2000; 85: 14–20.

Fang J, Shing Y, Wiederschain D, Yan L, Butterffield C, Jackson G, Harper J, Tamvakopoulos G, Moses MA. Matrix metalloproteinase-2 is required for the switch to the angiogenic phenotype in a tumor model. Proc Natl Acd Sci (USA) 2000; 97: 3884–3889.

Freije JMP, Diez-Itza I, Balbin M, Sanchez LM, Blasco R, Tolivia J, Lopez-Otin C. Molecular cloning and expression of collagenase-3 a novel human matrix metalloproteinase produced by breast carcinomas. J Biol Chem 1994; 269: 16766–16773.

73

Gilhardi G, Bioni ML, Mangoni J, Leviti S, DeMonti M, Guagnellini E, Scorza R. Matrix Metalloproteinase-1 promoter polymorphism 1G/2G is correlated with colorectal cancer invasiveness. Clin Cancer Res 2001; 7: 2344–2346.

Gilles C, Pollete M, Piette J, Munaut C, Thompson EW, Birembaut P, Foidart JM. High level of MT-MMP expression is associated with invasiveness of cervical cancer cells. Int J Cancer 1996; 65: 209–231.

Gilles C, Polette M, Birembaut P, Brunner N, Thompson EW. Expression of c-ets-1 mRNA is associated with an invasive EMT-derived phenotype in breast carcinoma lines. Clin Exp Metastasis 1997; 5: 519–526.

Ginestra A, La Placa MD, Saladino F, Cassara D, Nagase H, Vittorelli ML. The amount and proteolytic content of vesicles shed by human cancer cell lines correlates with their in vitro invasiveness. Anticancer Res 1998; 18: 3433–3437.

Ginestra A, Micell D, Dolo V, Romano FM, Vitorelli ML. Membrane vesicles in ovarian cancer fluids a new potential marker. Anticancer Res 1999; 19: 3439–3945.

Gomez DE, Alonso DF, Yoshiji H, Thorgeirsson U. Tissue inhibitors of metalloproteinases structure regulation and biologic functions. Eur J Cell Biol 1997; 7: 111–122.

Greenwald RA, Golub LM, Ramamurthy NS, Chowdhury M, Moak SA, Sorsa T. In vitro sensitivity of the three mammalian collagenases to tetracycline inhibition relationship to bone and cartilage degradation. Bone 1998; 22: 33–38.

Guo H, Zucker S, Gordon MK, Toole BP, Biswas C. Stimulation of matrix metalloproteinase production by recombinant extracellular matrix metalloproteinase inducer from transfected Chinese hamster ovary cells. J Biol Chem 1997; 272: 24–27.

Hanahan D, Folkman J. Patterns and emerging mechanisms of the angiogenic switch during tumorigenesis. Cell 1996; 86: 353–364.

Hanahan D, Weinberg RA. The hallmarks of cancer. Cell 2000; 100: 57–70.

Haq M, Shafli A, Zervos EE, Rosemurgy AS. Addition of matrix metalloproteinase inhibition to conventional cytotoxic therapy reduces tumor implantation and prolongs survival in a murine model of human pancreatic cancer. Cancer Res 2000; 60: 3207–3211.

Heimbrook DC, Oliff A. Therapeutic intervention and signaling. Current Opin Cell Biology 1998; 10: 284–288.

Heppner KJ, Matrisian LM, Jensen RA, Rodgers WH. Expression of most matrix metalloproteinase family members in breast cancer represents a tumor-induced host response. Am J Pathol 1996; 149: 273–282.

Hotary K, Allen E, Punturieri A, Yana I, Weiss SJ. Regulation of cell invasion and morphogenesis in a three-dimentional type I collagen matrix by membrane-type matrix metalloproteinases 1, 2 and 3. J Cell Biology 2000; 149: 309–1323.

Imamura T, Ohshio G, Mise M, Harada T, Suwa H, Wang Z, Yoshitomi S, Tanaka T, Sata S, Arii S, Seiki M, Imamura M. Expression of membrane-type matrix metalloproteinase-1 in human pancreatic adenocarcinomas. J Cancer Res Clin Oncol 1998; 124: 65–72.

Inoue T, Yashiro M, Nishimura S, Maeda K, Sawada T, Ogawa Y, Sowa M, Chung KH. Matrix metalloproteinase-1 expression is a prognostic factor for patients with advanced gastric cancer. Int J Mol Med 1999; 4: 73–77.

Ishigake S, Toi M, Ueno T, Matsumoto H, Muta M, KoikeM, Seiki M. Significance of membrane type I matrix metalloproteinase expression in breast cancer. Jpn J Cancer Res 1999; 90: 516–522.

Issing WJ, Wustrow TP. Expression of retinoic acid receptors in squamous cell carcinoma and their possible implications for chemoprevention. Anticancer Res 1996; 16: 2373–2377.

Ito T, Ito M, Shiozawa J, Naito S, Kanematsu T, Sekine I. Expression of the MMP-1 in human pancreatic carcinoma relationship with prognostic factor. Mod Pathol 1999; 12: 669–674.

74

Jimenez MJ, Balbin M, Lopez JM, Alvarez J, Komori T, Lopez-Otin C. Collagenase-3 is a target of Cbfa1 a transcription factor of the runt gene family involved in bone formation. Mol Cell Biol 1999; 19: 4431–4442.

Johansson N, Vaalamo M, Grenman S, Hietanen S, Klemi P, Saarialho-Kere U, Kahari VM. Collagenase-3 (MMP-13) is expressed by tumor cells in invasive squamous cell carcinomas. Am J Pathology 1999; 154: 469–480.

Kahari VM, Johansson N, Grenman R, Airola K, Saarialho-Kere U. Expression of collagenase-3 (MMP-13) by tumor cells in squamous cell carcinomas of the head and neck. Adv Exp Med Biol 1998; 451: 63–68.

Kanamori Y, Matsushima M, Minaguchi T, Kobayashi K, Sagae S, Kudo R, Terakawa N, Nakamura Y. Correlation between expression of the matrix metalloproteinase-1 gene in ovarian cancers and an insertion/deletion polymorphism in its promoter region. Cancer Res 1999; 59: 4225–4227.

Kim J, Yu W, Kovalski K, Ossowski L. Requirement for specific proteases in cancer cell intravasation as revealed by a novel semiquantitative PCR-based assay. Cell 1999; 94: 353–362.

Kitagawa Y, Kunimi K, Ito H, Sato H, Uchibayashi T, Okada Y, Seiki M, Namiki M. Expression and tissue localization of membrane-types 1, 2 and 3 matrix metalloproteinases in human urothelial carcinomas. J Urol 1998; 160: 1540–1545.

Kitagawa Y, Kunimi K, Uchibayashi T, Sato H, Namiki M. Expression of messenger RNAs for membrane-type 1, 2 and 3 matrix metalloproteinases in human renal cell carcinomas. J Urol 1999; 162: 905–909.

Kjellman M, Enberg U, Hoog A, Larsson C, Holst M, Farebo LO, Sato H, Backdahl M. Gelatinase A and membrane-type 1 matrix metalloproteinase mRNA expressed in adrenocortical cancers but not in adenomas. World J Surgery 1999; 23: 237–242.

Koblinski JA, Abrahram A, Sloane BF. Unraveling the role of proteases in cancer. Clin Chim Acta 2000; 291: 113–135.

Koochekpour S, Jeffers M, Wang PH, Gong C, Taylor GA, Roessler LM, Stearman R, Vasselli JR, Stetler-Stevenson WG, Kaelin WG, Linehan WM, Klausner RD, Gnarra JR, Vande Woude GF. The von-Hippel-Lindau tumor suppressor gene inhibits hepatocyte growth factor/scatter factor-induced invasion and branching morphogenesis in renal carcinoma cells. Mol Cell Biol 1999; 19: 5902–5912.

Kuniyasu H, Ellis LM, Evans DB, Abbruzzese JL, Fenoglio CJ, Bucana CD, Cleary KR, Tahara E, Fidler IJ. Relative expression of E-cadherin and type IV collagenase genes predicts disease outcome in patients with resectable pancreatic carcinoma. Clin Cancer Res 1999; 5: 23–33.

Kurahara S, Shinohara M, Ikebe T, Nakamura S, Beppu M, Hiraki A, Takeuchi H, Shirasuna K. Expression of MMPs MT-MMP and TIMPs in squamous cell carcinoma of the oral cavity correlation with tumor invasion and metastasis. Head Neck 1999; 21: 627–638.

Li H, Bauzon DE, Xu X, Tschesche H, Cao J, Sang QA. Immunological characterization of cell-surface and soluble forms of membrane type I matrix metalloproteinase in human breast cancer cells and in fibroblasts. Mol Carcinog 1998; 22: 84–89.

Lotan R. Retinoids and their receptors in modulation of differentiation development and prevention of head and neck cancers. Anticancer Res 1996; 16: 15–19.

Lovejoy B, Welch AR, Carr S, Luong C, Broka C, Hendricks RT, Campbell JA, Walker KAM, Martin R, Van Wort H, Browner MF. Crystal structures of MMP-1 and -13 reveal the structural basis for selectivity of collagenase inhibitors. Nature Struct Biol 1999; 6: 217–221.

Lui K, Wahlberg P, Ny T. Coordinated and cell-specific regulation of membrane type metalloproteinase 1 (MT1-MMP) and its substrate matrix metalloproteinase 2 (MMP-2) by physiologic signals during follicular development and ovulation. Endocrinology 1998; 139: 4735–4738.

75

Maniotis AJ, Folberg R, Hess A, Seftor EA, Gardner LMG, Peíer J, Trent JM, Meltzer PS, Hendrix MJC. Vascular channel formation by human melanoma cells in vivo and in vitro vasculogenic mimicry. Am J Pathol 1999; 155: 739–752.

McCawley LJ, Matrisian LM. Matrix metalloproteinases multifunctional contributors to tumor progression. Mol Med Today 2000; 6: 149–156.

Mengshol JA, Vincenti MP, Coon CI, Barchowsky A, Brinckerhoff CE. Interleukin-1 induction of collagenase 3 (matrix metalloproteinase 13) gene expression in chondrocytes requires p38 c-jun N-terminal kinase and nuclear factor kB. Arthritis Rheum 2000; 43: 801–811.

Mitchell PG, Magna HA, Reeves LM. Cloning expression and type II collagenolytic activity of matrix metalloproteinase13 from human osteoarthritic cartilage. J Clin Invest 1996; 97: 2011–2019.

Moser PL, Kieback DG, Hefler L, Tempfer C, Neunteufel W, Gitsch G. Immuno-histochemical detection of matrix metalloproteinases (MMP) 1 and 2 and tissue inhibitor of metalloproteinases 2 (TIMP 2) in stage I and II endometrial cancer. Anticancer Res 1999; 19: 236–2367.

Murray GI, Duncan ME, O'Neil P, Melvin WT, Fothergill JE. Matrix metalloproteinase-1 is associated with poor prognosis in colorectal cancer. Nature Med 1996; 2: 461–462.

Murray GI, Duncan ME, OÌNeil P, McKay JA, Melvin WT, Fothergill JE. Matrix metalloproteinase-1 is associated with poor prognosis in oesophageal cancer. J Pathol 1998p 185: 256–261.

Nagase H, Itoh Y, Binner S. Interaction of alpha$_2$ macroglobulin with matrix metalloproteinases and its use for identification of their active forms. Ann NY Acad Sci 1994; 6: 294–302.

Nagase H, Woessner JF Jr. Matrix Metalloproteinases. J Biol Chem 1999; 274: 21491–21492.

Nakopoulou L, Giannopoulou I, Gakiopoulou H, Liapis H, Tzonou A, Davaris PS. Matrix metalloproteinase-1 and -3 in breast cancer correlation with progesterone receptors and other clinicopathological feature. Hum Pathol 1999; 30: 436–442.

Nelson AR, Fingleton B, Rothenberg ML, Matrisian LM. Matrix metalloproteinases biologic activity and clinical implications. J Clin Oncol 2000; 18: 1135–1149.

Nishioka Y, Kobayashi K, Sagae S, Ishioka S, Nishikawa A, Matsushima M, Kanamori Y, Minaguchi T, Nakamura Y, Tokina T, Kudo R. A single nucleotide polymorphism in the matrix metalloproteinase-1 promoter in endometrial carcinomas. Jpn J Cancer Res 2000; 91: 612–615.

Noll WW, Belloni DR, Rutter JL, Storm CA, Schned AR, Titus-Ernstoff L, Ernstoff MS, Brinckerhoff CE. Loss of heterozygosity on chromosome 11q.22.23 in melanoma is associated with retention of the insertion polymorphism in the matrix metalloproteinase 1 promoter. Am J Pathol 2001; 158: 691–697.

Oberg A, Hoyhtya M, Tavelin B, Stenling R, Lindmark G. Limited value of preoperative serum analyses of matrix metalloproteinases (MMP-2 MMP-9) and tissue inhibitors of metalloproteinases (TIMP-1 TIMP-2) in colorectal cancer. Anticancer Res 2000; 20: 1085–1091.

O-Charoenrat P, Rhys-Evans P, Mldjtahedi H, Court W, Box G, Eccles S. Overexpression of epidermal growth factor receptor in head and neck squamous cell carcinoma cell lines correlates with matrix metallo-proteinase-9 expression and in vitro invasion. Int J Cancer 2000; 86: 307–317.

Ohishi K, Fujita N, Morinaga Y, Tsuruo T. H-32 human breast cancer cells stimulate type I collagenase production in osteoblast-like cells and induce bone resorption. Clin Exp Metastasis 1995; 13: 287–295.

Ohuchi E, Imai K, Fuji Y, Sato H, Seiko M, Okada Y. Membrane type I matrix metalloproteinase digest interstitial collagens and other extracellular matrix macromolecules. J Biol Chem 1997; 272: 2446–2451.

Parsons SL, Watson SA, Brown PD, Collins HM, Steele RJC. Matrix Metalloproteinases. Br J Surgery 1997; 84: 60–166.

Pei D. Identification and characterization of the fifth membrane-type matrix metalloproteinase MT5-MMP. J Biol Chem 1999; 274: 8925–8932.

Pendas AM, Balbin M, Llano E, Jimenez MG, Lopez-Otin C. Structural analysis and promoter characterization of the human collagenase-3 gene (MMP-13). Genomics 1997; 40: 222–233.

Pendas AM, Uria J, Jimenez MG, Balbin M, Freije JP, Lopez-Otin C. An overview of collagenase-3 expression in malignant tumors and analysis of its potential value as a target in anti-tumor therapies. Clin Chem Acta 2000; 291: 137–155.

Pickett KL, Harber GJ, DeCarlo AA, Louis P, Shaneyfelt S, Windsor LJ, Bodden MK. 72K-GL (MMP-9) and 92K-GL (MMP-2) are produced in vivo by human oral squamous cell carcinomas and can enhance FIB-CL (MMP-1) activity in vitro. J Dent Res 1999; 78: 1354–1361.

Polette M, Birembaut P. Membrane-type metalloproteinases in tumor invasion. Int J Biochem Cell Biochem 1998; 30: 1195–1202.

Ramos-deSimone N, Hahn-Dantona E, Sipley J, Nagase H, French DL, Quigley JP. Activation of matrix metalloproteinase-9 (MMP-9) via a converging plasmin/stromelysin-1 cascade enhances tumor cell invasion. J Biol Chem 1999; 274: 3066–13076.

Rasmussen HS, McCann PP. Matrix metalloproteinase inhibition as a novel anticancer strategy a review with special focus on Batimastat and Marimastat. Pharmacol Ther 1997; 75: 69–75.

Reboul P, Pelletier JP, Tardif G, Cloutier JM, Martel-Pelletier J. The new collagenase collagenase-3 is expressed and synthesized by human chondrocytes but not by synoviocytes. J Clin Invest 1996; 97: 2011–2019.

Remacle AG, Noel A, Duggan C, McDermott E, O'Higgins N, Foidart JM, Duffy MJ. Assay of matrix metalloproteinases types 1, 2, 3 and 9 in breast cancer. Br J Cancer 1998; 77: 926–931.

Rowinsky EK, Windle JJ, Von Hoff DD. Ras protein farnesyltransferase a strategic target for anticancer therapeutic development. J Clin Oncol 1999; 17: 3631–3652.

Rutter JL, Mitchell TI, Buttice G, Meyers J, Gusella JF, Ozelius LJ, Brinckerhoff CE. A single nucleotide polymorphism in the matrix metalloproteinase-1 promoter creates an Ets binding site and augments transcription. Cancer Res 1998; 58: 5321–5325.

Saez E, Rutberg SE, Mueller E, Oppenheim H, Smoluk J, Yuspa SH, Spiegelman BM. c-Fos is required for malignant progression of skin tumors. Cell 1995; 82: 721–732.

Sato T, Iwai M, Sakai T, Sato H, Seiki M, Mori Y, Ito A. Enhancement of membrane-type I-matrix metalloproteinase (MT1-MMP) production and subsequent activation of progelatinase A on human squamous cell carcinoma cells co-cultured with human dermal fibroblasts. Br J Cancer 1999; 80: 1137–1143.

Schadendorf D, Kern MA, Artuc M, Pahl HL, Rosenbach T, Fichtner I, Nurnberg W, Stuting S, von Stebut E, Worm M Makki A, Jurgovsky K, Kolde G, Benz BM. Treatment of melanoma cells with the synthetic retinoid CD437 induces apoptosis via activation of AP-1 in vitro and causes cell growth inhibition in xenografts in vivo. J Cell Biology 1996; 135: 1889–1898.

Schoenermark MP, Mitchell TI, Rutter JL, Reczek PR, Brinckerhoff CE. Retinoid-mediated inhibition of tumor invasion and matrix metalloproteinase synthesis. Ann NY Acad Sci 1999; 878: 466–486.

Schroen DJ, Brinckerhoff CE. Nuclear hormone receptors inhibit matrix metalloproteinase (MMP) gene expression through diverse mechanisms. Gene Expression 1997; 6: 197–207.

Seiki M. Membrane-type matrix metalloproteinases. APMIS 1999; 107: 137–143.

Shalinsky DR, Brekken J, Zou H, McDermott CD, Forsyth P, Edwards D, Margosiak S, Benber S, Truitt G, Wood A, Varki NM, Appelt K. Broad anti-tumor and anti-angiogenic activities of AG3340 a potent and selective MMP inhibitor undergoing advanced oncology clinical trials. Ann NY Acad Sci 1999; 878: 236–270.

Spanjaard RA, Ikeda M, Lee PJ, Charpentier B, Chin WW, Eberlein T. Specific activation of retinoic acid receptors (RARs) and retinoid X receptors reveals a unique role for RAR γ in induction of differentiation and apoptosis in S91 melanoma cells. J Biol Chem 1997; 27: 18990–18999.

Stetler-Stevenson WG. Matrix metalloproteinases in angiogenesis a moving target for therapeutic intervention. J Clin Invest 1999; 103: 1237–1241.

Tallman MS, Andersen JW, Schiffer CA, Appelbaum FR, Feusner JH, Ogden A, Shepherd L, Willman C, Bloomfield CD, Rowe JM, Wiernik PH. All-trans-retinoic acid in acute promyelocytic leukemia. N Eng J Med 1997; 337: 1021–1028.

Talvensaari-Mattila A, Paakko P, Hoyhtya M, Blanco-Sequeriros G, Turpeenniemi-Hujanen T. Matrix metalloproteinase-2 immunoreactive protein a marker of aggressiveness in breast carcinoma. Cancer 1998; 83: 1153–1162.

Tanney DC, Feng L, Pollock AS, Lovett DH. Regulated expression of matrix metalloproteinases and TIMP in nephrogenesis. Dev Dyn 1998; 213: 121–129.

Tardiff G, Pelletier J-P, Dupuis M, Hambor JE, Martel-Pelletier J. Cloning sequencing and characterization of the 5'-flanking region of the human collagenase-3 gene. Biochem J 1997: 32313–32316.

Tsukifuji R, Tagawa K, Hatamouchi A, Shinkai H. Expression of matrix metalloproteinase -1 -2 and -3 in squamous cell carcinoma and actinic keratosis. Br J Cancer 1999; 8: 10878–10891.

Uitto VJ, Airola K, Vaalamo M, Johansson N, Putnins EE, Firth JD, Salonen J, Lopez-Otin C, Saarialho-Kere U, Kahari VM. Collagenase-3 (matrix metalloproteinase-13) expression is induced in oral mucosal epithelium during chronic inflammation. Am J Pathol 1998; 152: 1489–1499.

Unemori EN, Ferrara N, Bauer EA, Amento EP. Vascular endothelial growth factor induces interstitial collagenase expression in human endothelial cells. J Cellular Physiol 1992; 153: 557–562.

Vaisanen A, Kallioinen M, Taskinen PJ, Turpeenniemi-Hujanen T. Prognostic value of MMP-2 immunoreactive protein (72 kD type IV collagenase) in primary skin melanoma. J Pathol 1998; 186: 51–58.

Vaisanen A, Kallioinen M, von Dickhoff K, Laatikainen L, Hoytya M, Turpeenniemi-Hujanen T. Matrix metalloproteinase-2 (MMP-2) immunoreactive protein – a new prognostic marker in uveal melanoma? J Pathol 1999; 188: 56–62.

Vaalamo M, Mattila L, Johansson N, Kariniemi AL, Kajalainen-Lindsberg ML, Kahari VM, Saarialho-Kere U. Distinct populations of stromal cells express collagenase-3 (MMP-13) and collagenase-1 (MMP-1) in chronic ulcers but not in normally healing wounds. J Invest Dermatol 1997; 109: 96–101.

Velesco G, Cal S, Merlos-Suarez A, Ferrando AA, Alverez S, Nakano A, Arribas J, Lopez-Otin C. Human MT6-matrix metalloproteinase identification progelatinase A activation and expression in brain tumors. Cancer Res 2000; 60: 877–882.

Vincenti MP, Clark IM, Brinckerhoff CE. Using inhibitors of metalloproteinases to treat arthritis easier said than done? Arthritis and Rheum 1994; 37: 1115–1126.

Vincenti MP, White LA, Schroen DJ, Benbow U, Brinckerhoff CE. Regulating expression of the gene for matrix metalloproteinase-1 (collagenase) mechanisms that control enzyme activity transcription and mRNA stability. Critical Reviews in Eucaryotic Gene Expression 1996; 6: 391–411.

Vincenti MP, Coon CI, Brinckerhoff CE. Nuclear factor kB/p50 activates an element in the distal matrix metalloproteinase 1 promoter in Interleukin-1? stimulated synovial fibroblasts. Arthritis Rheum 1998; 4: 1981–994.

Vu TH, Shipley JM, Bergers, Berger JE, Helms JA, Hanahan D, Shipiro SD, Senior RM, Werb Z. MMP-9/Gelatinase B is a key regulator of growth plate angiogenesis and apoptosis of hypertrophic chondrocytes. Cell 1998; 93: 411–422.

78

Wang H, Keiser J. Vascular endothelial growth factor upregulates the expression of matrix metalloproteinases in vascular smooth muscle. Circ Res 1998; 157: 5–12.

Wasylyk B, Hahn SL, Giovane A. The Ets family of transcription factors. Eur J Biochem 1993; 15: 7–18.

Wen W, Moses MA, Wiederschain D, Arbiser JL, Folkman J. The generation of endostatin is mediated by elastase. Cancer Res 1999; 59: 6052–6056.

Westermarck J, Kahari V-M. Regulation of matrix metalloproteinase expression in tumor invasion. FASEB J 1999; 13: 781–792.

White LA, Brinckerhoff CE. Two AP-1 elements in the collagenase promoter have differential effects on transcription and bind JunD c-Fos and Fra-2. Matrix Biology 1995; 14: 715–725.

Wojtowicz-Praga S, Low J, Marshall J, Ness E, Dickson R, Barter J, Sale M, McCann P, Moore J, Cole A, Hawkins MJ. Phase I trial of a novel matrix metalloproteinase inhibitor Batimastat (BB-94). Invest New Drugs 1996; 14: 193–202.

Wojtowicz-Praga S, Torri J, Johnson M, Steen V, Marshall J, Nese E, Dickson R, Sale M, Rasmussen HS, Chiodo TA, Hawkins MJ. Phase I trial of Marimastat a novel matrix metalloproteinase inhibitor administered orally to patients with advanced lung cancer. J Clin Oncol 1998; 16: 2150–2156.

Wosikowski K, Schuurhuis D, Geert JP, Kops JPL, Saceda M, Bates SE. Altered gene expression in drug-resistant human breast cancer cells. Clinical Cancer Res 1997; 3: 2405–2414.

Ye S, Dhillon S, Turner SJ, Bateman AC, Theaker JM, Pickering RM, Day I, Howell WM. Invasiveness of cutaneous malignant melanoma is influenced by Matrix Metalloproteinase 1 gene polymorphism. Cancer Res 2001; 61: 1296–1298.

Yoon S-S, Fidler I,J Beltran PJ, Bucana CD, Wang Y-F, Fan D. Intratumor heterogeneity for and epigenetic modulation of mdr-1 expression in murine melanoma. Melanoma Res 1997; 7: 275–287.

Zhang XK, Liu Y, Lee MO. Retinoic receptors in human lung cancer and breast cancer. Mutation Res 1996; 350: 267–277.

Zhu Y, Spitz MR, Lei L, Mills GB, Wu X. A single nucleotide polymorphism in the matrix metalloproteinase-1 (MMP-1) promoter enhances lung cancer susceptibility. Cancer Res 2001; 61: 7825–7829.

Zimmerman CM, Padgett RW. Transforming growth factor beta signaling mediators and modulators. Gene 2000; 16: 17–30.

Chapter 5

STROMELYSIN-3, A PARTICULAR MEMBER OF THE MATRIX METALLOPROTEINASE FAMILY

M.-C. Rio

U184 INSERM, UPR 6520 CNRS, Université Louis Pasteur, Institut de Génétique et de Biologie Moléculaire et Cellulaire, BP 163, 67404 Illkirch, France

1. INTRODUCTION

Matrix metalloproteinases (MMPs) are extracellular proteolytic enzymes. The MMP family that extends continuously contains to date over 20 members. Even if all these proteins share an intrinsic proteolytic activity against extracellular matrix (ECM) or matrix-associated components, they differ depending on the nature of their substrates, and their spatial and temporal patterns of expression. Therefore, they are involved in various biological processes and proliferative, invasive, pro-angiogenic and proapoptotic effects have been demonstrated for MMPs (Birkedal-Hansen, 1995; Blasi and Stoppelli, 1999; Noël et al, 1997; Moses, 1997). However, animals deficient for MMPs (Wilson et al, 1997; Itoh et al, 1997) can be devoid of obvious phenotypes, suggesting that MMP members may also share overlapping functions. MMP function is balanced *in vivo* by endogenous specific molecules, the tissue inhibitors of matrix metalloproteinases (TIMPs).

Numerous studies have provided evidence that, although the transformation of epithelial cells is the *sine qua non* condition for the development of carcinomas, the nature of the connective/stromal tissue environment is crucial for tumor progression (Raff, 1992; Lukashev and Werb, 1998). MMPs that interact with stromal components have been shown to contribute to malignancy in both the early and late stages of tumor progression in human (Basset et al, 1997; Coussens and Werb, 1996) and mouse (Rudolph-Owen and Matrisian, 1998; Lochter et al, 1998). Therefore their study is of interest to improve our understanding of malignant processes. In this context, the eleventh member of the MMP family (MMP11), also named stromelysin-3 (ST3), fulfiles this paradigm. It was discovered in 1990 because of its overexpression in a cDNA library established from a human breast cancer biopsy (Basset et al, 1990). Later on, clinical

J.-M. Foidart and R.J. Muschel (eds.), Proteases and Their Inhibitors in Cancer Metastasis, 81–107.

trials showed that high levels of ST3 expression correlated with a lower survival rate among patients with breast, head and neck, or colon cancer (Muller et al, 1993; Porte et al, 1995). Therefore, the possibility that ST3 might play a role during tumor progression, was promising for the diagnosis, prognosis and design of new treatment. During the past 10 years, numerous experiments have been performed to enhance the knowledge of the biological function of ST3, and to evaluate its clinical relevance.

In the present review, starting from the results of the literature, we will attempt to appreciate the participation of ST3 into non-cancerous and cancerous human diseases, and to draw a scheme of its cellular and molecular functions. From these data, ST3 appears to be an unique member of the MMP family exhibiting peculiar features and function.

2. ST3 IS A CONSTITUTIVELY ACTIVE MMP

Primary sequence analysis of the encoded ST3 protein leads to the definition of several protein domains shared by the members of the MMP protein family. The mouse homologue of ST3 is 89% similar to the human protein showing that ST3 is globally well-conserved between the 2 species (Lefebvre et al, 1992). Thus, ST3 contains a pre-domain corresponding to a signal peptide specific for the secreted proteins, a pro-domain that maintains the enzyme under an inactive form, a catalytic domain responsible of the enzymatic activity and an hemopexin-like domain that is supposed to be responsible for the specificity of the MMP substrates (Basset et al, 1990). In addition, ST3 shares with membrane type MMPs (MT-MMPs; MMP14, MMP15, MMP16 and MMP17) a cleavage site for the intracellular furin-type convertases, located between the pro-domain and the catalytic domain. Thus, the ubiquitously-expressed furin (Pei and Weiss, 1995; Santvicca et al, 1996) and to a lesser extent, PACE 4 (paired basic amino-acid-cleaving enzyme 4) (Santavicca et al, 1996; Bassi et al, 2000) intracellularly process the proST3 into its mature form within the trans-Golgi network. Similar motifs are found in some growth factors and adhesion molecules such as E-cadherin. Thus, ST3 activation is not dependent on the extracellular 'cysteine switch mechanism' usually involved in MMP activation (Pei and Weiss, 1995; Santvicca et al, 1996). Interestingly, it has been shown that PACE 4 overexpresssion can induce tumorigenesis in mice (Bassi et al, 2000), and is associated with increased cell invasivity (Hubbard et al, 1997).

Using Western blot analysis, the pro- and the mature forms of human ST3 are usually observed at about 56 and 47 kDa, respectively (Santavicca et al, 1996). However, several other forms of ST3 have been reported. In an *in vitro* stromal/epithelial cell co-culture model, a 35 kDa protein lacking enzymatic activity was found to be produced by normal pulmonary fibroblasts (Mari et al, 1998). Two forms of 35 kDa and 28 kDa were also observed in human atherosclerotic tissues (Schonbeck et al, 1999). Moreover, an additive 28 kDa form was seen after furin cleavage of human ST3 (Santavicca et al, 1996). The diversity of the observed forms of ST3 raises the question of the existence of possible various post-translational maturation of the ST3 protein.

Most of MMPs are able to cleave one or more major component(s) of the ECM. By contrast, ST3 was shown to be unable to cleave collagens, gelatins, casein, laminin, entactin or fibronectin putting into question the functionality of the ST3 catalytic domain. However, further data permitted to discard this hypothesis. The first evidence that ST3 had enzymatic activity was given by observation that a 28 kDa form of the mouse ST3 (but not of the human ST3) devoid of the 216 carboxy-terminal amino-acids has weak caseinolytic activity (Murphy et al, 1993). Moreover, in 1994, it was shown that the mature form of the human ST3 is a powerful endopeptidase since it was able to destroy the antiproteolytic function of alpha$_1$-proteinase inhibitor (α_1PI) by cleaving the antiproteinase at a distinct site within the reactive site loop between alanine 350 and methionine 351. ST3 also has the ability to cleave alpha$_2$-macroglobulin (α_2M) between phenylalanine 684 and tyrosine 685, a site identical to that recognized by stromelysin-1 (MMP3) (Pei et al, 1994). Moreover, it has been reported that IGFBP-1 (insulin-like growth factor binding protein 1) is a substrate of the human ST3 *in vitro* and *in vivo*. The cleavage occurs in the mid-region of IGFBP-1, at the histidine 140-valine 141 bond, and leads to decreased affinity of IGFBP-1 for IGF-1 and subsequently to the recovery of IGF1 biological activity (Manes et al, 1997). Very recently, a human mature form of ST3 synthesized in baculovirus-infected insect cells was shown to be active *in vitro* against casein and α_2M (Barbacid et al, 1998). It should be noted that all these substrates are not specific to ST3 since they are also cleaved by one or several other MMPs.

Thus, ST3 possesses all the features required to belong to the MMP family. However, whereas most other MMPs are activated extracellularly, ST3 is activated prior to secretion by Golgi-associated furin-like proteases. ST3 is thus a constitutively active MMP. The absence of post-translational activation suggests a decreased inertia leading to a shorter delay between ST3 expression and action. Finally, the hypothesis of the existence of highly specific ST3 substrate(s), in addition to the anti-proteinases α_1PI and α_2M, and the growth factor binding protein IGFBP-1, remains to be addressed.

3. THE ST3 GENE PROMOTER POSSESSES PARTICULAR REGULATORY ELEMENTS

The human ST3 gene is located on the long arm of chromosome 22 (22q11.2). This position differs from that reported on chromosomes 11, 14 and 16 for the other MMP genes, suggesting that ST3 could be the first member of a new MMP sub-family (Levy et al, 1992). The mouse ST3 gene is located to the C band of chromosome 10 showing a syntenic conservation during evolution (our unpublished results). General gene organization including 8 exons and 7 introns is well conserved between human, mouse, and xenopus ST3 (Lefebvre et al, 1992; Li et al, 1998).

Analysis of the 5′ region upstream of the TATA box shows several functional regulatory elements common to the human, mouse and/or xenopus ST3 genes. A cis-acting retinoic acid responsive element (RARE) of the DR1 type is present in the proximal region, and 2 RAREs of the DR2 type are found in the distal region of the human and mouse ST3 genes. The xenopus ST3 promoter is devoid of RARE elements. The proximal DR1 has been shown to be sufficient for ST3 promoter activity *in vitro*. This RARE may be responsible, at least partially, for the *in vivo* expression of ST3 since retinoic acid receptor beta and gamma (RARb and RARg) – deficient mice exhibit lower levels of ST3 (Dupe et al, 1999). Additional distal elements have been reported (Luo et al, 1999; Ludwig et al, 2000). An AP1-like responsive element is responsible for the basal human ST3 promoter activity. This element is not present in the mouse promoter. One (human) and 2 (mouse) CCAAT/enhancer binding protein (C/EBP)-binding sites that efficiently bind the C/EBPbeta transcription factor, are involved in the TPA-regulated induction of ST3 gene expression. The ST3 promoter contains also 1 (human and mouse) or 2 (xenopus) GAGA factor binding sites. Moreover, a thyroid hormone responsive element (TRE), shared by human, mouse and xenopus, is present in the distal region of the ST3 promoter. This TRE has been shown to be functional in frog, and ST3 is a direct immediate-early thyroid hormone (T3) responsive gene (Patterton et al, 1995). In contrast to the other MMPs, no proximal AP1-binding site was identified in the ST3 promoter in all the species studied (Luo et al, 1999; Ludwig et al, 2000). Finally, in xenopus, 2 transcription start sites (+1, −94) and a second TATA box (−87, −82) were reported, suggesting a possible second ST3 messenger RNA (Li et al, 1998). Similar organization leading to 2 types of messenger RNAs might also exist in the human ST3 gene (P. Anglard, personal communication).

Thus, ST3 differs from most of the other MMPs in the induction of its expression. Like most MMP genes, human and mouse ST3 are induced by TPA treatment. However, whereas MMPs are usually induced via their proximal AP1-binding sites, in ST3, this regulation is mediated by C/EBP binding sites.

Similarly, the TPA delayed response of the interstitial collagenase (MMP1) was shown to be controlled by C/EBPbeta (Doyle et al, 1997). Moreover, other MMPs are devoid of RAREs and, in contrast to ST3 that is positively regulated, they are down-regulated by retinoic acid treatment. Finally, to date, ST3 is the only MMP to possess a TRE. However, the biological relevance of this TRE in human and mouse remains to be established.

4. ST3 IS EXTENSIVELY EXPRESSED IN NORMAL CONDITIONS

ST3 is extensively expressed throughout embryogenesis. During human placentation, extravillous trophoblasts invading the maternal decidua produce ST3, and later on, ST3 is restricted to the syncytiotrophoblasts that line the intervillous vascular spaces (Maquoi et al, 1997). Similarly, trophoblast giant cells expressing ST3 were observed during mouse embryonic implantation (Lefebvre et al, 1995). During embryonic development, ST3 was first reported to be present in the mesoderm underlying the primitive epiderm in the interdigital region of the limb bud of 8-weeks-old human embryo (Basset et al, 1990). Extensive analysis of ST3 expression during mouse embryogenesis further showed transient ST3 expression in various tissues, including skin, lung, bone and intestine, indicating that ST3 participates in the ontogenesis of various organs (Lefebvre et al, 1995). During amphibian development, ST3 is present in regions of active morphogenesis (Ishizuya-Oka et al, 2000), such as the region where future hind limb buds develop, implicating a role of ST3 in tissue patterning. ST3 is also observed during xenopus tail elongation, and hindgut and proectoderm formation (Damjanovski et al, 2000).

Another biological event during which ST3 is expressed is tadpole metamorphosis (Patterton et al, 1995). ST3 is expressed in and surrounding resorbing epithelial and connective tissues throughout the entire tadpole. This ST3 up-regulation during metamorphosis is thyroid hormone-dependent, and thyroid hormone receptors are extensively expressed during these processes. Furthermore, it was shown that ST3 is crucial for resorption of larval tissues (Berry et al, 1998).

In the adult, several tissues undergoing cyclic or punctual breakdown and regeneration processes express ST3. The menstrual endometrium remodeling is controlled by ovarian steroids and local cytokines. Stromelysin-1, matrilysin (MMP7) and ST3 are expressed during menstrual breakdown and subsequent estrogen-mediated growth, but not during the secretory phase (Osteen et al, 1999). Intense ST3 expression was also reported during ovulation (Hagglund et al, 1999), and at the time of the post-partum regression of the uterus (Rio et al, 1996). Finally, whereas ST3 cannot be detected in virgin, pregnant or lactating mouse mammary glands, it is observed during post-weaning involution of the gland. ST3 expression starts 3 days after weaning in fibroblastic cells immediately surrounding degenerative ducts (Lefebvre et al, 1992).

Thus, like other MMPs, ST3 expression is observed throughout biological processes in various embryonic and adult tissues. This is true for human, mouse, and xenopus showing that ST3 expression and presumably function is evolutionary well conserved, at least in vertebrates. Together, these observations indicate that ST3 is mainly synthesized and secreted by cells of mesenchymal origin during tissue remodeling processes accompanying regression, extension, invasion, or differentiation of epithelial compartment. This extensive localization of ST3 suggests that it concerns a major biological program occurring throughout animal life.

5. ST3 IS EXTENSIVELY EXPRESSED IN PATHOLOGICAL CONDITIONS

ST3 is observed during repair processes such as skin wound-healing in man (Wolf et al, 1992). In a rat model of skin repair, ST3 is highly expressed from day 5 to 10 after cutaneous incision. ST3 RNAs are detected, similar to the human system, in stromal cells of the scar tissue, below the thickened epithelial cell layer (Okada et al, 1997).

ST3 expression is also observed in numerous human diseases. Whereas normal arteries do not express ST3, it is observed in human atherosclerotic plaques (Schonbeck et al, 1999). In ST3-null mice, vessel formation is normal. However, after electric injury, the femoral artery of ST3-null mice showed an accelerated neointima formation leading to increased thickness. Massive infiltration by polymorphonuclear (PMN) cells (CD45 positive) is present in these ST3-null lesions (Lijnen et al, 1999). These data show that ST3 is involved in injured vessel remodeling and therefore may contribute to luminal stenosis. ST3 is also expressed in human rheumatoid arthritis and in traumatic synovial membrane suggesting that ST3 may participate in physiological synovial tissue remodeling (Konttinen et al, 1999). Accordingly, similar results were observed in an *in vivo* model of knee joint collagen-induced arthritis in mice (Lubberts et al, 1999). Finally, very few cases of benign tumors have been shown to express ST3. However, surprisingly, it was reported that almost all dermatofibromas, which correspond to benign fibrous nodules, are ST3 positive, although ST3 is not expressed in malignant dermatofibrosarcomas (Unden et al, 1996; Thewes et al, 1999).

While only rare sarcomas present ST3 positivity, ST3 ectopic expression has been reported in fibroblasts surrounding malignant epithelial tumor cells

Table 1. In vivo ST3 expression during normal and pathologic tissue remodeling processes.

Time of expression	Cells/Tissues	Remodeling processes
Development	Invading trophoblasts	Embryonic implantation
	Syncytiotrophoblasts	Placentation
	Limb bud mesenchyme	Interdigitation
	Invading osteoblasts	Osteogenesis
	Neuroepithelial cells	Spinal cord morphogenesis
	Snout, tail mesenchyme	Epithelium growth
Metamorphosis	Tail	Larval tissue resorption
	Intestine	Morphogenesis
Adult tissues	Endometrium	Menstrual breakdown
	Uterus	Post-partum involution
	Ovary	Ovulation
	Mammary gland	Post-weaning involution
Non-malignant diseases	Atherosclerosis	Inflammation, repair
	Skin	Wound healing
	Arthritis	Inflammation
	Dermatofibroma	Benign tumor proliferation
Malignant tumors	Carcinomas, fibroblasts	Tissue invasion

of almost all types of carcinomas including breast, lung (squamous cells), ovary, prostate, small intestine, stomach, uterus, colon, larynx, esophagus, pancreas, bladder, skin, and head and neck. ST3 is rarely observed in liver, kidney and lung small cell carcinomas. Moreover, ST3 is more frequent in primary tumors (50% to 100%), than in secondary tumors (30% to 70%) (Rouyer et al, 1994; Rio et al, 1996). This may be due to the fact that in some metastases, cancer cells have acquired additional genetic alteration and can therefore survive and proliferate without sustaining help from stromal cells. In addition, high levels of ST3 are correlated with bad prognoses and pejorative patient outcomes. For example, ST3 has been shown to be a strong independent pronostic parameter for disease-free survival in breast cancers (Chenard et al, 1996; Ahmad et al, 1998). In invasive bladder carcinomas, ST3 is associated with a more aggressive tumor phenotype (Basset et al, 1993; Mueller et al, 2000), and overexpression of ST3 is related to the lymph node involvement in non-small cell lung cancer (Delebecq et al, 2000).

Thus, similar to normal conditions, ST3 expression is related to intense tissue remodeling in benign and malignant diseases. Moreover, clinical data strongly suggest that ST3 favors cancer progression in human. Finally, the observation of ST3 in diseases involving inflammatory processes leads to the question of possible ST3 involvement in immune and/or inflammatory responses.

6. ST3 EXHIBITS A PRECISE SPATIAL EXPRESSION PATTERN

Almost all cases in which cells expressing ST3 are not fibroblasts concern normal invasive processes occuring during development. In this context, ST3 may be observed in the invading cells themselves as is the case for trophoblastic giant cells and osteoblasts during embryonic implantation and osteogenesis, respectively. However, ST3 may also be synthesized by cells of the invaded tissue as reported for the neuroepithelial cells of the floor plate during spinal cord morphogenesis (Rio et al, 1996). These results suggest that, during development, ST3 may exert part of its biological function in an autocrine manner. This hypothesis is reinforced by the fact that, in experimental tumor models, ST3 expression by the cancer cells themselves leads to results similar to those obtained using cancer cells associated with ST3 expressing fibroblasts (see below).

Usually, ST3 is expressed by fibroblasts. However, this expression does not concern all fibroblasts but a few fibroblasts with a very precise spatial pattern of expression (Basset et al, 1990; Rio et al, 1996). Thus, during the mouse snout, limb and tail development, the ST3 positive fibroblasts constitute a thin layer of cells located just beneath the basement membrane lining the extending epithelium (Lefebvre et al, 1995). Similarly, during tissue regression events, ST3 is most often expressed by fibroblasts located in the vicinity of the dying epithelial cells (Lefebvre et al, 1992). The pattern of ST3 expression during limb bud development is more diffuse. This could be due to the fact that ST3 expressing fibroblasts belong to the dying connective compartment, since digitation occurs through the apoptosis of interdigital connective tissue (Basset et al, 1990). However, it should be noticed that close to the regression of the connective tissue, epithelial compartment has to extend dramatically to cover newly formed digits. In human carcinomas, ST3 is predominantly located in peritumoral fibroblasts with a decreasing gradient from the fibroblasts more proximal to the malignant cells to those located more distally which are ST3 negative (Basset et al, 1990).

Other MMPs are often co-expressed with ST3, but in different areas or by different cell types. Thus, several MMPs are released within the growth cone of commissural axons in order to generate extracellular spaces as they cross the floor plate that expresses ST3 (Lefebvre et al, 1995). In tadpole tissue resorption, both collagenase-3 (MMP13) and ST3 are extensively co-expressed. However, their spatial patterns are totally distinct and delineate 2 separate tissue-specific resorption programs (Berry et al, 1998). At the time of ovulation, proteolytic degradation of the follicular wall is required. In gonadotropin-induced ovulation in mice, ST3 has a distinct expression pattern since it is expressed by the granulosa cells of small and middle-size follicles, but not in the large preovulatory follicles expressing other MMPs, suggesting that ST3 is not involved in the follicle rupture (Hagglund et al, 1999). Finally, in human carcinomas, although the majority of expressed MMPs are fibroblastic, some of them may be observed in other cell types. Thus, matrilysin and stromelysin-2 (MMP10) are known to be expressed by cancer cells, and gelatinase B (MMP9) may be expressed by either fibroblastic, inflammatory or cancer cells (Noël et al, 1997).

Thus, in both normal and pathological events, cells expressing ST3 are usually of mesenchymal origin and most often they are fibroblasts. Moreover, ST3 expression is restricted to a fibroblast sub-population located at the vicinity of 'stressed' or malignant epithelial cells, notably when the integrity of the basement membrane, which separates epithelial cell com-partments from mesenchymal cells, is compromised, leading to normally 'illegitimate' epithe-lial/stromal cell communications and/or contacts. This highly precise ST3 location, suggests a drastic regulation of the ST3 gene *in vivo*, and a spatially restricted ST3 function. In this context, ST3 could help regulate the availability of proteins locally sequestered as inactive molecules in the extracellular matrix in order to act on surrounding epithelial cells.

7. ST3 EXHIBITS A SPECIFIC TEMPORAL EXPRESSION PATTERN

Besides its specific spatial pattern of expression, ST3 also exhibits a strict temporal expression pattern. In late murine placentation, expression of gelati-nase-A (MMP2) and TIMP1 is observed at 10.5 to 13.5 days post-coitum and decreases after (gelatinase-A) or remains constant (TIMP1), whereas ST3, TIMP2 and TIMP3 are only seen at 16.5 days. Thus, there is a very precise temporal regulation of the MMPs and inhibitors in the area of fetomaternal interfaces (Teesalu et al, 1999). Similarly, rat cutaneous wounding experiments show that from day 1 to 14 after incision, among the 6 MMPs expressed, ST3 is the most time restricted one. Its expression starts at day 5 whereas high levels of mRNA of stromelysin-1, gelatinase-B and collagenase-3 (MMP13) were already observed at day 1 and those of MT1-MMP and gelatinase-A at day 3 (Okada et al, 1997). In Xenopus, ST3 is likely to play a role in ECM remod-eling that facilitates apoptotic tissue remodeling or resorption, whereas colla-genase-3 and collagenase-4 (MMP18) appear to participate in earlier connective tissue degradation during development (Damjanovski et al, 2000). Accordingly,

ST3 is absent in intestinal explants from premetamorphic tadpoles cultured in the absence of thyroid hormone or at the onset of thyroid hormone treatment. After 3 days of treatment, ST3 was expressed in the fibroblasts underneath the larval epithelium that had begun the degeneration process, suggesting that ST3 favors adult epithelial morphogenesis ((Ishizuya-Oka et al, 2000). Finally, it has been shown *in vitro* that endometrial cells grown in culture medium supplemented with endometrial cytokines express first gelatinase-B, then interstitial collagenase and finally ST3 (Singer et al, 1999).

Few data are available concerning the precise relative order of MMP expression during carcinogenesis. It is likely that ST3 expression in human carcinomas occurs as a rather late event in the multistep process of carcinogenesis. This is consistent with the fact that high ST3 levels are observed in invasive tumors and has been associated with tumor invasion, constituting therefore, when observed in in situ carcinomas, a useful marker of an imminent progression to invasive cancer (Wolf et al, 1993; Munck-Wikland et al, 1998).

Thus, in normal and pathological conditions, the same tissue or cell type may express several MMPs during tissue remodeling, but the timing of their expression may dramatically differ. In these processes, ST3 is expressed later than most of the other co-expressed MMPs. This indicates that it is not involved in the initiation of the basement membrane breakdown and subsequent epithelial cell apoptosis, but later on, in downstream tissue remodeling events, at the time the connective compartment is transiently permissive for incoming epithelial cells. The fact that ST3 function is independent of the presence of additive extracellular proteinases since it is secreted directly under active form is consistant with such a local and punctuate function.

8. ST3 IS A KEY PLAYER IN TISSUE REMODELING PROCESSES, AT LEAST IN MALIGNANCY

Does ST3 actively participate in tissue remodeling processes? In order to address this question, several transgenic animal models were developed. No obvious phenotypes were observed in mice ectopically expressing ST3 in the mammary gland (WAP-ST3 mice), in fibroblastic cells (Vimentine-ST3 mice), or ubiquitously (CMV-ST3 mice), even during experimentally induced tissue remodeling processes (our unpublished results). In a similar manner, ST3-null mice were fertile and did not exhibit obvious alterations in appearance and behavior. Moreover, experimentally wounded skin and bone of ST3-null mice repair normally thereby suggesting the existence of com-pensatory/redundant mechanisms (Masson et al, 1998). Urokinase-type plasminogen activator (uPA) that exhibits a very similar expression pattern was proposed to play this role.

However this hypothesis is inaccurate since mice doubly deficient for ST3 and uPA are viable and fertile (Teesalu et al, 1999).

Comparison of developed tumors after subcutaneous injections to immuno-depressed nude mice of cancer cells transfected with sense or antisense ST3 cDNA to either express ST3 (i.e., in human MCF7 breast cancer cells) or inhibit constitutive ST3 expression (i.e. in mouse NIH-3T3 transformed cells), showed that ST3 expression by injected cancer cells is always correlated with a more rapid tumor appearance and higher tumor incidence and sizes (Noël et al, 1996). Moreover, since in human carcinomas ST3 is expressed by tumor stromal cells and not by the cancer cells themselves, another type of experimental tumors taken into account the ST3 status of connective tissue was designed to mimic human tumor development. Thus, the lack of ST3 in ST3-null mice resulted in a decreased DMBA- (Masson et al, 1998) or ras oncogene-induced tumori-genesis (our unpublished results). Thus, chemical or genetic *in vivo* transfor-mation of epithelial cells gave similar results indicating that ST3 is essential for optimal tumor development, and that it was not compensated for in ST3-null mice in malignant conditions. Finally, primary culture of fibroblasts were established from either wild type or ST3-null embryos. As expected from the previous *in vivo* data, ST3-null fibroblasts lost the capacity to promote implantation of MCF7 human malignant epithelial cells in nude mice (Masson et al, 1998).

Tumors that are obtained by sub-cutaneous injection of malignant cells should be regarded as a model for processes occurring during local invasion of primary tumors, with the exception of the steps of basement membrane effraction needed for in situ tumors to become invasive, since they are completely shunted by the injection of cancer cells directly into the connective tissue. Tumor devel-opment is therefore dependent upon the cell's capability to survive in host tissues, either on their own, or by the recruitment of required factors from their connective vicinity. In that context, in tumor models, ST3 represents a local stromal factor contributing to the survival and implantation of cancer cells. It appears reasonable to believe that, similarly, in human carcinomas, ST3 that is mainly produced and secreted by fibroblastic cells located in the vicinity of invasive cancer cells, acts as a paracrine factor contributing to cancer cell survival outside of their compartment of origin.

Thus, independently of the nature of the hits leading to epithelial cell trans-formation, tumorigenicity was always higher in wild type animals, indicating that ST3 is actually a key player during tissue remodeling processes occurring under malignant conditions. Together, these results show that ST3 is a stromal factor favoring the starting life of cancer cells in an aberrant cell environment, a process that occurs notably during local invasion when cancer cells reach adjacent connective tissues. A role for ST3 in favoring cell survival and tumor implantation, is consistent with observations that high ST3 expression levels were associated with metastatic propensity in human carcinomas.

9. ST3 FUNCTION IN TUMOR DEVELOPMENT REQUIRES A A FUNCTIONAL ST3 CATALYTIC DOMAIN AND ECM-ASSOCIATED FACTOR(S)

Since ST3 belongs to the MMP family, it was hypothesized that its capacity to enhance tumorigenesis *in vivo* may be dependent on its proteolytic activity. To test that possibility, MCF7 cells transfected with either wild type or the mutated catalytic domain of ST3 were sub-cutaneously implanted in nude mice. The ST3 mutation corresponded to the substitution of the active site glutamate of human and mouse ST3 with alanine by site-directed mutagenesis. These mutants are inactive against α_1PI *in vitro* (Noël et al, 1995). In a second set of experiments, a physiological inhibitor of MMPs was locally produced by infection of MCF7 cells with a retroviral vector bearing TIMP2 before their subcutaneous implantation in nude mice. Whatever the tumorigenesis model, human and mouse ST3 promotes tumor development only when the ST3 catalytic domain is functional, and in the absence of TIMP2. These results demonstrate that the function of ST3 in tumorigenesis is mediated through its enzymatic activity (Noël et al, 2000).

Since ST3 is devoid of catalytic activity against the major ECM components, it was checked if extracellular matrix (ECM)-associated molecules are required for ST3 function during tumorigenesis. MCF7 cells were therefore co-injected with wild type fibroblasts in the presence of either complete or depleted matrigel. The capacity to promote tumorigenesis was lost in presence of depleted matrix, as in presence of ST3-null fibroblasts (Masson et al, 1998; Noël et al, 2000). Thus, the most efficient tumor model mimicking human invasive carcinomas was reconstituted by associating complete matrigel to either cancer cells expressing ST3, or cancer cells devoid of ST3 expression but in the presence of wild type fibroblasts.

Thus, since, in human carcinomas, ST3 is expressed by fibroblasts located in the vicinity of cancer cells, ST3 function in tumor progression should require at least 3 partners: transformed epithelial cells, fibroblastic cells and ECM. Furthermore, the effect of ST3 is dependent on the functionality of its catalytic domain, and it may be hypothesized that ST3 substrates may be molecules associated with the ECM or minor ECM components or fragments.

10. ST3 ACTS AS AN ANTI-APOPTOTIC FACTOR IN MALIGNANT CONDITIONS

Tissue remodeling results from the successive and/or concomittent occurrence of numerous processes including protein degradation and deposition, epithelial cell proliferation, differentiation, migration and death, tissue neoangiogenesis, inflammatory and immune reaction. Besides their ability to digest ECM components, MMPs have been shown to favor neoangiogenesis and subsequent epithelial cell proliferation, to increase cell invasive capacity, and to exert pro-apoptotic function (Birkedal-Hansen, 1995; Coussens and Werb, 1996; Blasi, 1999; Noël et al, 1997), and similar functions were expected for ST3. However, ST3 is unable to increase cancer cell motility, invasive properties or proliferation (Masson et al, 1998; Noël et al, 1996; Boulay et al, 2001) in either *in vitro* co-culture and organoid assays, or in *in vivo* tumorigenesis models. These results are consistent with the absence of phenotype in transgenic mice over-expressing ST3, as is observed for some other MMPs. For exemple, stromelysin-1 overexpression in mammary gland leads to early budding and progression into mammary tumors (Lochter et al, 1997).

In all tumor models tested, palpable tumors developping in the presence or absence of ST3 were devoid of obvious histological differences, suggesting that ST3 may act early, before tumors became palpable. Studies were then performed using another tumor model that permits localization and analysis of nonpalpable microcarcinomas and has the advantage to use immuno-competent animals. This model consists of sub-cutaneous injections of syngeneic cancer cells in either wild type or ST3-null mice. Surprisingly very small tumors (< 0.40 mm^3) developping in ST3-null mice exhibited significantly higher number of vessels, indicating that ST3 is not a pro-angiogenic factor, and even suggesting that it may rather be a down-modulator of neoangiogenesis and/or vessel co-option (Boulay et al, 2001). Interestingly, a possible anti-angiogenic function has already been proposed for MMPs since the metalloelastase (MMP12) is able to process angiostatin (an inhibitor of angiogenesis) from plasminogen (Moses, 1997). Moreover, the ST3-null nonpalpable syngeneic tumors, although well vascularized, showed intense necrosis and PMN infiltration suggesting that ST3 might have a function related to cancer cell death and/or inflammatory processes. Accordingly, an increased number of apoptotic cancer cells was distributed throughout the ST3-null nonpalpable tumors, indicating that the lack of host ST3 leads to increased cancer cell apoptosis (Boulay et al, 2001). In this context, we note that mouse TIMP3, in contrast to TIMP1 and TIMP2 which exhibit anti-apoptotic features, promotes smooth muscle cell apoptosis (Baker et al, 1998). That ST3 might act at the opposite of other MMPs is not so surprising in regard to its specific features and spatio-temporal expression pattern.

In normal conditions, detached and misplaced epithelial cells, that are deprived of the specific signals required for their survival, die, leading to a correct tissue homeostasis. This apoptotic phenomenon referred to as anoïkis occurs at the time of alteration of the interaction between epithelial cells and their connective environment (i.e. tissue wounding) (Raff, 1992; Meredith et al, 1993; Frisch and Francis, 1994). However, in carcinomas during invasive processes, epithelial cells become refractory to extracellular apoptosis regulatory signals, and malignant epithelial cells survive in aberrant cell compartments. Acquisition of anchorage-independent growth during transformation would require that anoikis is abrogated, suggesting the existence of signals that inhibit cell death. Cancerous cells are more resistant to detachment-induced apoptosis in ST3 wild type than in ST3-null mice suggesting that ST3 is a stromal factor with anti-anoikis property (Figure 1). In this context, ST3 may help epithelial cells to circumvent homeostatic mechanisms and survive in an unusual and hostile environment. This is in agreement with the fact that ST3 is highly expressed by the invasive human carcinomas characterized by mixed epithelial and stromal cells, and that ST3 expression is significantly associated with poor patient outcome.

Thus, although essential for optimum tumor development, ST3 does not share any function with the other MMPs involved in malignant processes. ST3 is not able to digest any major ECM component, it does not modify epithelial cell proliferation nor motility, and it does not appear to be a pro-angiogenic or a pro-apoptotic factor. On the contrary, ST3 exhibits anti-apoptotic function, a new activity for a MMP.

11. ST3, A KEY REGULATOR OF EPITHELIUM HOMEOSTASIS?

Does ST3 exert a similar inhibitory function on apoptosis in normal conditions? Once the tissues have risen to their adult status, their size should remain constant, and epithelium homeostasis has been shown to require equilibrium between epithelial cells, stromal cells (fibroblasts, endothelial cells, inflammatory and immune cells) and the ECM. However, many life events lead to transient epithelial modification, and ST3 has been shown to be specifically expressed during these events (i.e., post-weaning mammary gland and post-partum uterus involution, wound healing), whereas the gene is silent in resting tissues (Rio et al, 1996). As during malignancy, normal tissue remodeling involves basement membrane alteration and the conversion of polarized epithelial cells to temporally invasive and/or mobile states, leading to transient epithelial/stromal communication or contacts.

Although a correlation can be drawn between ST3 expression and intense

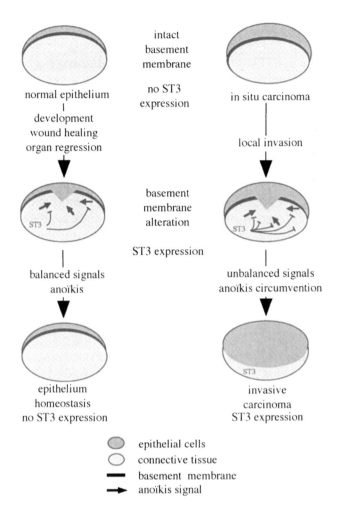

intact
basement
membrane

no ST3
expression

normal epithelium
|
development
wound healing
organ regression

in situ carcinoma

local invasion

basement
membrane
alteration

ST3 expression

balanced signals
anoïkis

unbalanced signals
anoïkis circumvention

epithelium
homeostasis
no ST3 expression

invasive
carcinoma
ST3 expression

epithelial cells
connective tissue
basement membrane
anoïkis signal

Figure 1. ST3 anti-apoptotic function in normal and malignant conditions. ST3 may prevent anoikis signals. Correct balance between ST3 and anoikis signals leads to correct tissue homeostasis, whereas in the presence of intense ST3 signals, anoikis is circumvented and tumors develop.

apoptosis during normal tissue remodeling processes, several data indicate that ST3 do not induce cell death nor act during the early steps of apoptosis. For example, in the post-weaning mouse mammary gland, ST3 starts to be expressed after the observation of early remodeling, and it continues to be present after acini breakdown, suggesting that it should be active during particular process(es) occurring during and after apoptosis itself. In this context, it has been shown that, subsequent to intense cell death, some epithelial cells survive, presumably through anti-apoptotic signals permitting them to escape cell death and to reconstitute new tissues (Raff et al, 1993). It is tempting to speculate that ST3 exerts such a function (Figure 1). Consistently, anoikis has been shown to play a role in governing epithelial cell survival after injury and in the maintenance of normal epithelium integrity (Raff, 1992; Meredith et al, 1993; Frisch and Francis, 1994).

Thus, in normal conditions, ST3 may transiently preserve the viability of regenerating cells during intense apoptotic processes occurring during tissue remodeling, and participate in the regulation of homeostasis of epithelial cell compartment. Corroborating this hypothesis, dermatofibromas that are the only benign tumors expressing high levels of ST3, show altered homeostasis since they are frequently accompanied by epithelial hyperplasia and annexogenesis (Unden et al, 1996; Thewes et al, 1999). Thus, during malignant invasive processes, epithelial cells may use ST3 to circumvent tissue homeostasis and anarchically proliferate.

12. NATURE OF THE ST3 EXPRESSION INDUCER(S)?

In vivo, ST3 expression is strictly regulated by the occurrence of remodeling process, suggesting that ST3 gene expression may result either from transient contact between cells of the epithelial and stromal compartments, from the action of a soluble factor specifically expressed at this time (i.e. growth factors, cytokines) or from the action of ECM degradation product(s) released during the early steps of tissue remodeling (i.e. basement membrane associated growth factors, fragments of ECM components). We note that a few in situ carcinomas have been shown to focally express ST3. Although it is assumed that the basement membrane integrity is conserved in these tumors, the presence of minor alterations cannot be excluded. Consistently, ST3 expressing in situ tumors have been associated with worse patient outcome (Wolf et al, 1993; Munck-Wikland et al, 1998). Electron microscopy examination remains to be performed to address this question.

In vitro, several factors have been tested for the induction of ST3 in normal fibroblasts of various origins. Basic fibroblastic growth factor (bFGF) and platelet-derived growth factor (PDGF) induce ST3 expression in normal human fetal and adult pulmonary fibroblasts. This induction is totally inhibited by all trans retinoic acid, a commonly used chemopreventive agent for aerodigestive tract malignancies (Anderson et al, 1995). bFGF modulates ST3 in the osteoblast cell line MC3T3 by controlling the stability of ST3 messenger RNA as well as increasing its transcriptional rate (Delany et al, 1998). In primary cultures of human endometrial fibroblasts, ST3 is selectively induced by insulin growth factor II (IGFII), epidermal growth factor (EGF), PDGF-BB, tumor necrosis factor alpha (TNFα) and interleukin1 alpha (IL1α) (Singer et al, 1999). Finally, the CD40 ligand, an inflammatory mediator localized in atheroma, induces ST3 expression in endothelial cells, smooth muscle cells and macrophages (Schonbeck et al, 1999).

In vivo, a statistical correlation ($P < 0.003$) was reported between bFGF and ST3 expression in the stromal compartment of breast carcinomas (Linder et al, 1998). Animals deficient for both RARb and RARg show a decrease of ST3 expression indicating that retinoic acid is responsible, at least partially, for *in vivo* induction of ST3. Similarly, xenopus ST3 can be induced by thyroid hormone *in vivo*. Interestingly, in mammals and xenopus, ST3 is expressed during limb bud development, a phenomenom dependent on retinoic acid in mammals (Dupe et al, 1999), and on thyroid hormone in xenopus (Li et al, 1998).

Numerous cancer/stroma cell co-culture models have been developed to test the efficiency of cell/cell contact to initiate ST3 expression, but most of them have been unsuccessful (our unpublished results). Certain breast cancer cells were shown to up-regulate reporter genes under the transcriptional control of a 3.4kb human 5′ flanking sequence of ST3 via a diffusible factor or a cell/cell contact mechanism (Ahmad et al, 1997). More recently, it has been shown that non-small cell lung cancer epithelial cells stimulate normal pulmonary fibroblasts to express and secrete ST3, suggesting that the organ origin of both cell types may be crucial to efficiently induce ST3 in a co-culture model. At the same time, release of extracellular bFGF was observed (Mari et al, 1998).

Thus *in vitro*, both soluble factors and cell/cell contact allow for the expression of ST3. However, besides retinoic acid and thyroid hormone, the nature of *in vivo* inducers involved in the tissue-specific ST3 expression remains to be established.

13. NATURE OF THE ST3 SIGNALING PATHWAY?

It is most likely that to exert its anti-apoptotic function, ST3 does not act directly (i.e. existence of specific ST3 receptors?) but indirectly, and should therefore interact with molecule(s) involved in pathways of programmed cell death. Although the number and nature of ST3 target(s) remain to be determined, several scenarios can be proposed for mediating ST3 function (Figure 2).

ST3 may regulate proteinase towards ECM. Thus, ST3 is able to cleave several proteinase inhibitors, namely the plasma $\alpha_2 M$, and the $\alpha_1 PI$ and alpha$_2$-antiplasmin ($\alpha_2 AP$) serine proteinase inhibitors (serpins) (Pei et al, 1994). $\alpha_1 PI$ is a membrane-bound antiproteinase, and its cleavage by ST3 can inactivate it and permit proteinase activity. Interestingly, $\alpha_1 PI$ is secreted by breast cancer

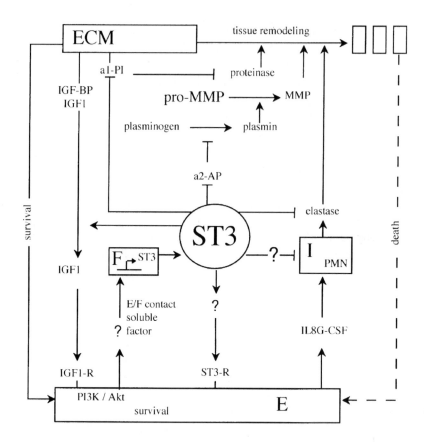

Figure 2. Putative pathways mediating the ST3 anti-apoptotic function.

cells and is present at the ECM. It may represent therefore a potential physiologic target of ST3 during ECM remodeling. ST3 also degrades α_2AP, prompting speculation that ST3 may indirectly increase local plasmin levels and promote plasmin-mediated conversion of additional pro-MMPs to their active forms in carcinomas. However, in these cases, the final effect will be increased apoptosis, which is contradictory with the observed anti-apoptotic ST3 function. In this context, we note that serpins are not ST3 specific substrates since they are also cleaved by other MMPs such as the interstitial collagenase and stromelysin-1. That ST3 cleaves serpins *in vivo*, and is the predominant regulator of serpin function at the tumor/stroma interface remain to be shown. However, ST3 has been shown to inhibit leukocytes/neutrophil elastase, a tissue-destructive proteinase released by neutrophils and monocytes (Schonbeck et al, 1999). This ST3 activity might lead to decreased ECM degradation and therefore contribute to the ST3 survival function.

ST3 can also mediate its function through down-regulation of the inflammatory tissue reaction. In fact, massive PMN tissue infiltration was observed in both vascular repair processes (Lijnen et al, 1999) and tumorigeneses (Boulay et al, 2001) in ST3-null but not in ST3 wild type mice. In tumor models, this infiltration can correspond to a tumor-induced non-specific inflammatory reaction due to the elevated number of dying cells. However, this phenomenom could also be ascribed to an increased availability of neutrophil-triggered factors such as interleukin-8 (IL8) (Gura, 1996) or granulocyte colony-stimulating factor (G-CSF) that have been shown to be ectopically expressed in some human malignant tumors. Interestingly, it has been reported that the anti-tumoral effect of G-CSF was mediated by recruitment and targeting of neutrophilic granulocytes to G-CSF-releasing tumor cells (Colombo et al, 1991). In this context, one of the functions of ST3 may be to inhibit the expression and/or activation of molecule(s) with chemoattractant properties for inflammatory cells. In this case, this would be a new link between MMPs and inflammatory reaction.

IGF-I would be another possible mediator. Like ST3, IGF-I is expressed in most tissues during embryogenesis, predominantly by cells of mesenchymal origin. It is present throughout the ECM, almost entirely bound to IGF binding proteins (IGF-BPs), constituting a pool of material available in stress conditions. Cleavage of IGF-BPs leads to the release of active IGF-I available for specific receptors (IGF-R) that are widely expressed. IGF-1 is a cell survival factor which activates the PI3K and Akt signaling pathway (Jones and Clemmons, 1995). Moreover, it has been reported that IGF-I can inhibit malignant cell apoptosis in a paracrine manner, and that it prevents ECM-induced apoptosis of mammary epithelial cells (Farrelly et al, 1999). Since *in vivo* ST3 function is dependent on factor(s) linked to the ECM (Masson et al, 1998), and since the ECM-linked IGF-BP1 is a substrate of ST3 (Manes et al, 1997) it is tempting to speculate that ST3 may inhibit epithelial cell apoptosis through regulating IGF-I bioavailability by proteolizing IGF-BPs. Finally, ST3 function may also be mediated through IGF-BP fragment(s) that can have IGF-independent cellular effects (Jones and Clemmons, 1995).

Thus, to date, available clues indicate that ST3 may either control proteinase activity, survival factor bioavailablity, or inflammatory reaction to favor cell survival in an environment initially not permissive for epithelial cell growth. However, it may be hypothesized that, besides proteinases, proteinase inhibitors, and IGF-BPs, ST3 may hydrolyze as yet uncharacterized specific substrate(s), and therefore act via other mechanism(s).

14. CLINICAL RELEVANCE OF ANTI-ST3 DRUG(S)

Together, these data give evidence that ST3 promotes tumorigenesis in a paracrine manner by favoring the homing and survival of malignant epithelial cells in connective tissues through anti-apoptotic function. Inhibition of apoptosis is an important feature of human neoplasia, potentially contributing to tumor progression and resistance to therapy (Thompson, 1995; Strasser, 1999). In this context, anti-ST3 treatments that may restore the ability to properly regulate cancer cell apoptosis could be of considerable benefit to the treatment of malignancies.

Most synthetic MMP inhibitors tested so far in clinical trials possess a zinc-binding function attached to a pseudo-peptide framework which binds to the primed regions of the enzyme catalytic site (Goss et al, 1998; Macaulay et al, 1999). The main problem concerns their specificity, and the occurrence of side effects (Tierney et al, 1999; Foda et al, 1999; Drummond et al, 1999). A new class of peptidic inhibitors was recently designed which contains a phosphinic group that mimics the substrate at the transition state (Cuniasse et al, 1995; Vassiliou et al, 1999). A strict binding stereoactivity and an absence of *in vivo* metabolism would be expected for these compounds (Dive et al, 1999). Preliminary results showed *in vitro* drug efficiency and *in vivo* decreased tumorigenicity (our unpublished results). The nature and the number of MMP(s) targeted *in vivo* by this new class of inhibitors remain to be established.

To design specific and potent ST3 inhibitors, the crystallographic structure of the mouse ST3 catalytic domain (Kannan et al, 1999) complexed to a phosphinic inhibitor was resolved (Gall et al, 2001). As observed for the already known structures of MMPs, the catalytic domain of ST3, is made up of 5-stranded beta-sheets and 3 alpha helices, and is a charged negatively globular protein containing several pockets. The major differences between MMPs lie in the S1′ subsite, a well defined hydrophobic pocket of variable depth depending on the nature of the amino acid at position 215. This amino acid is a leucine in gelatinase-A, collagenase-3, stromelysin-1 and MT1-MMP, a tyrosine in matrilysin and an arginine in collagenase-1. It has been shown *in vitro* that the S1′ pocket is crucial for the specificity of the enzymatic activity of MMPs. The S1′ ST3 pocket is larger than the corresponding one of the other MMPs due to the presence of a glutamine at position 215, leading to a very deep cavity allowing presumably the processing of larger substrate(s) (Gall et al, 2001; Holtz et al, 1999). Therefore synthetic substrates containing unusually long side chains in their P1′ positions were designed and tested on a panel of MMPs. Surprisingly, ST3 and MT1-MMP cleave these substrates more efficently than those containing the normal amino acids. This suggests that, *in vivo*, ST3 may also hydrolyze natural proteins containing long side chains, notably proteins undergoing post-translational modification (Mucha et al, 1998).

Thus, this characteristic of the ST3 protein structure should allow to design synthetic inhibitors exhibiting a longer chain in their P1′ position leading to a higher specificity against ST3 than other MMPs. ST3 therefore represents an appropriate target for specific inhibitor(s) in future cytostatic therapeutical approaches directed against the stromal compartment of human carcinomas.

15. CONCLUSION

Although numerous hypotheses remain to be addressed, several milestones can actually be drawn in the field of ST3: (a) ST3 acts at epithelial/stromal interfaces of remodeling tissues; (b) ST3 is involved in epithelium homeostasis; (c) malignant cancer cells subvert ST3 function in order to circumvent homeostasis and survive in connective host tissues; (d) ST3 is a peculiar MMP since it is the first found to exert anti-apoptotic function; (e) during cancer progression, MMPs can exert a dual effect, some MMPs leading to ECM-induced apoptosis, while others such as ST3 inhibit this ECM-induced apoptosis.

Thus, the future challenges in the study of ST3 will be: (a) to search for *in vivo* inducer(s) of ST3 expression; (b) to identify the *in vivo* substrate(s) of ST3; (c) to determine the direct or indirect mechanism(s) underlying the ST3 function; (d) to study the possible relationship between ST3 and tissue neoangiogenesis; (e) to study the possible relationship between ST3 and inflammatory tumor reaction; (f) to obtain highly specific and potent ST3 inhibitors.

ACKNOWLEDGMENTS

I would like to thank all my colleagues and collaborators who have participated to this work, and most notably Paul Basset who has initiated the ST3 research field 10 years ago. This work was supported by funds from the Institut National de la Santé et de la Recherche Médicale, the Centre National de la Recherche Scientifique, the Hôpital Universitaire de Strasbourg, the Bristol-Myers Squibb Pharmaceutical Research Institute, the Association pour la Recherche sur le Cancer, the Fondation de France, and the Ligue Nationale Française contre le Cancer and the Comités du Haut-Rhin et du Bas-Rhin (équipe labellisée).

REFERENCES

Ahmad A, Hanby A, Dublin E, Poulsom R, Smith P, Barnes D, Rubens R, Anglard P, Hart I. Stromelysin 3: an independent prognostic factor for relapse-free survival in node-positive breast cancer and demonstration of novel breast carcinoma cell expression. Am J Pathol 1998; 152: 721–728.

Ahmad A, Marshall JF, Basset P, Anglard P, Hart, IR. Modulation of human stromelysin 3 promoter activity and gene expression by human breast cancer cells. Int J Cancer 1997; 73: 290–296.

Anderson IC, Sugarbaker DJ, Ganju RK, Tsarwhas DG, Richards WG, Sunday M, Kobzik L, Shipp MA. Stromelysin-3 is overexpressed by stromal elements in primary non-small cell lung cancers and regulated by retinoic acid in pulmonary fibroblasts. Cancer Res 1995; 55: 4120–4126.

Baker AH, Zaltsman AB, George SJ, Newby AC. Divergent effects of tissue inhibitor of metal-loproteinase-1, -2, or -3 overexpression on rat vascular smooth muscle cell invasion, prolif-eration, and death in vitro. TIMP-3 promotes apoptosis. J Clin Invest 1998; 101: 1478–1487.

Barbacid MM, Fernandez-Resa P, Buesa JM, Marquez G, Aracil M, Mira E. Expression and purification of human stromelysin 1 and 3 from baculovirus-infected insect cells. Protein Expr Purif 1998; 13: 243–250.

Basset P, Bellocq J. P, Lefebvre O, Noël A, Chenard M. P, Wolf C, Anglard P, Rio MC. Stromelysin-3: a paradigm for stroma-derived factors implicated in carcinoma progression. Crit Rev Oncol Hematol 1997; 26: 43–53.

Basset P, Bellocq JP, Wolf C, Stoll I, Hutin P, Limacher JM, Podhajcer OL, Chenard MP, Rio MC, Chambon P. A novel metallo-proteinase gene specifically expressed in stromal cells of breast carcinomas. Nature 1990; 348: 699–704.

Basset P, Wolf C, Chambon P. Expression of the stromelysin-3 gene in fibroblastic cells of invasive carcinomas of the breast and other human tissues: a review. Breast Cancer Res Treat 1993; 24: 185–193

Bassi DE, Mahloogi H, Klein-Szanto AJ. The proprotein convertases furin and PACE4 play a significant role in tumor progression. Mol Carcinog 2000; 28: 63–69.

Berry DL, Rose CS, Remo BF, Brown DD. The expression pattern of thyroid hormone response genes in remodeling tadpole tissues defines distinct growth and resorption gene expression programs. Dev Biol 1998; 203: 24–35.

Birkedal-Hansen H. Proteolytic remodeling of extracellular matrix. Curr Opin Cell Biol 1995; 7: 728–735.

Blasi F and Stoppelli MP. Proteases and cancer invasion: from belief to certainty. AACR meeting on proteases and protease inhibitors in cancer, Nyborg, Denmark, 14–18 June 1998. Biochim Biophys Acta 2000; 1423: R35–44.

Boulay A, Masson R, Chenard MP, El Fahime M, Cassard L, Bellocq JP, Sautès-Fridman C, Basset P, Rio MC. High cancer cell death in syngeneic tumors developed in host mice deficient for the stromelysin-3 matrix metalloproteinase. Cancer Res 2001; 61: 2189–2193.

Chenard MP, O'Siorain L, Shering S, Rouyer N, Lutz Y, Wolf C, Basset P, Bellocq JP, Duffy MJ. High levels of stromelysin-3 correlate with poor prognosis in patients with breast carcinoma. Int J Cancer 1996; 69: 448–451.

Colombo MP, Ferrari G, Stoppacciaro A, Parenza M, Rodolfo M, Mavilio F, Parmiani G. Granulocyte colony-stimulating factor gene transfer suppresses tumorigenicity of a murine adenocarcinoma in vivo. J Exp Med 1991; 173: 889–897.

Coussens LM, Werb Z. Matrix metalloproteinases and the development of cancer. Chem Biol 1996; 3: 895–904.

Cuniasse P, Raynal I, Lecoq A, Yiotakis A, Dive V. Three-dimensional structure of cyclohexa-peptides containing a phosphinic bond in aqueous solution: a template for zinc metalloprotease inhibitors. A NMR and restrained molecular dynamics study. J Med Chem 1995; 38: 553–564.

Damjanovski S, Puzianowska-Kuznicka M, Ishuzuya-Oka A, Shi YB. Differential regulation of three thyroid hormone-responsive matrix metalloproteinase genes implicates distinct functions during frog embryogenesis. FASEB J 2000; 14: 503–510.

Delany AM, Canalis E. Dual regulation of stromelysin-3 by fibroblast growth factor-2 in murine osteoblasts. J Biol Chem 1998; 273: 16595–16600.

Delebecq TJ, Porte H, Zerimech F, Copin MC, Gouyer V, Dacquembronne E, Balduyck M, Wurtz A, Huet G. Overexpression level of stromelysin 3 is related to the lymph node involvement in non-small cell lung cancer. Clin Cancer Res 2000; 6: 1086–1092.

Dive V, Cotton J, Yiotakis A, Michaud A, Vassiliou S, Jiracek J, Vazeux G, Chauvet MT, Cuniasse P, Corvol P. RXP 407, a phosphinic peptide, is a potent inhibitor of angiotensin I converting enzyme able to differentiate between its two active sites. Proc Natl Acad Sci (USA) 1999; 96: 4330–4335.

Doyle GA, Pierce RA, Parks WC. Transcriptional induction of collagenase-1 in differentiated monocyte-like (U937) cells is regulated by AP-1 and an upstream C/EBP-beta site. J Biol Chem 1997; 272: 11840–11849.

Drummond AH, Beckett P, Brown PD, Bone EA, Davidson AH, Galloway WA, Gearing AJ, Huxley P, Laber D, McCourt M, Whittaker M, Wood LM, Wright A. Preclinical and clinical studies of MMP inhibitors in cancer. Ann NY Acad Sci 1999; 878: 228–235.

Dupe V, Ghyselinck NB, Thomazy V, Nagy L, Davies PJ, Chambon P, Mark M. Essential roles of retinoic acid signaling in interdigital apoptosis and control of MMP-7 expression in mouse autopods. Dev Biol 1999; 208: 30–43.

Farrelly N, Lee YJ, Oliver J, Dive C, Streuli CH. Extracellular matrix regulates apoptosis in mammary epithelium through a control on insulin signaling. J Cell Biol 1999; 144: 1337–1348.

Foda HD, Rollo EE, Brown P, Pakbaz H, Berisha H, Said SI, Zucker S. Attenuation of oxidant-induced lung injury by the synthetic matrix metalloproteinase inhibitor BB-3103. Ann NY Acad Sci 1999; 878: 650–653.

Frisch SM, Francis H. Disruption of epithelial cell-matrix interactions induces apoptosis. J Cell Biol 1994; 124: 619–626.

Gall AL, Ruff M, Kannan R, Cuniasse P, Dive V, Rio MC, Basset P, Moras D. Crystal structure of the stromelysin-3 (MMP11) catalytic domain complexed with a phosphinic inhibitor mim-icking the transition-state. J Mol Biol 2001; 307: 577–586.

Goss KJ, Brown PD, Matrisian LM. Differing effects of endogenous and synthetic inhibitors of metalloproteinases on intestinal tumorigenesis. Int J Cancer 1998; 78: 629–635.

Gura T. Chemokines take center stage in inflammatory ills. Science 1996; 272: 954–956.

Hagglund AC, Ny A, Leonardsson G, Ny T. Regulation and localization of matrix metallo-proteinases and tissue inhibitors of metalloproteinases in the mouse ovary during gonadotropin-induced ovulation. Endocrinology 1999; 140: 4351–4358.

Holtz B, Cuniasse P, Boulay A, Kannan R, Mucha A, Beau F, Basset P, Dive V. Role of the S1′ subsite glutamine 215 in activity and specificity of stromelysin-3 by site-directed mutagen-esis. Biochemistry 1999; 38: 12174–12179.

Hubbard FC, Goodrow TL, Liu SC, Brilliant MH, Basset P, Mains RE, Klein-Szanto AJ. Expression of PACE4 in chemically induced carcinomas is associated with spindle cell tumor conversion and increased invasive ability. Cancer Res 1997; 57: 5226–5231.

Ishizuya-Oka A, Li Q, Amano T, Damjanovski S, Ueda S, Shi YB. Requirement for matrix metallo-proteinase stromelysin-3 in cell migration and apoptosis during tissue remodeling in Xenopus laevis. J Cell Biol 2000; 150: 1177–1188.

Itoh T, Ikeda T, Gomi H, Nakao S, Suzuki T, Itohara S. Unaltered secretion of beta-amyloid precursor protein in gelatinase A (matrix metalloproteinase 2)-deficient mice. J Biol Chem 1997; 272: 22389–22392.

Jones JI, Clemmons DR. Insulin-like growth factors and their binding proteins: biological actions. Endocr Rev 1995; 16: 3–34.

Kannan R, Ruff M, Kochins JG, Manly S, Stoll I, El Fahime M, Noël A, Foidart JM, Rio MC, Basset P. Purification of active matrix metalloproteinase catalytic domains and its use for screening of specific stromelysin-3 inhibitors. Prot Expres Purif 1999; 16: 76–83.

Konttinen YT, Ainola M, Valleala H, Ma J, Ida H, Mandelin J, Kinne RW, Santavirta S, Sorsa T, Lopez-Otin C, Takagi M. Analysis of 16 different matrix metalloproteinases (MMP-1 to MMP-20) in the synovial membrane: different profiles in trauma and rheumatoid arthritis. Ann Rheum Dis 1999; 58: 691–697.

Lefebvre O, Regnier C, Chenard MP, Wendling C, Chambon P, Basset P, Rio MC. Developmental expression of mouse stromelysin-3 mRNA. Development 1995; 121: 947–955.

Lefebvre O, Wolf C, Limacher JM, Hutin P, Wendling C, LeMeur M, Basset P, Rio MC. The breast cancer-associated stromelysin-3 gene is expressed during mouse mammary gland apoptosis. J Cell Biol 1992; 119: 997–1002.

Levy A, Zucman J, Delattre O, Mattei MG, Rio MC, Basset P. Assignment of the human stromelysin 3 (STMY3) gene to the q11.2 region of chromosome 22. Genomics 1992; 13: 881–883.

Li J, Liang VC, Sedgwick T, Wong J, Shi YB. Unique organization and involvement of GAGA factors in transcriptional regulation of the Xenopus stromelysin-3 gene. Nucleic Acids Res 1998; 26: 3018–3025.

Lijnen HR, Van Hoef B, Vanlinthout I, Verstreken M, Rio MC, Collen D. Accelerated neointima formation after vascular injury in mice with stromelysin-3 (MMP-11) gene inactivation. Arterioscler Thromb Vasc Biol 1999; 19: 2863–2870.

Linder C, Bystrom P, Engel G, Auer G, Aspenblad U, Strander H, Linder S. Correlation between basic fibroblast growth factor immunostaining of stromal cells and stromelysin-3 mRNA expression in human breast carcinoma. Br J Cancer 1998; 77: 941–945.

Lochter A, Srebrow A, Sympson CJ, Terracio N, Werb Z, Bissell MJ. Misregulation of stromelysin-1 expression in mouse mammary tumor cells accompanies acquisition of stromelysin-1-dependent invasive properties. J Biol Chem 1997; 272: 5007–5015.

Lochter A, Sternlicht MD, Werb Z, Bissell MJ. The significance of matrix metalloproteinases during early stages of tumor progression. Ann NY Acad Sci 1998; 857: 180–193.

Lubberts E, Joosten LA, van Den Bersselaar L, Helsen MM, Bakker AC, van Meurs JB, Graham FL, Richards CD, van Den Berg WB. Adenoviral vector-mediated overexpression of IL-4 in the knee joint of mice with collagen-induced arthritis prevents cartilage destruction. J Immunol 1999; 163: 4546–4556.

Ludwig MG, Basset P, Anglard P. Multiple regulatory elements in the murine stromelysin-3 promoter. Evidence for direct control by CCAAT/enhancer-binding protein beta and thyroid and retinoic receptors. J Biol Chem 2000; 275: 39981–39990.

Lukashev ME, Werb Z. ECM signalling: orchestrating cell behaviour and misbehaviour. Trends Cell Biol 1998; 8: 437–441.

Luo D, Guerin E, Ludwig MG, Stoll I, Basset P, Anglard P. Transcriptional induction of stromelysin-3 in mesodermal cells is mediated by an upstream CCAAT/enhancer-binding protein element associated with a DNase I-hypersensitive site. J Biol Chem 1999; 274: 37177–37185.

Macaulay VM, O'Byrne KJ, Saunders MP, Braybrooke JP, Long L, Gleeson F, Mason CS, Harris

AL, Brown P, Talbot DC. Phase I study of intrapleural batimastat (BB-94), a matrix metalloproteinase inhibitor, in the treatment of malignant pleural effusions. Clin Cancer Res 1999; 5: 513–520.

Manes S, Mira E, Barbacid MM, Cipres A, Fernandez-Resa P, Buesa JM, Merida I, Aracil M, Marquez G, Martinez AC. Identification of insulin-like growth factor-binding protein-1 as a potential physiological substrate for human stromelysin-3. J Biol Chem 1997; 272: 25706–25712.

Maquoi E, Polette M, Nawrocki B, Bischof P, Noël A, Pintiaux A, Santavicca M, Schaaps, JP, Pijnenborg, R, Birembaut P, Foidart JM. Expression of stromelysin-3 in the human placenta and placental bed. Placenta 1997; 18: 277–285.

Mari BP, Anderson IC, Mari SE, Ning Y, Lutz Y, Kobzik L, Shipp MA. Stromelysin-3 is induced in tumor/stroma cocultures and inactivated via a tumor-specific and basic fibroblast growth factor-dependent mechanism. J Biol Chem 1998; 273: 618–626.

Masson R, Lefebvre O, Noël A, Fahime ME, Chenard MP, Wendling C, Kebers F, LeMeur M, Dierich A, Foidart JM, Basset P, Rio MC. In vivo evidence that the stromelysin-3 metalloproteinase contributes in a paracrine manner to epithelial cell malignancy. J Cell Biol 1998; 140: 1535–1541.

Meredith JE, Fazeli B, Schwartz MA. The extracellular matrix as a cell survival factor. Mol Biol Cell 1993; 4: 953–961.

Moses MA. The regulation of neovascularization of matrix metalloproteinases and their inhibitors. Stem Cells 1997; 15: 180–189.

Mucha A, Cuniasse P, Kannan R, Beau F, Yiotakis A, Basset P, Dive V. Membrane type-1 matrix metalloprotease and stromelysin-3 cleave more efficiently synthetic substrates containing unusual amino acids in their P1' positions. J Biol Chem 1998; 273: 2763–2768.

Mueller J, Steiner C, Hofler H. Stromelysin-3 expression in noninvasive and invasive neoplasms of the urinary bladder. Hum Pathol 2000; 31: 860–865.

Muller D, Wolf C, Abecassis J, Millon R, Engelmann A, Bronner, G, Rouyer N, Rio MC, Eber M, Methlin G, et al. Increased stromelysin 3 gene expression is associated with increased local invasiveness in head and neck squamous cell carcinomas. Cancer Res 1993; 53: 165–169.

Munck-Wikland E, Heselmeyer K, Lindholm J, Kuylenstierna R, Auer G, Engel G. Stromelysin-3 mRNA expression in dysplasias and invasive epithelial cancer of the larynx. Int J Oncol 1998; 12: 859–864.

Murphy G, Segain JP, O'Shea M, Cockett M, Ioannou C, Lefebvre O, Chambon P, Basset P. The 28-kDa N-terminal domain of mouse stromelysin-3 has the general properties of a weak metalloproteinase. J Biol Chem 1993; 268: 15435–15441.

Noël AC, Lefebvre O, Maquoi E, VanHoorde L, Chenard MP, Mareel M, Foidart JM, Basset P, Rio MC. Stromelysin-3 expression promotes tumor take in nude mice. J Clin Invest 1996; 97: 1924–1930.

Noël A, Boulay A, Kebers F, Kannan R, Hajitou A, Calberg-Bacq CM, Basset P, Rio MC, Foidart JM. Demonstration in vivo that stromelysin-3 functions through its proteolytic activity. Oncogene 2000; 19: 1605–1612.

Noël A, Gilles C, Bajou K, Devy L, Kebers F, Lewalle JM, Maquoi E, Munaut C, Remacle A, Foidart JM. Emerging roles for proteinases in cancer. Invasion Metastasis 1997; 17: 221–239.

Noël A, Santavicca M, Stoll I, L'Hoir C, Staub A, Murphy G, Rio MC, Basset P. Identification of structural determinants controlling human and mouse stromelysin-3 proteolytic activities. J Biol Chem 1995; 270: 22866–22872.

Okada A, Saez S, Misumi Y, Basset P. Rat stromelysin 3: cDNA cloning from healing skin wound, activation by furin and expression in rat tissues. Gene 1997; 185: 187–193.

105

Okada A, Tomasetto C, Lutz Y, Bellocq JP, Rio MC, Basset P. Expression of matrix metallo-proteinases during rat skin wound healing: evidence that membrane type-1 matrix metallo-proteinase is a stromal activator of pro-gelatinase A. J Cell Biol 1997; 137: 67–77.

Osteen KG, Keller NR, Feltus FA, Melner MH. Paracrine regulation of matrix metalloproteinase expression in the normal human endometrium. Gynecol Obstet Invest 1999; 48: 2–13.

Patterton D, Hayes WP, Shi YB. Transcriptional activation of the matrix metalloproteinase gene stromelysin-3 coincides with thyroid hormone-induced cell death during frog metamorphosis. Dev Biol 1995; 167: 252–262.

Pei D, Weiss SJ. Furin-dependent intracellular activation of the human stromelysin-3 zymogen. Nature 1995; 375: 244–247.

Pei D, Majmudar G, Weiss SJ. Hydrolytic inactivation of a breast carcinoma cell-derived serpin by human stromelysin-3. J Biol Chem 1994; 269: 25849–25855.

Porte H, Chastre E, Prevot S, Nordlinger B, Empereur S, Basset P, Chambon P, Gespach C. Neoplastic progression of human colorectal cancer is associated with overexpression of the stromelysin-3 and BM-40/SPARC genes. Int J Cancer 1995; 64: 70–75.

Raff MC. Social controls on cell survival and cell death. Nature 1992; 356: 397–400.

Raff MC, Barres BA, Burne JF, Coles HS, Ishizaki Y, Jacobson MD. Programmed cell death and the control of cell survival: lessons from the nervous system. Science 1993; 262: 695–700.

Rio MC, Lefebvre O, Santavicca M, Noël A, Chenard MP, Anglard P, Byrne JA, Okada A, Regnier CH, Masson R, Bellocq JP, Basset P. Stromelysin-3 in the biology of the normal and neoplastic mammary gland. J Mammary Gland Biol Neoplasia 1996; 1: 231–240.

Rouyer N, Wolf C, Chenard MP, Rio MC, Chambon P, Bellocq JP, Basset P. Stromelysin-3 gene expression in human cancer: an overview. Invasion Metastasis 1994; 14: 269–275

Rudolph-Owen LA, Matrisian LM. Matrix metalloproteinases in remodeling of the normal and neoplastic mammary gland. J Mammary Gland Biol Neoplasia 1998; 3: 177–189.

Santavicca M, Noël A, Angliker H, Stoll I, Segain JP, Anglard P, Chretien M, Seidah N, Basset P. Characterization of structural determinants and molecular mechanisms involved in pro-stromelysin-3 activation by 4-amino-phenylmercuric acetate and furin-type convertases. Biochem J 1996; 315: 953–958.

Schonbeck U, Mach F, Sukhova GK, Atkinson E, Levesque E, Herman M, Graber P, Basset P, Libby P. Expression of stromelysin-3 in atherosclerotic lesions: regulation via CD40-CD40 ligand signaling in vitro and in vivo. J Exp Med 1999; 189: 843–853.

Singer CF, Marbaix E, Lemoine P, Courtoy PJ, Eeckhout Y. Local cytokines induce differential expression of matrix metalloproteinases but not their tissue inhibitors in human endometrial fibroblasts. Eur J Biochem 1999; 259: 40–45.

Strasser A. Dr Josef Steiner Cancer Research Prize Lecture: the role of physiological cell death in neoplastic transformation and in anti-cancer therapy. Int J Cancer 1999; 81: 505–511.

Teesalu T, Masson R, Basset P, Blasi F, Talarico D. Expression of matrix metalloproteinases during murine chorioallantoic placenta maturation. Dev Dyn 1999; 214: 248–258.

Thewes M, Worret WI, Engst R, Ring J. Stromelysin-3 (ST-3): immunohistochemical charac-terization of the matrix metalloproteinase (MMP)-11 in benign and malignant skin tumours and other skin disorders. Clin Exp Dermatol 1999; 24: 122–126.

Thompson CB. Apoptosis in the pathogenesis and treatment of disease. Science 1995; 267: 1456–1462.

Tierney GM, Griffin NR, Stuart RC, Kasem H, Lynch KP, Lury JT, Brown PD, Millar AW, Steele RJ, Parsons SL. A pilot study of the safety and effects of the matrix metalloproteinase inhibitor marimastat in gastric cancer. Eur J Cancer 1999; 35: 563–568.

Unden AB, Sandstedt B, Bruce K, Hedblad M, Stahle-Backdahl M. Stromelysin-3 mRNA associated with myofibroblasts is overexpressed in aggressive basal cell carcinoma and in dermatofibroma but not in dermatofibrosarcoma. J Invest Dermatol 1996; 107: 147–153.

Vassiliou S, Mucha A, Cuniasse P, Georgiadis D, Lucet-Levannier K, Beau F, Kannan R, Murphy G, Knauper V, Rio MC, Basset P, Yiotakis A, Dive V. Phosphinic pseudo-tripeptides as potent inhibitors of matrix metalloproteinases: a structure-activity study. J Med Chem 1999; 42: 2610–2620.

Wilson CL, Heppner KJ, Labosky PA, Hogan BL, Matrisian LM. Intestinal tumorigenesis is suppressed in mice lacking the metalloproteinase matrilysin. Proc Natl Acad Sci (USA) 1997; 94: 1402–1407.

Wolf C, Chenard MP, Durand de Grossouvre P, Bellocq JP, Chambon P, Basset P. Breast-cancer-associated stromelysin-3 gene is expressed in basal cell carcinoma and during cutaneous wound healing. J Invest Dermatol 1992; 99: 870–872.

Wolf C, Rouyer N, Lutz Y, Adida C, Loriot M, Bellocq JP, Chambon P, Basset P. Stromelysin 3 belongs to a subgroup of proteinases expressed in breast carcinoma fibroblastic cells and possibly implicated in tumor progression. Proc Natl Acad Sci (USA) 1993; 90: 1843–1847.

107

Chapter 6

MEMBRANE-TYPE MATRIX METALLOPROTEINASES

Yoshifumi Itoh and Motoharu Seiki
Department of Cancer Cell Research, Institute of Medical Science, The University of Tokyo, 4-6-1 Shirokane-dai, Minato-ku, Tokyo 108-8639, Japan

1. INTRODUCTION

Matrix metalloproteinases (MMPs) can be divided into two groups; the membrane bound or membrane-type MMPs (MT-MMPs), and the soluble MMPs (Seiki, 1999; Nagase and Woessner, 1999). MT-MMPs have a membrane-anchoring sequence at the carboxyl terminus leading to the expection that they would degrade extracellular matrix (ECM) at the periphery of cells whereas soluble MMPs might be capable of degrading ECM distant from the producer cells in the tissue. Tissues are comprised of cells embedded in a framework of ECM in which the cells and the ECM are attached through cell surface adhesion molecules. The cells in tissue may need to modify the pericellular ECM environment for cellular functions, such as proliferation, migration or the alteration of cell morphology. An association of MMPs with the cell surface may facilitate the ECM remodeling associated with such cell functions (Werb, 1997; Murphy and Gavrilovic, 1999).

Malignant cancer cells are characterized by their ability to invade into surrounding tissue and finally metastasize to distant organ. MMPs are the major players for the ECM degradation associated with cancer cell invasion (Stetler-Stevenson et al, 1993; McCawley and Matrisian, 2000). Many MMPs are expressed at high levels in cancer tissues and they collectively contribute to the proliferation of the tumor cells and invasion into surrounding tissue. Particularly, MMPs associated with the cancer cell surface are expected to play important roles during such processes. In this review, we summarize recent information about MT1-MMP and other MT-MMPs.

J.-M. Foidart and R.J. Muschel (eds.), Proteases and Their Inhibitors in Cancer Metastasis, 109–124.

2. STRUCTURE OF MT-MMPS

Among the over 25 mammalian MMPs, six are MT-MMPs having an anchoring device to the plasma membrane at the C-terminus (Figure 1). All the six MT-MMPs have common structural characteristics. Adjacent to the cysteine switch in the propeptide, MT-MMPs have a multi-basic amino acid motif containing a recognition site for proprotein convertases such as furin and its related proteinases (Hosaka et al, 1991). Some soluble MMPs, MMP-11 (stromelysin 3), and MMP-23 also have this motif (Nagase and Woessner, 1999). The presence of this motif leads to the expectation that proMT-MMPs will be activated intracellularly and delivered to the cell surface as an active enzyme. MT-MMPs have catalytic and hemopexin-like domains in common with the soluble MMPs.

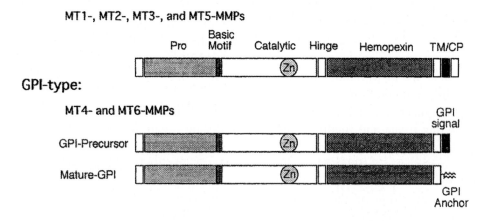

Figure 1. Domain structure of MT-MMP. MT-MMPs are unique among MMP family members in that they have a plasma membrane anchoring device at the carboxyl terminus They also have a multi-basic motif at the cleavage site for the processing of propeptide by subtilisin family proteinases The multi-basic motif is also present in MMP-11, and MMP-23 The C-terniminal hydrophobic stretch of proMT4-MMP and proMT6-MMP are cleaved off during secretion and transferred to glycosylphosphatidyl inositol (GPI). anchor Pro; propeptide, Catalytic; catalytic domain, Hemopexin; Hemopexin-like domain.

At the carboxy-terminus, there is a hydrophobic amino acid stretch that acts as an anchoring device to the plasma membrane. The C′ terminal hydrophobic sequences of MT1-MMP, MT2-MMP, MT3-MMP, and MT5-MMP act as a transmembrane domain as was demonstrated for MT1-MMP by Cao et al. (1995). The transmembrane domain extends into a short cytoplasmic tail of 20 amino acids. Since the cytoplasmic sequence of these MT-MMPs retains some conserved motifs, there is a possibility that the cytoplasmic domain plays a role in their regulation or function. In contrast to these four MT-MMPs, the hydrophobic C′ region of MT4-MMP and MT6-MMP is located at the most distal end of the carboxy-terminus. This region of MT4-MMP and MT6-MMP is a signal for cleavage and transfer to a glycosylphosphatidyl inositol (GPI) anchor (Itoh et al, 1999; Kojima et al, 2000). Thus, MT-MMPs can be further subgrouped into transmembrane-types and GPI-types.

3. SUBSTRATES OF MT-MMPS

Recombinant enzymes expressed as truncated soluble forms were used in biochemical studies to determine substrate specificity. rMT1-MMP cleaves type I and III collagen (into 3/4 and 1/4 fragments) (d'Ortho et al, 1997; Ohuchi et al, 1997) and other ECM components such as fibronectin, vitronectin, laminin, cartilage proteoglycan (Ohuchi et al, 1997; Pei and Weiss, 1996; Kishikawa et al, 2000) including aggrican (d'Ortho et al, 1997; Fosang et al, 1998). rMT2-MMP also has activity against fibronectin, tenascin, laminin, aggrecan and perlecan (d'Ortho et al, 1997). rMT3-MMP degrades type III collagen and fibronectin (Matsumoto et al, 1997). rMT4-MMP was demonstrated to have gelatinolytic and TNF-alpha converting activities (English et al, 2000). rMT5-MMP degrades gelatin and proteoglycans. MT6-MMP can also degrade gelatin (Pei, 1999).

In addition to the activity against ECM components, MT-MMPs activate some soluble proMMPs on the cell surface. MT1-MMP was originally reported as an activator of proMMP-2 (pro-gelatinase A) (Sato et al, 1994), and later it was shown also to activate proMMP-13 (pro-collagenase 3) (Knauper et al, 1996). Other MT-MMPs were reported to activate proMMP-2 at least *in vitro* (Wang Y et al, 1999; Wang X et al, 1999; Llano et al, 1999; Hotary et al, 2000; Velasco et al, 2000), but conflicting results have been reported for MT4-MMP (English et al, 2000; Kolkenbrock et al, 1999) and MT6-MMP (Kojima et al, 2000).

4. CELL-MEDIATED ACTIVATION OF PROMMPS

The activation of proMMP-2 is mediated on the cell surface by MT1-MMP (Seiki, 1999; Nagase and Woessner, 1999; Stetler-Stevenson, 1993). MT1-MMP plays two different roles in the activation process (Figure 2). First it is a cell surface receptor for proMMP-2 and second it activates proMMP-2 through enzymatic cleavage. However, MT1-MMP cannot bind proMMP-2 directly. Instead tissue inhibitor of metalloproteinases-2 (TIMP-2) a specific inhibitor of MT1-MMP acts as an adapter molecule to mediate proMMP-2 binding by forming a ternary complex. The N-terminal domain of TIMP-2 binds to the catalytic domain of MT1-MMP and inhibits it, while the C-terminal domain

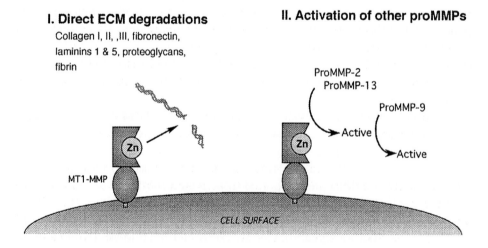

Figure 2. Cell surface activity of MT1-MMP. In the left, direct activities of MT-MMPs against ECM components are presented In the right, other MMP activities controlled by MT1-MMP are summarized FN; fibronectin, TN; tenescin, LN; laminin, GelA; gelatinase A (MMP-2); Col-3; collagenase 3 (MMP-13); GelB; gelatinase B (MMP-9).

binds specifically to the hemopexin-like domain (PEX) of proMMP-2 (Strongin et al, 1995; Butler et al, 1998). Since MT1-MMP is tethered to the cell membrane, TIMP-2 then acts as a bridge linking proMMP-2 to the surface of the cell. MT1-MMP when in the complex with TIMP-2 and proMMP-2 cannot cleave the propeptide of proMMP-2 for activation (Kinoshita et al, 1998). Activation of proMMP-2 in the complex occurs only when free MT1-MMP is available nearby (Kinoshita et al, 1998). Thus, cell-mediated activation of proMMP-2 requires at least two MT1-MMP molecules close enough to carry out the reaction.

MT2-MMP, MT3-MMP and MT5-MMP have similar activities to MT1-MMP in the activation of proMMP-2. Since MMP-2 activation by fibroblasts and embryonic tissues is hardly detectable in *mt1-mmp* knockout mice, MT1-MMP seems to be the major activator of proMMP-2 *in vivo* (Zhou et al, 2000) (our unpublished observation).

MT1-MMP also activates proMMP-13 in a cell-mediated manner (Knauper et al, 1996; Cowell et al, 1998). However, proMMP-13 can also be activated by MMP-3 (stromelysin 3), plasmin or trypsin (Knauper, 1996). It is not clear whether activation of proMMP-13 is disturbed in the *mt1-mmp* knockout mice as well.

5. ACTIVATION OF PROMT-MMPS

Because of the presence of the multi-basic motif immediately upstream of the putative processing site, proMT1-MMP was postulated to be activated intra-cellularly by a furin-like proprotein convertase that processes secretory pre-cursor proteins in a trans-Golgi network (Sato et al, 1994). Recombinant soluble proMT1-MMP must be processed by cleavage of the propeptide by furin or trypsin for the generation of enzymatic activity (Sato et al, 1996). A soluble mutant MT1-MMP generated by a expression vector coding for MT1-MMP lacking the transmembrane region was processed in a similar fashion (Pei and Weiss, 1996).

There are conflicting data on the requirement for this processing on the ultimate activation of proMMP-2 (Cao et al, 1996); mutations introduced into the muti-basic motif did not affect activation of proMMP-2 by MT1-MMP leading to the conclusion that MMP-2 activation does not require processing of the MT1-MMP propeptide. Yana and Weiss tried to address this problem recently and identified a secondary proprotein convertase-sensitive site in the propeptide (Yana and Weiss, 2000). In addition to the previously reported [108]RRKR, they identified [89]RRPR. The majority of processing occurs at [108]RRKR from the N-terminal amino acid of the mature enzyme (Strongin et al, 1995;

Imai et al, 1996). However, when the major site was mutated, substantial amount of processing was observed at the secondary site and the processed MT1-MMP activated proMMP-2. Mutation of both sites abolished processing of proMT1-MMP and activation of proMMP-2 as well (Yana and Weiss, 2000). Thus, cleavage of the propeptide must occur for MT1-MMP to function, but this cleavage can occure at two different sites. This conclusion is consistent with the *in vitro* study using recombinant proMT1-MMP (Sato et al, 1996).

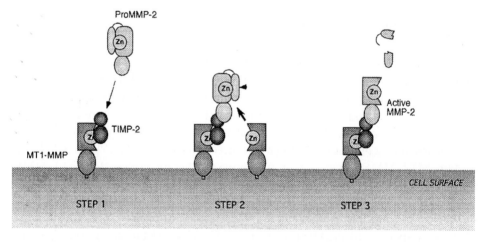

Figure 3. Mechanism of the cell-mediated activation of proMMP-2. MT1-MMP plays two different roles in activation of proMMP-2 on the cell surface. One is as a receptor and the other is as an activator for proMMP-2. ProMMP-2 binds to TIMP-2 and forms an inhibitor-enzyme complex with MT1-MMP on the cell surface that acts as a platform to bind proMMP-2. Thus, complex formation with TIMP-2 differentiates the roles of MT1-MMP. Processing of proMMP-2 in the complex can be carried out by TIMP-2-free MT1-MMP by nearby proMMP-2; pro-gelatinase A, Zn; zinc atom at the catalytic site, Hx; hemopexin-like domain, C; carboxy-terminal domain, N; amino terminal domain.

The proprotein convertases responsible for proMT1-MMP processing are likely to be furin and/or PC6, members of subtilisin family of serine proteinases (Yana and Weiss, 2000). Among the four members of the mammalian subtilisin-family proprotein convertases (furin, PACE4, PC6, and PC7), furin and PC6 are the most widely expressed. Lovo cells are known to lack both furin and PC6, and proMT1-MMP failed to be processed in the cells. Expression of furin by transfection restored the processing activity. Another mutant cell line, RPE.40, which lacks furin but expresses PC6, was able to process proMT1-MMP.

6. FATE OF MT1-MMP ON THE CELL SURFACE

ProMT1-MMP is processed intracellularly and appears on the cell surface as an active 60 kDa enzyme. Then, what is the fate of the enzyme? Some fraction of the enzyme can be inhibited by TIMP-2, allowing it to act as an acceptor for proMMP-2. After proMMP-2 activation, MT1-MMP may be internalized together with TIMP-2. Maquoi et al. reported recently that the TIMP-2 bound to HT1080 or MT1-MMP-expressing A2058 cells was internalized and degraded in a bafilomycin A1-sensitive manner (Maquoi et al, 2000).

The enzyme can be inactivated by proteolysis as well. In HT1080 cells that express MT1-MMP at high levels, a 43–45 kDa degraded form can be detected in addition to the 60 kDa mature enzyme (Stanton et al, 1998; Lehti et al, 1998). It is a result of proteolytic cleavage between the Ala255-Ile bond located at the end of the catalytic domain of MT1-MMP by the action of either MT1-MMP itself or MMP-2 activated by MT1-MMP. Thus, the 43–45 kDa cleavage product remaining on the cell surface is the PEX fragment.

Interestingly, similar proteolytic cleavage of MMP-2 releasing the MMP-2 PEX fragment occurs in tissues during angiogeneis (Brooks et al, 1998). The PEX fragment of MMP-2 is known to inhibit cell-mediated activation of proMMP-2 (Strongin et al, 1993). It also competes with the binding of MMP-2 to $\alpha v \beta 3$ integrin on endothelial cells and inhibits angiogenesis (Brooks et al, 1998). By analogy it is interesting to speculate that the PEX fragment of MT1-MMP may also have some negative regulatory roles against the biological roles mediated by MT1-MMP.

7. BIOLOGICAL SIGNIFICANCE OF PERICELLULAR ECM REMODELING BY MT1-MMP

ECM remodeling at the periphery of cells is important for various cell functions in tissue. A recent comparative study of MT-MMPs and soluble MMPs in reconstituted tissue models clearly demonstrated the importance of MT1-MMP in invasion and tubular formation of MDCK cells (Hotary et al, 2000). MDCK cells retain a well-differentiated epithelial cell phenotype and are able to form a branched tubular structure in response to HGF in three dimensional gels composed of type I collagen or Matrigel. Enforced expression of soluble MMPs (MMP-1, MMP-2, MMP-3, MMP-7, MMP-9, MMP-11, and MMP-13) did not affect the phenotype of the cells, but expression of MT1-MMP rendered the cells invasive when cells were cultivated atop type I collagen gel regardless of the presence or absence of HGF. Branching tubulogenesis was also disturbed possibly by the extensive type I collagen degrading activity of the MT1-MMP. MDCK cells also express endogenous MT1-MMP when they are growing in the type I collagen gel. HGF-induced morphogenesis can be inhibited by TIMP-2 but not TIMP-1 (Kadono et al, 1998). MT1-MMP is inhibited by TIMP-2, but not TIMP-1. Hence the TIMP-2-sensitive proteinase, most likely MT1-MMP, is important for the tubulogenesis of the MDCK cells. Thus, the balance between pericellular proteolysis and cell adhesion is important for regulated morphogenesis in the ECM matrix. The result also suggests a key role of MT1-MMP in cancer cell invasion in stroma where type I collagen is the major scaffold.

MT1-MMP may also play a role in cell migration in addition to degradation of barrier ECM (Murphy and Gavrilovic, 1999). Cells have to adhere to and detach from ECM during migration. Many ECM components can support cell migration providing footholds for movement. Laminin-5 is one such ECM component of the basement membrane that supports cell migration. Recently, MMP-2 was reported to enhance the cell migration on laminin-5. At the same time, MMP-2 cleaved laminin-5, suggesting the importance of the cleavage for migration (Giannelli et al, 1997). Koshikawa et al. demonstrated that MT1-MMP also cleaves laminin-5 and stimulates cell migration (Kishikawa et al, 2000). Since MMP-2 needs MT1-MMP for activation, MT1-MMP can initiate both MMP-2-dependent and -independent processes. Treatment of the cells with antisense oligonucleotide against the *mt1-mmp* gene inhibited cell migration in spite of the production of proMMP-2 (Kishikawa et al, 2000).

The importance of MT1-MMP in the formation and maintenance of tissue was also demonstrated in MT1-MMP null mice (Zhou et al, 2000; Brooks et al, 1998). Although these mice are viable, they have marked abnormalities especially in the hard tissues of the skeleton manifested by craniofacial dysmorphism, dwarfism, osteopenia, fibrosis, and impaired ossification. These tissues normally are rich in type I collagen. Fibroblasts isolated from the skeletal tissue of the MT1-MMP deficient mice were defective in degrading type I collagen. Since *mmp-2* knockout mice do not show such defects, this phenotype can be attributed to the lack of MT1-MMP itself. Thus, the accumulating evidence suggests that MT1-MMP is responsible for type I collagen turnover at the periphery of cells in tissue.

8. EXPRESSION OF MT-MMPS IN TUMORS

Expression of MT1-MMP confers invasive activity to cells. Thus, aberrant expression of MT1-MMP in tumor cells is thought to play an important role in invasion and metastasis. In addition, MT1-MMP was originally identified as an activator of proMMP-2 on cancer cell surface. Since MMP-2 has a type IV collagenase activity, MT1-MMP is believed to be the key enzyme for cancer cells to invade basement membrane. MMP-2 is expressed in a variety of cancer tissues mainly by the fibroblasts surrounding the cancer cells. Expression of active MMP-2 in tumor tissue correlates well with invasive and metastasis and with the expression levels of MT1-MMP (Seiki, 1999). Expression of MT1-MMP was detected in many types of tumors by immunostaining, such as lung (Sato et al, 1994; Tokuraku et al, 1995; Polett et al, 1996; Nawrocki et al, 1997), gastric (Nomura et al, 1995; Mori et al, 1997), colon (Okada et al, 1995; Ohtani et al, 1996), liver (Harada et al, 1998), breast (Polette et al, 1996; Okada et al, 1995; Ueno et al, 1997; Ishigaki et al, 1999), bladder (Kanayama et al, 1998), head and neck (Okada et al, 1995; Yoshizaki et al, 1997), thyroid (Nakamura et al, 1999), ovarian (Afzal et al, 1998; Fishman et al, 1996), and cervical carcinomas (Gilles et al, 1996) and brain tumors (Yamamoto et al, 1996; Nakada et al, 1999; Forsyth et al, 1999). The signals were both in tumor cells and adjacent stromal cells. Transcripts were also detected in tumor cells and stromal cells (Okada et al, 1995; Ohtani et al, 1996; Afzal et al, 1998; Heppner et al, 1996). However, the intensity of the signals in the tumor cells varies depending on tumor types. For example, relatively stronger signals in tumor cells compared with the surrounding stroma cells were detected in colon, gastric and ovarian carcinomas (Ohtani et al, 1996; Afzal et al, 1998) but the signal was weaker in breast carcinomas (Okada et al, 1995; Heppner et al, 1996; Chenard et al, 1999).

In normal tissue, expression of MT1-MMP is rarely detectable in epithelial cells even during wound healing (Okada et al, 1997), but it can be seen in carcinoma cells. Thus, expression of MT1-MMP may be a direct or indirect consequence of the genetic changes in the transformed cells. Indeed, transformation of MDCK cells by v-src oncogene up-regulated expression of MT1-MMP, and at the same time, it enhanced the umorigenic and metastatic ability of the cells when they were implanted in nude mouse (Kadono et al, 1998).

Expression levels of MT1-MMP in tumor cell lines correlated with the malignant nature of the cells as well. Weakly tumorigenic and poorly invasive human breast carcinoma cell lines, such as MCF-7, T47D, MDA-MB 468, ZR-75-1 cells, do not express MT1-MMP nor MMP-2, but invasive and metastatic ones, MDA-MB-231, MDA-MB-435, BT-549, Hs578T cells, express MT1-MMP (Pulyaeva et al, 1997). Expression levels of MT1-MMP in the cells correlated with the loss of the epithelial phenotype and acquisition of mesenchymal characteristics such as expression of vimentin. A similar correlation of MT1-MMP expression with invasiveness was reported for human cervical carcinoma cell lines (Gilles et al, 1996).

Only limited information is available for expression of other MT-MMPs in human cancers. MT1-MMP was the more frequently expressed compared to MT2-MMP and MT3-MMP in breast carcinomas (Ueno et al, 1997), urothelial carcinomas (Kitagawa et al, 1998), thyroid carcinomas (Nakamura et al, 1999). MT4-MMP is expressed in breast carcinoma cell lines (Puente et al, 1996; Kajita et al, 1999), MT5-MMP in brain tumor cell lines (Llano et al, 1999), and MT6-MMP in colon and brain tumor cell lines (Llano et al, 1999). However, more extensive evaluation using clinical samples needs to be done to understand the exact relevance to tumors.

9. LOCALIZATION OF MT1-MMP DURING TUMOR CELL INVASION

Activation of proMMP-2 requires at least two MT1-MMP molecules, one to function as a receptor and one as an activator. These two molecules must be close to carry out the activation reaction. The odds favoring this condition will be increased with increased concentrations of the enzyme. This may be enhanced by localization of the enzyme to a discrete location. Mosky et al. demonstrated that many proteases including MMP-2 were localized to specialized cell surface protrusions called invadopodia (Monsky et al, 1993). MT1-MMP was also shown to localize at protrusions and lamellipodia (Monsky et al, 1993). Nakahara et al. pointed out the importance of transmembrane and cytoplasmic domains of MT1-MMP for the localization and degradation of pericellular ECM (Monsky et al, 1993). However, the importance of the cytoplasmic tail was not evident in other assays, including tubular formation by MDCK cells (Hotary et al, 2000; Hiraoka et al, 1998).

10. REGULATION OF GENE EXPRESSION

During mouse development, MT1-MMP expression can be seen mainly in the cells of mesenchymal origin (Kinoh et al, 1996; Apte et al, 1997), though some epithelial cells do express it (Apte et al, 1997; Ota et al, 1998). Thus, expression of MT1-MMP is regulated according to a cell type specific manner in the developmental program.

Promoter sequences of mouse and human MT1-MMP genes have been reported recently (Haas et al, 1999; Lohi et al, 2000). Comparison of the 5′ upstream sequences between the species revealed the existence of some conserved *cis*-elements. There is a common sequence containing overlapping Sp-1 and Egr-1 binding sites immediately upstream from the multiple transcription start sites. The Sp-1 binding site was identified as an important cis-element for basal transcription activity in HT1080 cells (Lohi et al, 2000), while Egr-1 but not Sp-1 was critical in endothelial cells when cultivated in collagen gel (Haas et al, 1999). These promoters lack TATA-box and growth factor responsive transcription binding sites such as TRE. It is not yet clear how MT1-MMP expression is regulated in a cell type specific manner and how transformation up-regulates gene expression.

11. FUTURE DIRECTIONS

MT1-MMP expressed in tumors is believed to contribute to degradation of the basement membrane by activating proMMP-2 and thereby to facilitate the tumor cells ability to migrate across type I collagen rich connective tissues. However, it is unclear whether the MT1-MMP and MMP-2 system contributes to the tumor cell growth, invasion or metastasis, and raises the question of whether inhibition of MT1-MMP for cancer treatment would be effective. Over-expression of MT1-MMP certainly enhances the rate of experimental metastasis (Tsunezuka et al, 1996), however we do not know what happens when MT1-MMP expression is down-regulated in invasive cancers. Although it would be interesting to test the malignant behavior of tumors in MT1-MMP knockout mice, this is difficult because of the early death of the mice. Experiments using cell lines established from the null mouse may be useful for addressing these questions. In the MMP-2 null mutant mice, the rate of growth and experimental metastasis of implanted tumors was significantly reduced compared to that in the wild type mice (Itoh et al, 1998). Tumor-induced angiogenesis was also suppressed in the mutant mice. Since MT1-MMP is the most important physiological activator of proMMP-2, the results support the importance of MT1-MMP and MMP-2 system in cancer.

MMP-2 null mice grow normally, but MT1-MMP null mice show severe phenotype in skeletal tissues. The phenotype is similar to the side effects observed in patients who received relatively high doses of wide spectrum MMP inhibitors. Thus, extensive inhibition of MT1-MMP in normal tissue may disturb type I collagen turnover and results in musculo-skeletal side effects. This may also raise some constraints upon the use of these inhibitors as therapeutic agents.

REFERENCES

Afzal S, Lalani EN, Poulsom R, Stubbs A, Rowlinson G, Sato H, Seiki M, Stamp GW. MT1-MMP and MMP-2 mRNA expression in human ovarian tumors: possible implications for the role of desmoplastic fibroblasts. Hum Pathol 1998; 29: 155–165.

Apte SS, Fukai N, Beier DR, Olsen BR. The matrix metalloproteinase-14 (MMP-14). gene is structurally distinct from other MMP genes and Is Co-expressed with the TIMP-2 gene during mouse embryogenesis, J Biol Chem 1997; 272: 25511–25517.

Brooks PC, Silletti S, von T, Friedlander M, Cheresh DA. Disruption of angiogenesis by PEX, a non-catalytic metalloproteinase fragment with integrin binding activity. Cell 1998; 92: 391–400.

Butler GS, Butler MJ, Atkinson SJ, Will H, Tamura T, van Westrum SS, Crabbe T, Clements J, Pia d'Ortho M, Murphy G. The TIMP2 membrane type 1 metalloproteinase 'receptor' regulates the concentration and efficient activation of progelatinase A. A kinetic study. J Biol Chem 1998; 273: 871–880.

Cao J, Sato H, Takino T, Seiki M. The C-terminal region of membrane type matrix metalloproteinase is a functional transmembrane domain required for pro-gelatinase A activation. J Biol Chem 1995: in press.

Cao J, Rehemtulla A, Bahou W, Zucker S. Membrane type matrix metalloproteinase 1 activates pro-gelatinase A without furin cleavage of the N-terminal domain. J Biol Chem 1996; 271: 30174–30180.

Chenard MP, Lutz Y, Mechine-Neuville A, Stoll I, Bellocq JP, Rio MC, Basset P. Presence of high levels of MT1-MMP protein in fibroblastic cells of human invasive carcinomas. Int J Cancer 1999; 82: 208–812.

Cowell S, Knauper V, Stewart ML, D'Ortho MP, Stanton H, Hembry RM, Lopez-Otin C, Reynolds JJ, Murphy G. Induction of matrix metalloproteinase activation cascades based on membrane-type 1 matrix metalloproteinase: associated activation of gelatinase A, gelatinase B and collagenase 3. Biochem J 1998; 331: 453–458.

d'Ortho MP, Will H, Atkinson S, Butler G, Messent A, Gavrilovic J, Smith B, Timpl R, Zardi L, Murphy G. Membrane-type matrix metalloproteinases 1 and 2 exhibit broad-spectrum proteolytic capacities comparable to many matrix metalloproteinases. Eur J Biochem 1997; 250: 751–757.

English WR, Puente XS, Freije JM, Knauper V, Amour A, Merryweather A, Lopez-Otin C, Murphy G. Membrane type 4 matrix metalloproteinase (MMP17) has tumor necrosis factor-alpha convertase activity but does not activate pro-MMP2. J Biol Chem 2000; 275: 14046–14055.

Fishman DA, Bafetti LM, Stack MS. Membrane-type matrix metalloproteinase expression and matrix metalloproteinase-2 activation in primary human ovarian epithelial carcinoma cells. Invasion Metastasis 1996; 16: 150–159.

Forsyth PA, Wong H, Laing TD, Rewcastle NB, Morris DG, Muzik H, Leco KJ, Johnston RN, Brasher PM, Sutherland G, Edwards DR. Gelatinase-A (MMP-2). gelatinase-B (MMP-9) and membrane type matrix metalloproteinase-1 (MT1-MMP) are involved in different aspects of the pathophysiology of malignant gliomas. Br J Cancer 1999; 79: 1828–1835.

Fosang AJ, Last K, Fujii Y, Seiki M, Okada Y. Membrane-type 1 MMP (MMP-14) cleaves at three sites in the aggrecan interglobular domain. FEBS Lett 1998; 430: 186–190.

Giannelli G, Falk-Marzillier J, Schiraldi O, Stetler-Stevenson WG, Quaranta V. Induction of cell migration by matrix metalloprotease-2 cleavage of laminin-5. Science 1997; 277: 225–228.

Gilles C, Polette M, Piette J, Munaut C, Thompson EW, Birembaut P, Foidart JM. High level of MT-MMP expression is associated with invasiveness of cervical cancer cells. Int J Cancer 1996; 65: 209–213.

Haas TL, Stitelman D, Davis SJ, Apte SS, Madri JA. Egr-1 mediates extracellular matrix-driven transcription of membrane type 1 matrix metalloproteinase in endothelium. J Biol Chem 1999; 274: 22679–22685.

Harada T, Arii S, Mise M, Imamura T, Higashitsuji H, Furutani M, Niwano M, Ishigami S, Fukumoto M, Seiki M, Sato H, Imamura M. Membrane-type matrix metalloproteinase-1 (MT1-MTP) gene is over-expressed in highly invasive hepatocellular carcinomas. J Hepatol 1998; 28: 231–239.

Heppner KJ, Matrisian LM, Jensen RA, Rodgers WH. Expression of most matrix metallo-proteinase family members in breast cancer represents a tumor-induced host response. Am J Pathol 1996; 149: 273–282.

Hiraoka N, Allen E, Apel IJ, Gyetko MR, Weiss SJ. Matrix metalloproteinases regulate neo-vascularization by acting as pericellular fibrinolysins. Cell 1998; 95: 365–377.

Holmbeck K, Bianco P, Caterina J, Yamada S, Kromer M, Kuznetsov SA, Mankani M, Robey PG, Poole AR, Pidoux I, Ward J M, Birkedal-Hansen H. MT1-MMP-deficient mice develop dwarfism, osteopenia, arthritis, and connective tissue disease due to inadequate collagen turnover. Cell 1999; 99: 81–92.

Hosaka M, Nagahama M, Kim WS, Watanabe T, Hatsuzawa K, Ikemizu J, Murakami K, Nakayama K. Arg-X-Lys/Arg-Arg motif as a signal for precursor cleavage catalyzed by furin within the constitutive secretory pathway. J Biol Chem 1991; 266; 12127–12130.

Hotary K, Allen E, Punturieri A, Yana I, Weiss SJ. Regulation of cell invasion and morphogen-esis in a three-dimensional type I collagen matrix by membrane-type matrix metalloproteinases 1, 2, and 3. J Cell Biol 2000; 149: 1309–1323.

Imai K, Ohuchi E, Aoki T, Nomura H, Fujii Y, Sato H, Seiki M, Okada Y. Membrane-type matrix metalloproteinase 1 is a gelatinolytic enzyme and is secreted in a complex with tissue inhibitor of metallo-proteinases 2. Cancer Res 1996; 56: 2707–2710.

Ishigaki S, Toi M, Ueno T, Matsumoto H, Muta M, Koike M, Seiki M. Significance of membrane type 1 matrix metalloproteinase expression in breast cancer. Jpn J Cancer Res 1999; 90: 516–522.

Itoh T, Tanioka M, Yoshida H, Yoshioka T, Nishimoto H, Itohara S. Reduced angiogenesis and tumor progression in gelatinase A-deficient mice. Cancer Res 1998; 58: 1048–1051.

Itoh Y, Kajita M, Kinoh H, Mori H, Okada A, Seiki M. Membrane type 4 matrix metallo-proteinase (MT4-MMP, MMP-17) is a glycosylphosphatidylinositol-anchored proteinase. J Biol Chem 1999; 274: 34260–34266.

Kadono Y, Shibahara K, Namiki M, Watanabe Y, Seiki M, Sato H. Membrane type 1-matrix

121

metalloproteinase is involved in the formation of hepatocyte growth factor/scatter factor-induced branching tubules in madin-darby canine kidney epithelial cells. Biochem Biophys Res Commun 1998; 251: 681–687.

Kajita M, Kinoh H, Ito N, Takamura A, Itoh Y, Okada A, Sato H, Seiki M. Human membrane type-4 matrix metalloproteinase (MT4-MMP) is encoded by a novel major transcript: isolation of complementary DNA clones for human and mouse mt4-mmp transcripts. FEBS Lett 1999; 457: 353–356.

Kanayama H, Yokota K, Kurokawa Y, Murakami Y, Nishitani M, Kagawa S. Prognostic values of matrix metalloproteinase-2 and tissue inhibitor of metalloproteinase-2 expression in bladder cancer. Cancer 1998; 82: 1359–1366.

Kinoh H, Sato H, Tsunezuka Y, Takino T, Kawashima A, Okada Y, Seiki M. MT-MMP, the cell surface activator of proMMP-2 (pro-gelatinase A) is expressed with its substrate in mouse tissue during embryogenesis. J Cell Sci 1996: 953–959.

Kinoshita T, Sato H, Okada A, Ohuchi E, Imai K, Okada Y, Seiki M. TIMP-2 promotes activation of progelatinase A by membrane-type 1 matrix metalloproteinase immobilized on agarose beads. J Biol Chem 1998; 273: 16098–16103.

Kitagawa Y, Kunimi K, Ito H, Sato H, Uchibayashi T, Okada Y, Seiki M, Namiki M. Expression and tissue localization of membrane-types 1, 2, and 3 matrix metalloproteinases in human urothelial carcinomas. J Urol 1998; 160: 1540–1545.

Knauper V, Lopez-Otin C, Smith B, Knight G, Murphy G. Biochemical characterization of human collagenase-3. J Biol Chem 1996; 271: 1544–1550.

Knauper V, Will H, Lopez OC, Smith B, Atkinson SJ, Stanton H, Hembry RM, Murphy G. Cellular mechanisms for human procollagenase-3 (MMP-13) activation Evidence that MT1-MMP (MMP-14) and gelatinase a (MMP-2) are able to generate active enzyme. J Biol Chem 1996; 271: 17124–17131.

Kojima S, Itoh Y, Matsumoto S, Masuho Y, Seiki, M. Membrane-type 6 matrix metalloproteinase (MT6-MMP, MMP-25) is the second glycosyl-phosphatidyl inositol (GPI)-anchored MMP. FEBS Lett 2000: in press.

Kolkenbrock H, Essers L, Ulbrich N, Will H. Biochemical characterization of the catalytic domain of membrane-type 4 matrix metalloproteinase. Biol Chem 1999; 380: 1103–1108.

Koshikawa N, Giannelli G, Cirulli V, Miyazaki K, Quaranta V. Role of cell surface metallprotease MT1-MMP in epithelial cell migration over laminin-5. J Cell Biol 2000; 148: 615–624.

Lehti K, Lohi J, Valtanen H, Keski-Oja J. Proteolytic processing of membrane-type-1 matrix metalloproteinase is associated with gelatinase A activation at the cell surface, Biochem J 1998; 334, 345–353.

Llano E, Pendas AM, Freije JP, Nakano A, Knauper V, Murphy G, Lopez-Otin C. Identification and characterization of human MT5-MMP, a new membrane-bound activator of progelatinase a overexpressed in brain tumors. Cancer Res 1999; 59: 2570–2576.

Lohi J, Lehti K, Valtanen H, Parks WC, Keski-Oja J. Structural analysis and promoter characterization of the human membrane-type matrix metalloproteinase-1 (MT1-MMP) gene. Gene 2000; 242: 75–86.

Maquoi E, Frankenne F, Baramova E, Munaut C, Sounni NE, Remacle A, Noel A, Murphy G, Foidart JM. Membrane type 1 matrix metalloproteinase-associated degradation of tissue inhibitor of metalloproteinase 2 in human tumor cell lines. J Biol Chem 2000; 275: 11368–11378.

Matsumoto S, Katoh M, Saito S, Watanabe T, Masuho Y. Identification of soluble type of membrane-type matrix metalloproteinase-3 formed by alternatively spliced mRNA. Biochim Biophys Acta 1997; 1354: 159–170.

McCawley LJ, Matrisian LM. Matrix metalloproteinases: multifunctional contributors to tumor progression. Mol Med Today 2000; 6: 149–156.

Monsky WL, Kelly T, Lin C-Y, Yeh Y, Stetler-Stevenson WG, Mueller SC, Chen W-T. Binding and localization of Mr 72,000 matrix metalloproteinase at cell surface invadopondia. Cancer Res 1993; 53: 3159–3164.

Mori M, Mimori K, Shiraishi T, Fujie T, Baba K, Kusumoto H, Haraguchi M, Ueo H, Akiyoshi T. Analysis of MT1-MMP and MMP2 expression in human gastric cancers. Int J Cancer 1997; 74: 316–321.

Murphy G, Gavrilovic J. Proteolysis and cell migration: creating a path? Curr Opin Cell Biol 1999; 11: 614–621.

Nagase H, Woessner JF Jr. Matrix metalloproteinases. J Biol Chem 1999; 274: 21491–21494.

Nakada M, Nakamura H, Ikeda E, Fujimoto N, Yamashita J, Sato H, Seiki M, Okada Y. Expression and tissue localization of membrane-type 1, 2, and 3 matrix metalloproteinases in human astrocytic tumors. Am J Pathol 1999; 154: 417–428.

Nakahara H, Howard L, Thompson EW, Sato H, Seiki M, Yeh Y, Chen WT. Transmembrane/cytoplasmic domain-mediated membrane type 1-matrix metalloprotease docking to invadopodia is required for cell invasion. Proc Natl Acad Sci (USA) 1997; 94: 7959–7964.

Nakamura H, Ueno H, Yamashita K, Shimada T, Yamamoto E, Noguchi M, Fujimoto N, Sato H, Seiki M, Okada Y. Enhanced production and activation of progelatinase A mediated by membrane-type 1 matrix metalloproteinase in human papillary thyroid carcinomas. Cancer Res 1999; 59: 467–473.

Nawrocki B, Polette M, Marchand V, Monteau M, Gillery P, Tournier JM, Birembaut P. Expression of matrix metalloproteinases and their inhibitors in human bronchopulmonary carcinomas: quantificative and morphological analyses. Int J Cancer 1997; 72: 556–564.

Nomura H, Sato H, Seiki M, Mai M, Okada Y. Expression of membrane-type matrix metalloproteinase in human gastric carcinomas. Cancer Research 1995; 55: 3263–3266.

Ohtani H, Motohashi H, Sato H, Seiki M, Nagura H. Dual over-expression pattern of membrane-type metalloproteinase-1 in cancer and stromal cells in human gastrointestinal carcinoma revealed by in situ hybridization and immunoelectron microscopy. Int J Cancer 1996; 68: 565–570.

Ohuchi E, Imai K, Fujii Y, Sato H, Seiki M, Okada Y. Membrane type 1 matrix metalloproteinase digests interstitial collagens and other extracellular matrix macromolecules. J Biol Chem 1997; 272: 2446–2451.

Okada A, Bellocq JP, Rouyer N, Chenard MP, Rio MC, Chambon P, Basset P. Membrane-type matrix metalloproteinase (MT-MMP) gene is expressed in stromal cells of human colon, breast, and head and neck carcinomas. Proc Natl Acad Sci (USA) 1995; 92: 2730–2734.

Okada A, Tomasetto C, Lutz Y, Bellocq JP, Rio MC, Basset P. Expression of matrix metalloproteinases during rat skin wound healing: evidence that membrane type-1 matrix metalloproteinase is a stromal activator of pro-gelatinase A. J Cell Biol 1997; 137: 67–77.

Ota K, Stetler-Stevenson WG, Yang Q, Kumar A, Wada J, Kashihara N, Wallner EI, Kanwar YS. Cloning of murine membrane-type-1-matrix metalloproteinase (MT-1-MMP) and its metanephric developmental regulation with respect to MMP-2 and its inhibitor. Kidney Int 1998; 54: 131–142.

Pei D, Weiss SJ. Transmembrane-deletion mutants of the membrane-type matrix metalloproteinase-1 process progelatinase A and express intrinsic matrix-degrading activity. J Biol Chem 1996; 271; 9135–9140.

Pei D. Leukolysin/MMP25/MT6-MMP: a novel matrix metalloproteinase specifically expressed in the leukocyte lineage. Cell Res 1999; 9: 291–303.

Polette M, Nawrocki B, Gilles C, Sato H, Seiki M, Tournier JM, Birembaut P. MT-MMP expression and localisation in human lung and breast cancers. Virchows Arch 1996; 428: 29–35.

Puente XS, Pendas AM, Llano E, Velasco G, Lopez OC. Molecular cloning of a novel membrane-type matrix metalloproteinase from a human breast carcinoma. Cancer Res 1996; 56: 944–949.

Pulyaeva H, Bueno J, Polette M, Birembaut P, Sato H, Seiki M, Thompson EW. MT1-MMP correlates with MMP-2 activation potential seen after epithelial to mesenchymal transition in human breast carcinoma cells. Clin Exp Metastasis 1997; 15: 111–120.

Sato H, Takino T, Okada Y, Cao J, Shinagawa A, Yamamoto E, Seiki M (1994) A matrix metalloproteinase expressed on the surface of invasive tumor cells. *Nature* **370**, 61–65.

Sato H, Kinoshita T, Takino T, Nakayama K, Seiki M. Activation of a recombinant membrane type 1 matrix metalloproteinase (MT1-MMP) by furin and its interaction with tissue inhibitor of metalloproteinases (TIMP-2). FEBS Lett 1996; 393: 101–104.

Seiki M. Membrane-type matrix metalloproteinases. Apmis 1999; 107: 137–143.

Stanton H, Gavrilovic J, Atkinson SJ, d'Ortho MP, Yamada KM, Zardi L, Murphy G. The activation of ProMMP-2 (gelatinase A) by HT1080 fibrosarcoma cells is promoted by culture on a fibronectin substrate and is concomitant with an increase in processing of MT1-MMP (MMP-14) to a 45 kDa form. J Cell Sci 1998; 111: 2789–2798.

Stetler-Stevenson WG, Liotta LA, Kleiner DJ. Extracellular matrix 6: role of matrix metalloproteinases in tumor invasion and metastasis. FASEB J 1993; 7: 1434–1441.

Strongin AY, Marmer BL, Grant GA, Goldberg GI. Plasma membrane-dependent activation of the 72-kDa type IV collagenase is prevented by complex formation with TIMP-2. J Biol Chem 1993; 268: 14033–14039.

Strongin, AY, Collier I, Bannikov G, Marmer BL, Grant GA, Goldberg GI. Mechanism of cell surface activation of 72-kDa type IV collagenase – Isolation of the activated form of the membrane metalloprotease. J Biol Chem 1995; 270: 5331–5338.

Tokuraku M, Sato H, Murakami S, Okada Y, Watanabe Y, Seiki M. Activation of the precursor of gelatinase A/72 kDa type IV collagenase/MMP-2 in lung carcinomas correlates with the expression of membrane-type matrix metalloproteinase (MT-MMP) and with lymph node metastasis. Int J Cancer 1995; 64: 355–359.

Tsunezuka Y, Kinoh H, Takino T, Watanabe Y, Okada Y, Shinagawa A, Sato H, Seiki M. Expression of membrane-type matrix metalloproteinase 1 (MT1-MMP) in tumor cells enhances pulmonary metastasis in an experimental metastasis assay, Cancer Res 1996; 56: 5678–5683.

Ueno H, Nakamura H, Inoue M, Imai K, Noguchi M, Sato H, Seiki M, Okada Y. Expression and tissue localization of membrane-types 1, 2, and 3 matrix metalloproteinases in human invasive breast carcinomas. Cancer Res 1997; 57: 2055–2060.

Velasco G, Cal S, Merlos-Suarez A, Ferrando AA, Alvarez S, Nakano A, Arribas J, Lopez-Otin C. Human MT6-matrix metalloproteinase: identification, progelatinase A activation, and expression in brain tumors. Cancer Res 2000; 60: 877–882.

Wang X, Yi J, Lei J, Pei D. Expression, purification and characterization of recombinant mouse MT5-MMP protein products. FEBS Lett 1999; 462: 261–266.

Wang Y, Johnson AR, Ye QZ, Dyer RD. Catalytic activities and substrate specificity of the human membrane type 4 matrix metalloproteinase catalytic domain. J Biol Chem 1999; 274: 33043–33049.

Werb Z. ECM and cell surface proteolysis: regulating cellular ecology. Cell 1997; 91: 439–442.

Yamamoto M, Mohanam S, Sawaya R, Fuller GN, Seiki M, Sato H, Gokaslan ZL, Liotta LA, Nicolson GL, Rao JS. Differential expression of membrane-type matrix metalloproteinase and its correlation with gelatinase A activation in human malignant brain tumors in vivo and in vitro. Cancer Res 1996; 56: 384–392.

Yana I, Weiss SJ. Regulation of membrane type-1 matrix metalloproteinase activation by pro-protein convertases. Mol Biol Cell 2000; 11: 2387–2401.

Yoshizaki, T Sato H, Maruyama Y, Murono S, Furukawa M, Park CS, Seiki M. Increased expression of membrane type 1-matrix metalloproteinase in head and neck carcinoma. Cancer 1997; 79: 139–144.

Zhou Z, Apte SS, Soininen R, Cao R, Baaklini GY, Rauser RW, Wang J, Cao Y, Tryggvason K. Impaired endochondral ossification and angiogenesis in mice deficient in membrane-type matrix metalloproteinase I. Proc Natl Acad Sci (USA) 2000; 97: 4052–4057.

Chapter 7

3D STRUCTURE AND DRUG DESIGN

J. Schröder, H. Wenzel and H. Tschesche
*Universität Bielefeld, Fakultät für Chemie, Biochemie I, Universitätsstr. 25,
D-33615 Bielefeld, Germany*

Abstract

Matrix metalloproteinases (MMPs) are involved in extracellular matrix degradation. Their proteolytic activity must be precisely regulated by their endogenous protein inhibitors, the tissue inhibitors of metalloproteinases (TIMPs). Experimental evidence confirms that MMPs play a decisive role in a wide variety of pathologic conditions that involve connective tissue destruction such as arthritis, tumor growth and metastasis. Modulation of MMP regulation is possible at several biochemical sites, but direct inhibition of enzyme action provides a particularly attractive target for therapeutic intervention. To date the main focus of the therapeutic applications of MMP inhibitors (MMPIs) has been in the areas of cancer and arthritis. One key issue in their clinical development relates to whether broad spectrum inhibitors, active against a range of different enzymes, or selective inhibitors targeted against a particular subset of the MMPs, represents the optimal strategy. Some orally active compounds for the treatment of cancer and/or arthritis are currently under clinical investigations. Representative examples include succinamides (Marimastat), linear sulfonamides (CGS-27023A), heterocyclic sulfonamides (Prinomastat) and biphenylbutyric acid derivatives (BAY-129566). However, since their inception during the eighties, MMPIs have gone through several cycles of metamorphosis. From this, two important approaches to the design, synthesis, and biological evaluation of MMPIs are highlighted: 1. the invention of alternatives to hydroxamic acid zinc chelators and 2. the construction of nonpeptide scaffolds. One current example from our own work in each of these two approaches is described.

1. INTRODUCTION

The matrix metalloproteinases (MMPs, matrixins) form a subfamily of the metzincins and are structurally and functionally related zinc endopeptidases. They are able to degrade *in vitro* and *in vivo* all kinds of extracellular matrix proteins such as basement and interstitial collagens, proteoglycans, fibronectin, laminin, and also plasma proteins (Curran and Murray, 1999). Thus, these enzymes are involved not only in connective tissue remodelling processes like wound healing, growth, embryonic development, implantation a.o. (Woessner, 1991), but also in pathological situations, such as rheumatoid- and osteoarthritis, atherosclerosis, fibrosis, and tumor growth and metastasis (Chambers and Matrisian, 1997; Coussens and Werb, 1996; Johnson et al, 1998; Nagase et al,

J.-M. Foidart and R.J. Muschel (eds.), Proteases and Their Inhibitors in Cancer Metastasis, 127–150.
© 2002 *Kluwer Academic Publishers. Printed in the Netherlands.*

1997; Yong et al, 1998). All but one of the so far discovered two dozen MMPs have similar domain structures including as major domains an N-terminal prodomain (present in the zymogen, i.e. the latent enzyme), the catalytic domain and a hemopexin domain (not present in matrilysin, MMP-7) in some MMPs involved in substrate specificity (Murphy et al, 1992; Schnierer et al, 1993) (Figure 1).

The MMPs are synthesized as zymogens in which the prodomain with its strongly conserved cysteine coordinates to the catalytic zinc ion. They are activated by proteolytic or autolytic removal of the prodomain that can also be

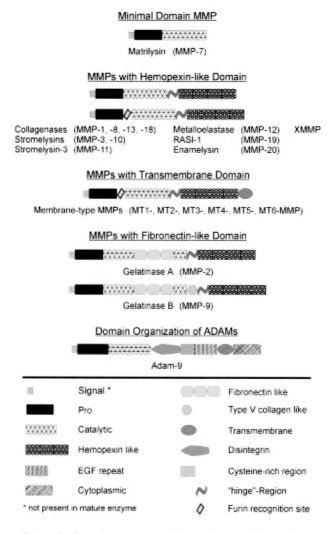

Figure 1. Domain structure of the matrix metalloproteinases.

128

dislocated from the zinc atom by organomercuric agents that attach to the coordinating cysteine. This activation mechanism is designated as the cysteine switch mechanism of activation (Van Wart and Birkedal-Hansen, 1990).

The three-dimensional structures of the catalytic domains all follow the same folding pattern. The spherical molecule contains a flat active-site cleft separating the smaller C-terminal part from the larger N-terminal part, which is built of a central, highly twisted five-stranded β-sheet, flanked by an S-shaped double loop and two additional bridging loops on its convex side and two long α-helices on its concave side. The catalytic zinc ion is located at the bottom of the active site cleft and is coordinated by the N-atoms of three histidins within the HEXXHXXGXXH zinc binding consensus sequence. The active site helix contains His, Glu and His and extends to Gly, where the polypeptide chain turns away from the helix axis towards the third His zinc ligand (Bode et al, 1994) (Figure 2).

A water molecule between the zinc ion and the active site Glu serves as a nucleophil in the catalytic steps of proteolytic substrate cleavage. The subsites of the individual enzymes determine the varying substrate specificities of the MMPs (Bode et al, 1999a). These are mainly determined by the S_1' specificity pocket, which in size and shape considerably differs among the various MMPs,

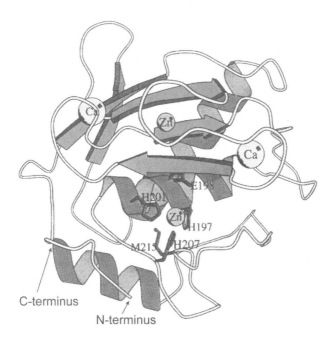

Figure 2. Ribbon plot of the catalytic domain of human neutrophil collagenase.

129

and the almost hydrophobic S_3 pocket. The S_2 site is a shallow depression followed from the S_1 surface groove, which accommodates longer side chains of P_1 residues (in collagen cleavage sites mostly a Gly) of differing size and polarity. The P_2' side chains extend away from the surface and can contribute varying strength of interaction depending on the nature of the exposed residue. Further, to the right side the molecular surface again presents a hydrophobic/polar groove, which could accommodate P_3' side chains of differing nature.

Further examples of metalloproteinases include the reprolysin or adamalysin (ADAM) family, which includes the secretases and sheddases; the astacin family, which includes enzymes such as procollagen processing proteinase (PCP); and other metalloproteinases such as aggrecanase, the endothelin converting enzyme family and the angiotensin converting enzyme family. ADAM-17, also known as tumor necrosis factor-alpha converting enzyme (TACE), is the best known ADAM. ADAM-17 is responsible for cleavage of cell bound tumor necrosis factor-alpha (TNF-α). TNF-α is recognized to be involved in many infectious and autoimmune diseases. Furthermore, TNF-α is the prime mediator of the inflammatory response seen in sepsis and septic shock (Friers, 1991). Other ADAMs that have shown expression in pathological situations include ADAM TS-1, and ADAM-10, -12 and -15 (Kuno et al, 1997; Wu, Croucher and KcKie, 1997). As knowledge of the expression, physiological substrates and disease implication of the ADAMs increases, the full significance of the role of inhibition of this class of enzymes will be appreciated.

The degradative potential of the MMPs is normally controlled by the endogenous specific tissue inhibitors of metalloproteinases (TIMPs) and the more general, non-specific large protein inhibitor, α_2-macroglobulin. The TIMPs associate with the MMPs in a 1:1 stoichiometric manner. The X-ray structural analysis of TIMP/ MMP-complexes (Fernandez-Catalan et al 1998; Gomis-Rüth et al, 1997) have revealed that the TIMPs bind with their edge into the active-site cleft of their cognate MMPs under removal of about 1300 Å^2 surfaces of each molecule from contact with bulk water and some rigidification of the participating loops upon complex formation (Bode et al, 1999b; Musket et al, 1998) (Figure 3). The first five N-terminal TIMP residues Cys1 to Pro5 bind to the active-site cleft in a substrate- or product-like manner, that is similar to P_1, P_1', P_2', P_3', and P_4' peptide substrate residues, forming five intermolecular inter-chain hydrogen bonds. The Cys1 is located directly above the catalytic zinc, coordinating it with its N-terminal α-amino nitrogen and its carbonyl oxygen atoms together with the three imidazole rings from the cognate MMP. Thus, inhibition by stoichiometric inhibitor binding requires zinc complex coordination and substrate analogous binding as well as additional participation of the sA-sB loop and the sC-connector loop in intermolecular contacts for protein-protein association (Fernandez-Catalan et al 1998; Gomis-Rüth et al, 1997).

130

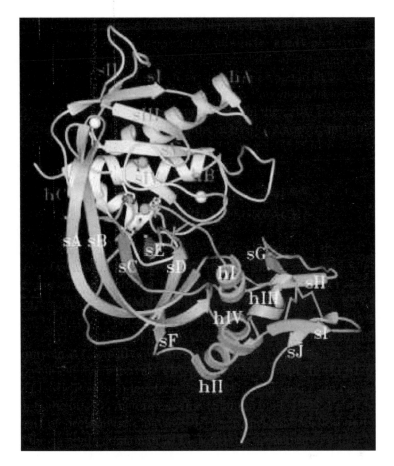

Figure 3. X-ray structure of the catalytic domain of human membrane-type-1 MMP (cdMMP-14), white, complexed with bovine tissue inhibitor of metalloproteinases (TIMP-2), grey.

These facts provide a structural basis for design of synthetic inhibitors based on the tertiary structures of the MMP-proteins as target enzymes.

2. DEVELOPMENT OF SYNTHETIC MATRIX METALLOPROTEINASE INHIBITORS

Two approaches to the identification of MMP inhibitors have been followed: substrate-based design of pseudopeptide derivatives and random screening of compound libraries and natural products. The design of early MMP inhibitors was based on the scissile site sequence of peptide substrates (Figure 4).

This is the sequence around the glycine-isoleucine and glycine-leucine

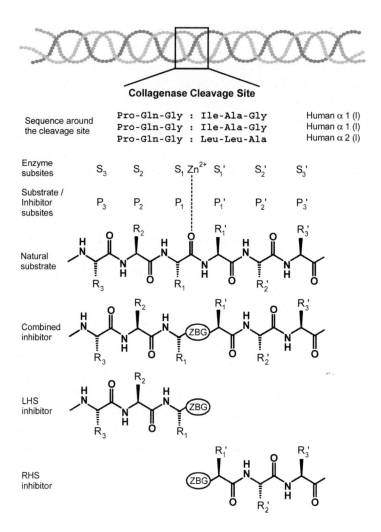

Figure 4. Design of matrix metalloproteinase inhibitors based on the cleavage site of collagen.

cleavage sites in the collagen molecules that are hydrolysed by collagenase. The key to obtain potent enzyme inhibition has been the incorporation of a zinc-binding group (ZBG), to chelate the active-site zinc(II) ion, into peptide analogues of the sequence on either the left-hand side (LHS) or the right-hand side (RHS), or both sides of the cleavage site. At an early stage, it was found that RHS inhibitors featuring a hydroxamic acid ZBG, are particularly potent in terms of their *in vitro* activity (Dickens et a, 1988). Considerable insight into MMP-ligand interactions has been obtained from the study of inhibitor structure-activity relationships (SARs) (Johnson, Robert and Borkakoti, 1987;

132

Schwartz and Van Wart, 1992). Now, however, the use of high-resolution X-ray crystallography (Bode et al, 1994; Borkakoti et al, 1994; Browner, Smith and Castelhano, 1995; Grams et al, 1995a; Lovejoy et al, 1994; Spurlino et al, 1994; Stams et al, 1994) and NMR spectroscopy (Gooley et al, 1994) in the elucidation of structures is providing new paradigms for the design of inhibitors in general and selective inhibitors in particular.

As the number of pharmaceutical companies with an interest in MMPIs has increased, the family of MMP enzymes has grown dramatically. Furthermore, it is now apparent that certain known MMPIs inhibit the production of tumor necrosis factor-alpha (TNF-α). There are two forms of TNF-α, a type II membrane protein of molecular mass 26 kD and a soluble 17 kD form generated from the cell bound protein by specific proteolytic cleavage. The soluble 17 kD form is released by the cell and is associated with the deleterious effects of TNF-α. This form is also capable of acting at sites distant from the site of synthesis. The metalloproteinase ADAM-17 (TACE) is responsible for cleavage of cell bound TNF-α. Thus, inhibitors of TACE prevent the formation of soluble TNF-α and prevent the deleterious effects of the soluble factor. However, it is recognized that different combinations of MMPs and ADAMs are expressed in different pathological situations. According to this, inhibitors with specific selectivities for individual ADAMs and/or MMPs may be preferred for individual diseases. For example, rheumatoid arthritis is an inflammatory joint disease characterized by excessive TNF-α levels and the loss of joint matrix constituents. In this case, a compound that inhibits TACE as well as MMPs such as collagenase-3 (MMP-13) may be preferred for therapeutical use. In contrast, in less inflammatory joint disease such as osteoarthritis, compounds that inhibit matrix degrading MMPs such as MMP-13 but not TACE may be preferred (Reiter, 2000).

From X-ray crystallographic analysis and homology modeling, the MMPs may be classified as falling into two broad structural classes dependent on the depth of the S_1' pocket. This selectivity pocket is relatively deep for the majority of the enzymes like gelatinase A (MMP-2), stomelysin-1 (MMP-3) or collagenase-3 (MMP-13), but for certain enzymes like human fibroblast collagenase (MMP-1) or matrilysin (MMP-7) it is partially or completely occluded due to an increase in size of the side-chain or one of the amino acid residues that forms the pocket (Bode et al, 1999a).

Consequently, the main type of selectivity that has been obtained is for the inhibition of the deep pocket enzymes over the short pocket enzymes. This is achieved by the incorporation of an extended P_1' group, whereas the presence of smaller P_1' groups generally leads to broad spectrum inhibition. The following types of MMPI structures are actually under development: succinyl hydroxamates, sulfonamide hydroxamates and non-hydroxamates (Beckett and

Whittaker, 1998). This classification for MMPIs further includes the so-called first generation MMPIs, which are pseudopeptide derivatives based on the structure of the collagen molecule at the site of initial cleavage by interstitial collagenase, and the next generation MMPIs, which are compounds with good oral bioavailability and with selective inhibitory activity against individual MMPs.

3. ZINC-BINDING GROUPS

The selection of suitable ZBGs has been the subject of intense interest within the research groups. Several different zinc chelators like hydroxamate, carboxylate, sulfhydryl, sulfodiimide and derivatives of phosphorous acid have been identified (Broadhurst et al, 1988; Brown, 1994; Darlak et al, 1990; Marwell, Hunter and Ward, 1989, 1993, Odake et al., 1994) (Figure 5).

Pseudopeptides, containing a derivative of phosphorous acid as the ZBG, first represented an interesting inhibitor design alternative. In contrast to peptidic inhibitors containing a thiol or a carboxylate function, these inhibitors act as good mimics of the substrate in the transition state, providing interaction with both the primed and unprimed side of the active site cleft. In this respect, the design of inhibitors using a phosphinate chelating group included in the peptide backbone seems to be more convenient. This property can be exploited to optimize inhibitor selectivity (Gavuzzo et al, 2000; Vassiliou et al, 1999).

However, the hydroxamates have proved to be the most useful ones and the majority of inhibitors currently under clinical investigation contain this group. The hydroxamate acts as a bidentate ligand with each oxygen at an optimum distance (1.9–2.3 Å) from the active-site zinc(II) ion. The position of the hydroxamate nitrogen suggests that it is protonated and forms a hydrogen bond with a carbonyl oxygen of the enzyme backbone (Grams et al, 1995b). As shown in Figure 6, the hydroxamic acid unit with at least 4-point attachments truly

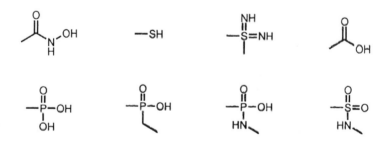

Figure 5. Different zinc chelators used in MMP inhibitor templates.

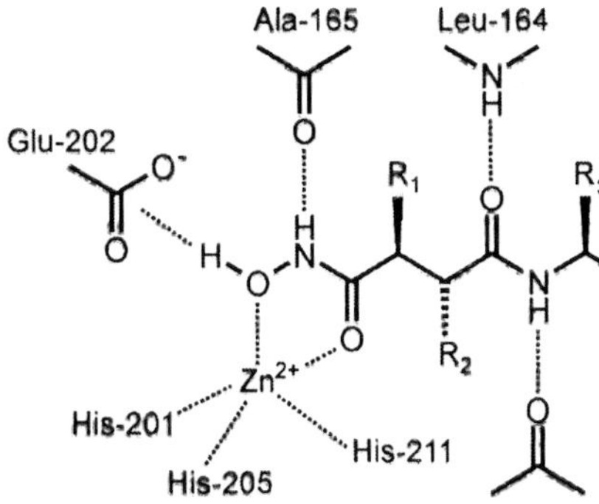

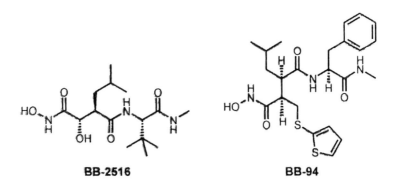

Figure 6. Overview of key enzyme-inhibitor interactions of succinyl RHS-hydroxamates (active site of stromelysin).

behaves like a molecular magnet, a significance which becomes clear as one converts this group to its corresponding carboxylic acid with a concomitant 100–1000-fold loss in binding potency. The remaining residues (R_1, R_2 etc.) play a significant role in filling specific pockets, endowing the individual inhibitors with unique potency and selectivity (Babine and Bender, 1999).

4. First generation MMP inhibitors

Representative examples of this series of MMPIs featuring a succinyl scaffold are the broadspectrum hydroxamates batimastat (BB-94) and marimastat (BB-2516) developed by British Biotech (Rasmussen and McCann, 1997) (Figure 7).

Batimastat was the first compound to enter clinical investigation because of

BB-2516   **BB-94**

Figure 7. Structures of marimastat and batimastat.

135

its ability to inhibit primary tumor growth, metastatic spread, and secondary tumor growth *in vivo*. In animal studies using either murine B16 melanoma cells, human ovarian cancer cells or human colon cancer xenografts, investigators found that batimastat inhibited lung colonisation and significantly affected the growth of the primary tumor and the size of spontaneous metastasis (Chirivi et al, 1994; Eccles et al, 1996; Taraboletti et al, 1995; Vincenti, Clark and Brinckerhoff, 1994; Watson et al, 1996; Wang et al, 1994). However, treatment with batimastat did not cause any significant reduction in the number of metastases formed from a primary tumor. Despite the effectiveness of batimastat the development of this agent was discontinued because of its low oral bioavailability. The compound's utility is further limited by poor water solubility, which requires intraperitoneal administration (Berattie and Smyth, 1998; Parsons, Watson and Steele, 1997). Latest data seem to indicate that batimastat as a hydroxamate-type MMPI promotes liver metastasis (Krüger et al, 2001). Structural modification of batimastat resulted in the synthesis of marimastat, which retains the activity of its predeccessor but has excellent oral bioavailability. It is a potent and reversible inhibitor of MMPs, exhibiting K_i values in the nanomolar range against MMP-1, MMP-2, MMP-3, MMP-7, MMP-9 and MMP-12. It has little or no activity against unrelated metalloproteinases such as enkephalinase. Using animal cancer models, marimastat has been observed to inhibit tumor growth and metastasis (Brown, 1997; Nemunaitis et al, 1998). Administration of the compound to healthy volunteers suggested a rapidly absorbed and well tolerated drug, with pharmacokinetic data indicating that total daily doses of 50–100 mg would achieve blood levels greater than 40 µg/l (Millar et al, 1998). Unfortunately, the development of marimastat was problematic in that, as an anti-tumor drug, it was not expected to induce the reduction in tumor size associated with conventional cytotoxic drugs (Steward, 1999).

Batimastat and marimastat are examples of RHS inhibitors with the ZBG on the left end, which has prompted several research groups to establish SAR considerations for this type of MMPIs. Figure 8 shows the summary of SARs, which apply to most MMPIs with a succinyl scaffold (Beckett et al, 1996).

These inhibitors are clearly different from LHS inhibitors like the Spilburg inhibitor (Moore and Spilburg, 1986) composed of Pro-Leu-Gly-NHOH and carrying the ZBG on the right end. From this, we undertook additional efforts to develop hydroxamate derivatives of substrate-analogous peptides that carry the ZBG in the middle (Krumme, Wenzel and Tschesche, 1998). The precursor of the hydroxamate ZBG is an aminomalonic acid in position P_1 (Figure 9).

This new scaffold allows the addition of various substituents to gain maximum attachment to the entire binding sites of the target enzyme. The most important feature of this type of inhibitor is the peptide backbone built up by

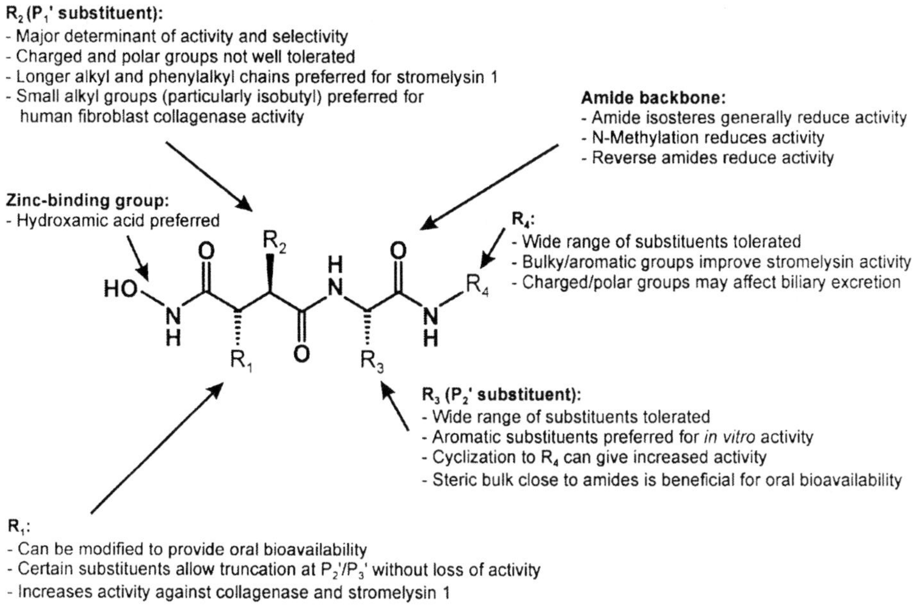

R$_2$ (P$_1$' substituent):
- Major determinant of activity and selectivity
- Charged and polar groups not well tolerated
- Longer alkyl and phenylalkyl chains preferred for stromelysin 1
- Small alkyl groups (particularly isobutyl) preferred for human fibroblast collagenase activity

Amide backbone:
- Amide isosteres generally reduce activity
- N-Methylation reduces activity
- Reverse amides reduce activity

Zinc-binding group:
- Hydroxamic acid preferred

R$_4$:
- Wide range of substituents tolerated
- Bulky/aromatic groups improve stromelysin activity
- Charged/polar groups may affect biliary excretion

R$_3$ (P$_2$' substituent):
- Wide range of substituents tolerated
- Aromatic substituents preferred for *in vitro* activity
- Cyclization to R$_4$ can give increased activity
- Steric bulk close to amides is beneficial for oral bioavailability

R$_1$:
- Can be modified to provide oral bioavailability
- Certain substituents allow truncation at P$_2$'/P$_3$' without loss of activity
- Increases activity against collagenase and stromelysin 1

Figure 8. Summary of structure-activity relationships for right-hand side MMP inhibitors.

α-amino acids to comprise the positions P3 to P$_3$' at least, giving these compounds the same basic frame as a peptide substrate. In agreement with the specifity of the tested MMPs, the P$_3$ position of these inhibitors is occupied by a proline and the P$_2$ position is an aliphatic amino acid, whereby leucine or alanine is preferred. The best inhibitory properties were obtained with the bulky tyrosyl benzylether moiety in the P$_1$' position (Figures 9 and 10).

Inhibitor no. 4, for example, shows a nearly 400-fold inhibitory discrimination between MMP-9 and the catalytic domain of human neutrophil collagenase (cdMMP-8). Other derivatives of this series of MMPIs discriminate between MMP-9 and cdMT1-MMP by three to four orders of magnitude (Tschesche and Krumme, 2000). Despite their peptide character these inhibitors are resistant to hydrolysis by proteinases. Testing of these compounds in animal models of human cancer is under way.

5. NEXT GENERATION MMP-INHIBITORS

In order to develop selective MMPIs with good oral bioavailability, a new concept of inhibitor design has been followed. The discovery and disclosure of CGS-27023A, a small non peptidic MMP inhibitor at Ciba-Geigy in the mid-

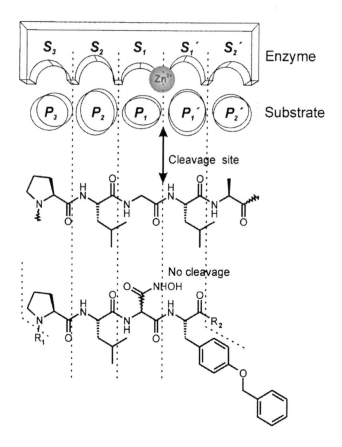

Figure 9. Design of combined left/right-hand side MMP inhibitors derived from aminomalonic acid.

1990's represented a major advance with this concept (Lombard et al, 1998; MacPherson et al, 1997) (Figure 11).

The obvious potential of a small molecule inhibitor to overcome the pharmacokinetic problems associated with peptides, such as poor absorption and metabolic lability, attracted the interest of a large number of research groups and has led to several promising compounds based on the sulfonylamino hydroxamic acid scaffold. Related compounds have also been independently identified by other research groups through high throughput screening. In general, these inhibitors have a ZBG like hydroxamic acid, carboxylic acid or thiol and a group capable of acting as a hydrogen bond acceptor (HBA) like sulfone, ether or ketone spaced apart by two atoms (Figure 12).

The HBA group is typically substituted with an aryl group (AG) which interacts with the S_1' site. In general the size of the P_1' substituent determines

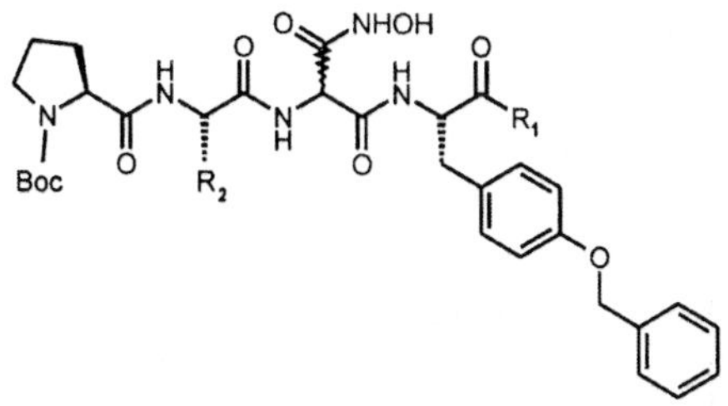

Compound no.	R₁	R₂	MMP-9	cdMMP-8
1	NH-R-CH(Ph)CH$_3$	H	4.0×10^{-7}	6.5×10^{-6}
2	NH-S-CH(Ph)CH$_3$	H	$>10^{-7}$	1.8×10^{-5}
3	NH-R-CH(c-C$_6$H$_{11}$)CH$_3$	H	$>10^{-7}$	1.4×10^{-5}
4	NH-S-CH(Ph)CH$_3$	CH$_3$	5.0×10^{-9}	1.9×10^{-6}
5	NH-R-CH(Ph)CH$_3$	CH$_2$-CH(CH$_3$)$_2$	5.0×10^{-9}	8.0×10^{-7}
6	NH-S-CH(Ph)CH$_3$	CH$_2$-CH(CH$_3$)$_2$	5.0×10^{-9}	8.0×10^{-7}
7	NH-R-CH(c-C$_6$H$_{11}$)CH$_3$	CH$_2$-CH(CH$_3$)$_2$	1.8×10^{-8}	2.5×10^{-6}

Figure 10. MMP inhibition data (K$_i$ values in mol/l) for aminomalonic acid derivatives.

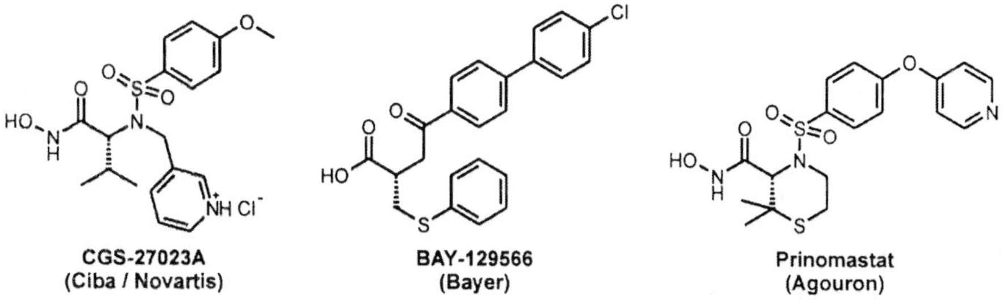

Figure 11. MMP inhibitors reported to be evaluated in clinical trials.

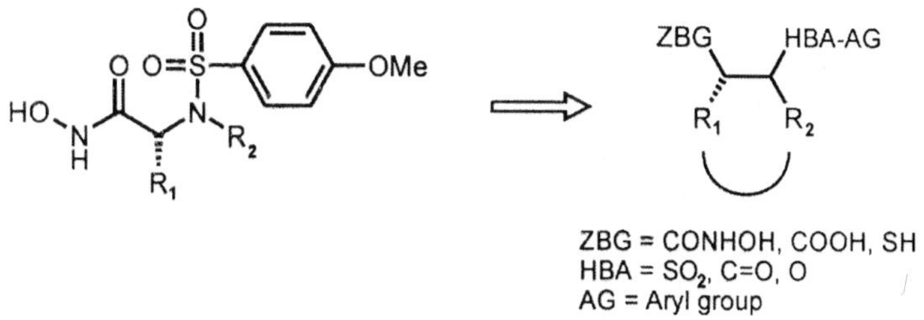

ZBG = CONHOH, COOH, SH
HBA = SO$_2$, C=O, O
AG = Aryl group

Figure 12. Development of non-peptidic MMP inhibitors.

139

selectivity, with monophenyl groups usually resulting in broad spectrum inhibition and with larger biaryls which are often linked through an oxygen providing selectivity over MMP-1 and MMP-7 (Michaelides and Curtin, 1999). Exceptions from this trend also exist.

Representative examples of this series of MMPIs are the biphenylbutyric acid derivative (BAY-129566) and the heterocyclic sulfonamide Prinomastat (AG-3340), (Figure 11). Researchers at Bayer developed a unique series of γ-keto carboxylic acids leading to the clinical candidate BAY-129566. As with the sulfonamide CGS-27023A, the key to the discovery of this breakthrough series was high throughput screening, which identified a fenbufen derivative as a micromolar MMP-3 inhibitor. An exhaustive examination of the SARs of the α-position and the terminal phenyl substitution led to BAY-129566. This is the only MMP inhibitor under clinical investigation that is a carboxylic acid. In preclinical studies, the inhibitory activities in both *in vitro* and *in vivo* models of matrix invasion, malignant angiogenesis and tumor growth were noteable (Nelson et al, 2000). The compound was active in various models of tumor metastases. In a subcutaneously implanted Lewis Lung carcinoma that spontaneously metastasized to the lungs daily oral treatment of mice with this inhibitor beginning 3 days after implantation delayed the growth of primary tumors by 50% and reduced the total number of lung metastases and lung lesions by up to 90%. The agent also inhibited the growth of well-established subcutaneous xeno-grafts of human colon carcinomas. Preclinical pharmacologic studies in mice, rats, guinea pigs and dogs indicated that BAY-129566 is highly bioavailable after oral administration, with peak plasma concentrations attained by 0.5 to 2 hours. Hepatotoxicity, characterized by reversible elevations in serum transaminases, was the principal toxic effect of the compound in both rodents and dogs (Gatto et al, 1999). It is further noteable, that the recommended dose for subsequent disease-directed studies is 800 mg twice daily to achieve biologically relevant pharmacologic profiles. Unfortunately, further development of BAY-129566 was abandoned because no positive effects could be revealed in humans in a clinical phase III trial (Nelson, 1998).

The discovery of CGS-27023A has provided the drive to design more potent non-peptide inhibitors of MMP-3, the gelatinases (MMP-2, MMP-9) and collagenase-3 (MMP-13). Agouron has disclosed a series of related aryloxy-phenyl-sulfonyl compounds that display selectivity for certain MMPs (Zook et al, 1997). X-ray crystallographic analysis of the Novartis compound CGS-25966, a close analogue of CGS-27023A, complexed to the catalytic domain of MMP-1 revealed two opportunities for structural modification. Firstly, the D-valine side-chain and the benzyl group could be replaced by a six-membered ring, thereby introducing a beneficial ligand pre-organisation. Secondly, the 4-methoxyphenyl-sulfonyl group that occupies the S_1' pocket is sub-optimal in other members of the MMP family and addition of a second aromatic ring in place of the methyl group resulted in increased potency and selectivity. The unique combination of the described modifications led to the development of Agouron's compound Prinomastat (AG-3340) (Bender, 1997) (Figure 11). Ultimately, the choice of AG-3340 over other candidates was based on pharmacokinetic properties and efficiacy in animal models of cancer (Santos et al, 1997; Shalinsky et al, 1999). When administered intraperitoneally in the Lewis Lung carcinoma model, the compound abolished primary tumor growth in 4 out of 6 mice. In addition, the formation of secondary tumors greater than 5 mm in diameter was reduced by 90%. Clinical studies with this compound are under way.

6. ALTERNATIVE CHELATORS

Several studies suggest that the hydroxamate function is the best zinc-chelating group for the development of potent inhibitors of MMPs. However, concerns about the unfavorable pharmacokinetics of hydroxamates, poor solubility, and potential for chronic toxicities arising from metabolic activation of the hydrox-amate group have stimulated the development of MMP inhibitors based on other zinc-chelating groups. Pharmacia and Upjohn has identified a series of MMP-3 inhibitors with a 5-amino-1,3,4-thiadiazole-2-thione zinc binding group linked to the peptide fragment by a urea moiety (Jacobsen et al, 1999). The compounds were moderately effective stromelysin inhibitors with K_i values between 0.3 and 1.0 µM. The most effective analogues utilized an L-phenylalanine as the amino acid component. Stromelysin inhibition was further improved using a pentafluorophenylalanine substituent. The SARs for analogues described within this series can be rationalized through a recently attained stromelysin/inhibitor X-ray structure. As showed in Figure 13 the compound binds to stromelysin completely on the unprimed side of the enzyme substrate binding cleft. The thiocarbonyl group interacts with the catalytic zinc with the remainder of the inhibitor located towards the S_1 to S_3 portion of stromelysin. The NH group on the thiadiazole core participates in a bifurcated hydrogen bond to the carboxy-late of glutamate 202. The other thiadiazole nitrogen accepts a hydrogen bond from alanine 167. Furthermore, both urea hydrogens participate in a hydrogen bond to the carbonyl of alanine 167 on the stromelysin backbone (Finzel et al, 1998). Clinical studies with this series of MMPIs have not been published.

As part of a collaborative effort, we have undertaken the structure-based design and synthesis of potent matrix metalloproteinase inhibitors derived from a thiadiazine scaffold (Schröder et al, 2001). A series of chiral 6-methyl-1,3,4-thiadiazines previously reported (Jira et al, 1994; Pfeiffer, Dilk and Bulka, 1977, 1978; Szulzewsky et al, 1993) were assayed with the catalytic domain of neu-

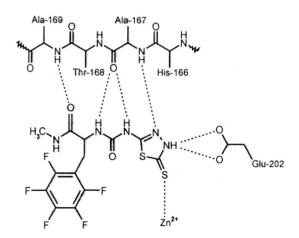

Figure 13. Hydrogen bonding between a thiadiazole-2-thione inhibitor and the stromelysin active site.

trophil collagenase (cdMMP-8) as the screening enzyme. From this, a small number of compounds were determined to be competitive inhibitors with weak (K_i > 40 μM) inhibitory activity (Figure 14).

Further chemical modifications, including lack of the 6-methyl group, resulted in novel 6H-1,3,4-thiadiazine derivatives, which are potent inhibitors of matrix metalloproteinases with an exceptional binding mode to the active site. As a first approach we focused on preparing 5-substituted-6H-1,3,4-thia-diazine-2-amides with a sulfonamide moiety to improve primed site activity. The promising concept of these novel sulfonamide inhibitors prompted us to establish SAR considerations which apply to most of the 6H-1,3,4-thiadiazines tested as MMPIs (Figure 15).

The class in general inhibits cdMMP-2, cdMMP-8, MMP-9 and cdMMP-14 selectively in the nanomolar range. Depending on functional group manipulations within the compound series the inhibition of these MMPs showed great variability. On the other hand, the inhibition of MMP-1 and cdMMP-12 was less potent relative to the other enzymes and demonstrated very few variations

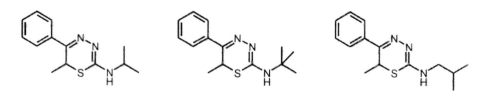

Figure 14. Chiral thiadiazine-based screening leads.

142

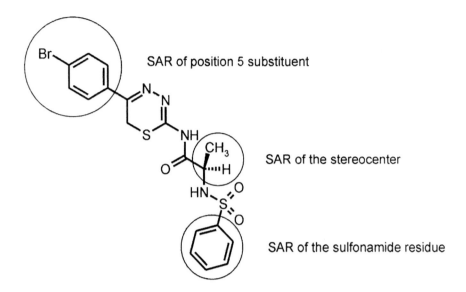

Figure 15. Optimized result of structure-activity relationship studies on thiadiazine-based MMP inhibitors.

in potency as functional groups were altered. Surprisingly the inhibition of cdMMP-13, in general, occurs in the micromolar to submicromolar range within the tested 6*H*-1,3,4-thiadiazine series. The unique combination of the observed SARs produced the best selective inhibitor (2R)-N-[5-(4-bromophenyl)-6*H*-1,3,4-thiadiazin-2-yl]-2-[(phenylsulfonyl)amino]propanamide with high affinity for MMP-9 (K_i = 40 nM), (Figure 15). A crystal structure of the catalytic domain of human neutrophil collagenase (cdMMP-8) complexed with N-allyl-5-(4-chlorophenyl)-6*H*-1,3,4-thiadiazin-2-amine hydrobromide was determined (Schröder et al, 2001) (Figure 16). This structure has provided insight into the key enzyme-inhibitor interactions which played a role in the exceptional binding of 6*H*-1,3,4-thiadiazine based MMP inhibitors.

In contrast to the established MMP-inhibitors which exclusively bind to the primed side, the compounds described interact with both the primed and the unprimed side of the MMP. Furthermore, the conformational rigidity of the series may be advantageous as a means to obtain the observed selectivity. Studies of thiadiazine-based MMPIs in a syngenetic mouse-lymphoma model are under way.

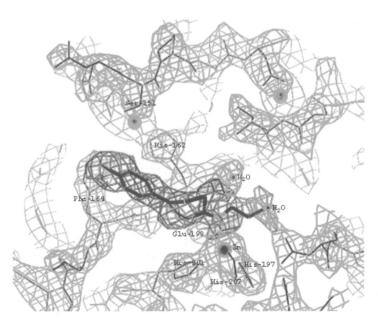

Figure 16. View of the electron density at the active site of the catalytic domain of human neutrophil collagenase (cdMMP-8) complexed with N-allyl-5-(4-chlorophenyl)-6*H*-1,3,4-thiadiazin-2-amine.

7. ALTERNATIVE APPROACHES TO THE DEVELOPMENT OF MMP INHIBITORS

Several alternative strategies exist for the development of synthetic MMP inhibitors. One of these approaches is based on the cysteine switch mechanism of the MMPs, in which proforms of these enzymes are inhibited by a highly conserved sequence in the prosegment, which is cleaved on activation (Stetler-Stevenson et al, 1989; Van Wart and Birkedal-Hansen, 1990). This sequence contains a cysteine residue that is believed to coordinate the active site zinc atom, thereby maintaining enzyme latency. This linear peptide sequence (MRKPRCGN/VPDV) has been shown to exhibit inhibitory activity against gelatinase A and stromelysin and to inhibit the MMP-dependent invasion of tumor cells through a reconstituted basement membrane *in vitro* (Melchiori et al, 1992; Stetler-Stevenson et al, 1991). The peptide has also been shown to block neurite outgrowth on reconstituted extracellular matrix, as well as endothelial cell invasion in models of Kaposi's sarcoma (Benelli et al, 1994; Muir, 1994).

Irreversible MMP-inhibitors (Ghosh and Mosbashery, 1991), peptidic ketomethylene isostere-based collagenase inhibitors (Wallace et al, 1986), non-peptide inhibitors of MMP-8 and bacterial collagenases, based on tetracyclines, anthraquinones and aranciamycin (Bols et al, Golub et al, 1987, Greenwald et al, 1992, Tanaka et al, 1990) have also been reported. Although the activities are generally very weak in comparison to many of the inhibitors described in this review, these compounds may provide leads for drug design work.

8. CONCLUSION

The design and synthesis of inhibitors of matrix metalloproteinases continues to be a prominent area of pharmaceutical research. Both peptide- and nonpeptide-based inhibitors are in clinical studies for various indications. The concept of antiproteolytic tumor therapy has not yet been fully exploited. The open question remaining is whether inhibitors of broadspectrum specificity are preferred over more specific and selective MMP (or ADAM) inhibitors for individual malignant and degenerative diseases. There are some indications for the latter approach. It is important to realize that tumors from different tissues are different in enzyme expression and regulation and obviously require different therapeutic approaches. At the time it is still unclear, if suppression of the activity of one or more proteolytic enzymes by physiological or synthetic inhibitors could stimulate genetic expression of other substitute enzymes. The search for new and improved alternatives to the hydroxamic acid zinc chelator continues. Numerous classes of surrogates have been exploited with varying success. In the present case, syntheses of a series of 6H-1,3,4-thiadiazines have been accomplished to furnish nanomolar MMPIs.

REFERENCES

Babine RE, Bender SL. Molecular recognition of protein-ligand complexes: applications to drug design. Chem Rev 1997; 97: 1359–1472.

Beattie GJ, Smyth JF. Phase I study of intraperitoneal metalloproteinase inhibitor BB94 in patients with malignant ascites. Clin Cancer Res 1998; 4: 1899–1902.

Beckett RP, Davidson AH, Drummond AH, Huxley P, Whittaker M. Recent advances in matrix metalloproteinase inhibitor research. Drug Disc Today 1996; 1: 16–26.

Beckett RP, Whittaker M. Matrix metalloproteinase inhibitors 1998. Exp Opin Ther Patents 1998; 8: 259–282.

Bender SL. Structure-based design of MMP inhibitors: discovery and development of AG-3340. 214th ACS Meeting, Las Vegas, 7–11 September 1997, MEDI 108.

Benelli R, Adatia R, Ensoli B, Stetler-Stevenson WG, Santi L, Albini A. Inhibition of AIDS-Kaposi's sarcoma cell induced endothelial cell invasion by TIMP-2 and a synthetic peptide from the metalloproteinase propeptide: implications for an anti-angiogenic therapy. Oncol Res 1994; 6: 251–257.

Bode W, Reinemer P, Huber R, Kleine T, Schnierer S, Tschesche H. The X-ray crystal structure of the catalytic domain of human neutrophil collagenase inhibited by a substrate analogue reveals the essentials for catalysis and specificity. EMBO J 1994; 13: 1263–1269.

Bode W, Fernandez-Catalan C, Tschesche H, Grams F, Nagase H, Maskos K. Structural properties of matrix metalloproteinases. Cell Mol Life Sci 1999a; 55: 639–652.

Bode W, Fernandez-Catalan C, Grams F, Gomis-Rüth FX, Nagase H, Tschesche H, Maskos K. Insights into MMP-TIMP interactions. Ann NY Acad Sci 1999b; 878: 73–91.

Bols M, Binderup L, Hansen J, Rasmussen P. Inhibition of collagenase by aranciamycin and aranciamycin derivatives. J Med Chem 1992; 35: 2768–2771.

Borkakoti N, Winkler FK, Williams DH, D'Arcy A, Broadhurst MJ, Brown PA, Johnson WH, Murray EJ. Structure of the catalytic domain of human fibroblast collagenase complexed with an inhibitor. Nat Struct Biol 1994; 1: 106–110.

Broadhurst MJ, Johnson WH, Lawton G, Handa BK, Machin PJ. Phosphinic acid derivatives. European Patent EP0276436, 1988.

Brown PD. Clinical trials of a low molecular weight matrix metalloproteinase inhibitor in cancer. Ann NY Acad Sci 1994; 732: 217–221.

Brown PD. Matrix metalloproteinase inhibitors in the treatment of cancer. Med Oncol 1997; 14: 1–10.

Browner MF, Smith WW, Castelhano AL. Matrilysin-inhibitor complexes: common themes among metalloproteases. Biochemistry 1995; 34: 6602–6610.

Chambers AF, Matrisian LM. Changing views of the role of matrix metalloproteinases in metastasis. J Natl Cancer Inst 1997; 89: 1260–1270.

Chirivi RG, Garofalo A, Crimmin MJ, Bawden LJ, Stoppacciaro A, Brown PD, Giavazzi R. Inhibition of the metastatic spread and growth of B16-BL6 murine melanoma by a synthetic matrix metalloproteinase inhibitor. Int J Cancer 1994; 58: 460–464.

Coussens LM, Werb Z. Matrix metalloproteinases and the development of cancer. Chem Biol 1996; 3: 895–904.

Curran S, Murray GI. Matrix metallo-proteinases in tumour invasion and metastasis. J Pathol 1999; 189: 300–308.

Darlak K, Miller RB, Stack MS, Spatola AF, Gray RD. Thiol-based inhibitors of mammalian collagenase. Substituted amide and peptide derivatives of the leucine analogue, 2-[(R,S)-mercaptomethyl]-4-methylpentanoic acid. J Biol Chem 1990; 265: 5199–5205.

Dickens JP, Donald DK, Kneen G, Mckay WR. Hydroxamic acid based collagenase inhibitors. European Patent EP0214639, 1988.

Eccles SA, Box GM, Court WJ, Bone EA, Thomas W, Brown PD. Control of lymphatic and hematogenous metastasis of a rat mammary carcinoma by the matrix metalloproteinase inhibitor batimastat (BB-94). Cancer Res 1996; 56: 2815–2822.

Fernandez-Catalan C, Bode W, Huber R, Turk D, Calvete JJ, Lichte A, Tschesche H, Maskos K. Crystal structure of the complex formed by the membrane type 1-matrix metalloproteinase with the tissue inhibitor of metalloproteinases-2, the soluble progelatinase A receptor. EMBO J 1998; 17: 5238–5248.

Finzel BC, Baldwin ET, Bryant GL Jr, Hess GF, Wilks JW, Trepod CM, Mott JE, Marshall VP, Petzold GL, Poorman RA, O'Sullivan TJ, Schostarez HJ, Mitchell MA. Structural characterizations of nonpeptidic thiadiazole inhibitors of matrix metalloproteinases reveal the basis for stromelysin selectivity. Protein Sci 1998; 7: 2118–2126.

Friers W. Tumor necrosis factor: characterization at the molecular, cellular and in vivo level. FEBS Lett 1991; 285: 199–212.

Gatto C, Rieppi M, Borsotti P, Innocenti S, Ceruti R, Drudis T, Scanziani E, Casazza AM,

146

Taraboletti G, Giavazzi R. BAY 12-9566, a novel inhibitor of matrix metalloproteinases with antiangiogenic activity. Clin Cancer Res 1999; 5: 3603–3607.

Gavuzzo E, Pochetti G, Mazza F, Gallina C, Gorini B, D'Alessio S, Pieper M, Tschesche H, Tucker PA. Two crystal structures of human neutrophil collagenase, one complexed with a primed- and the other with an unprimed-side inhibitor: implications for drug design. J Med Chem 2000; 43: 3377–3385.

Ghosh SS, Mobashery S. N-acyl peptide metalloproteinase inhibitors and methods of using the same. World Patent WO9105555, 1991.

Golub LM, McNamara TF, D'Angelo G, Greenwald RA, Ramamurthy NS. A non-antibacterial chemically-modified tetracycline inhibits mammalian collagenase activity. J Dent Res 1987; 66: 1310–1314.

Gomis-Rüth FX, Maskos K, Betz M, Bergner A, Huber R, Suzuki K, Yoshida N, Nagase H, Brew K, Bourenkov GP, Bartunik H, Bode W. Mechanism of inhibition of the human matrix metalloproteinase stromelysin-1 by TIMP-1. Nature 1997; 389: 77–81.

Gooley PR, O'Connell JF, Marcy AI, Cuca GC, Salowe SP, Bush BL, Hermes JD, Esser CK, Hagmann WK, Springer JP, et al. The NMR structure of the inhibited catalytic domain of human stromelysin-1. Nat Struct Biol 1994; 1: 111–118.

Grams F, Crimmin M, Hinnes L, Huxley P, Pieper M, Tschesche H, Bode W. Structure determination and analysis of human neutrophil collagenase complexed with a hydroxamate inhibitor. Biochemistry 1995b; 34: 14012–14020.

Grams F, Reinemer P, Powers JC, Kleine T, Pieper M, Tschesche H, Huber R, Bode W. X-ray structures of human neutrophil collagenase complexed with peptide hydroxamate and peptide thiol inhibitors. Implications for substrate binding and rational drug design. Eur J Biochem 1995a; 228: 830–841.

Greenwald RA, Moak SA, Ramamurthy NS, Golub LM. Tetracyclines suppress matrix metalloproteinase activity in adjuvant arthritis and in combination with flurbiprofen, ameliorate bone damage. J Rheumatol 1992; 19: 927–938.

Jacobsen EJ, Mitchell MA, Hendges SK, Belonga KL, Skaletzky LL, Stelzer LS, Lindberg TJ, Fritzen EL, Schostarez HJ, O'Sullivan TJ, Maggiora LL, Stuchly CW, Laborde AL, Kubicek MF, Poorman RA, Beck JM, Miller HR, Petzold GL, Scott PS, Truesdell SE, Wallace TL, Wilks JW, Fisher C, Goodman LV, Kaytes PS, et al. Synthesis of a series of stromelysin-selective thiadiazole urea matrix metalloproteinase inhibitors. J Med Chem 1999; 42: 1525–1536.

Jira T, Pfeiffer WD, Lachmann K, Epperlein U. Syntheses and HPLC separation of chiral 1,3,4-thiadiazines and 1,3,4-selenadiazines. Pharmazie 1994; 49: 401–406.

Johnson LL, Dyer R, Hupe DJ. Matrix metalloproteinases. Curr Opin Chem Biol 1998; 2: 466–471.

Johnson WH, Roberts NA, Borkakoti N. Collagenase inhibitors: their design and potential therapeutic use. J Enzyme Inhib 1987; 2: 1–22.

Krüger A, Soeltl R, Sopov I, Kopitz C, Arlt M, Magdolen V, Harbeck N, Gänsbacher B, Schmitt M. Hydroxamate-type matrix metalloproteinase inhibitor batimastat promotes liver metastasis. Cancer Res 2001; 4: 1272–1275.

Krumme D, Wenzel H, Tschesche H. Hydroxamate derivatives of substrate-analogous peptides containing aminomalonic acid are potent inhibitors of matrix metalloproteinases. FEBS Lett 1998; 436: 209–212.

Kuno K, Kanada N, Nakashima E, Fujiki F, Ichimura, F, Matsushima K. Molecular cloning of a gene encoding a new type of metalloproteinase-disintegrin family protein with thrombospondin motifs as an inflammation associated gene. J Biol Chem 1997; 272: 556–562.

147

Lombard MA, Wallace TL, Kubicek MF, Petzold GL, Mitchell MA, Hendges SK, Wilks JW. Synthetic matrix metalloproteinase inhibitors and tissue inhibitor of metalloproteinase (TIMP)-2, but not TIMP-1, inhibit shedding of tumor necrosis factor-alpha receptors in a human colon adenocarcinoma (Colo 205) cell line. Cancer Res 1998; 58: 4001–4007.

Lovejoy B, Cleasby A, Hassell AM, Longley K, Luther MA, Weigl D, McGeehan G, McElroy AB, Drewry D, Lambert MH, et al. Structure of the catalytic domain of fibroblast collagenase complexed with an inhibitor. Science 1994; 263: 375–377.

MacPherson LJ, Bayburt EK, Capparelli MP, Carroll BJ, Goldstein R, Justice MR, Zhu L, Hu S, Melton RA, Fryer L, Goldberg RL, Doughty JR, Spirito S, Blancuzzi V, Wilson D, O'Byrne EM, Ganu V, Parker DT. Discovery of CGS 27023A, a non-peptidic, potent, and orally active stromelysin inhibitor that blocks cartilage degradation in rabbits. J Med Chem 1997; 40: 2525–2532.

Markwell RE, Hunter DJ, Ward RW. Peptides with collagenase inhibiting activity. European Patent EP0320118, 1989.

Markwell RE, Ward RW, Hunter DJ. Phosphonopeptides with collagenase inhibiting activity. World Patent WO9309136, 1993.

Melchiori A, Albini A, Ray JM, Stetler-Stevenson WG. Inhibition of tumor cell invasion by a highly conserved peptide sequence from the matrix metalloproteinase enzyme prosegment Cancer Res 1992; 52: 2353–2356.

Michaelides MR, Curtin ML. Recent advances in matrix metalloproteinase inhibitors research. Curr Pharm Design 1999; 5: 787–819.

Millar AW, Brown PD, Moore J, Galloway WA, Cornish AG, Lenehan TJ, Lynch KP. Results of single and repeat dose studies of the oral matrix metalloproteinase inhibitor marimastat in healthy male volunteers. Br J Clin Pharmacol 1998; 45: 21–26.

Moore WM, Spilburg CA. Purification of human collagenases with a hydroxamic acid affinity column. Biochemistry 1986; 25: 5189–5195.

Muir D. Metalloproteinase-dependent neurite outgrowth within a synthetic extra-cellular matrix is induced by nerve growth factor. Exp Cell Res 1994; 210: 243–252.

Murphy G, Allan JA, Willenbrock F, Cockett MI, O'Connell JP, Docherty AJ. The role of the C-terminal domain in collagenase and stromelysin specificity. J Biol Chem 1992; 267: 9612–9618.

Muskett FW, Frenkiel TA, Feeney J, Freedman RB, Carr MD, Williamson RA. High resolution structure of the N-terminal domain of tissue inhibitor of metalloproteinases-2 and characterization of its interaction site with matrix metalloproteinase-3. J Biol Chem 1998; 273: 21736–21743.

Nagase H, Das SK, Dey SK, Fowlkes JL, Huang W, Brew K. In: Hawkes SP, Edwards DR, Khokha R (eds), Inhibitors of Metalloproteinases in Development and Disease. Harwood, Lausanne, 1997.

Nelson AR, Fingleton B, Rothenberg ML, Matrisian LM. Matrix metalloproteinases: biologic activity and clinical implications. J Clin Oncol 2000; 18: 1135–1149.

Nelson NJ. Inhibitors of angiogenesis enter phase III testing. J Natl Cancer Inst 1998; 90: 960–963.

Nemunaitis J, Poole C, Primrose J, Rosemurgy A, Malfetano J, Brown P, Berrington A, Cornish A, Lynch K, Rasmussen H, Kerr D, Cox D, Millar A. Combined analysis of studies of the effects of the matrix metalloproteinase inhibitor marimastat on serum tumor markers in advanced cancer: selection of a biologically active and tolerable dose for longer-term studies. Clin Cancer Res 1998; 4: 1101–1109.

Odake S, Morita Y, Morikawa T, Yoshida N, Hori H, Nagai Y. Inhibition of matrix metalloproteinases by peptidyl hydroxamic acids. Biochem Biophys Res Comm 1994; 199: 1442–1446.

Parsons SL, Watson SA, Steele RJ. Phase I/II trial of batimastat, a matrix metalloproteinase inhibitor, in patients with malignant ascites. Eur J Surg Oncol 1997; 23: 526–531.

Pfeiffer WD, Dilk E, Bulka E. Über die Umsetzung von 4-Alkyl-thiosemicarbaziden mit α-Halogenketonen. Z Chem 1977; 17: 218–220.

Pfeiffer WD, Dilk E, Bulka E. Zur Reaktivität von 2-tert. Butylamino- und 2-(2,2,4-Trimethyl-pent-4-yl)amino-1,3,4-thiadiazinen. Z Chem 1978; 18: 65–66.

Rasmussen HS, McCann PP. Matrix metalloproteinase inhibition as a novel anticancer strategy: a review with special focus on batimastat and marimastat. Pharmacol Therapeut 1997; 75: 69–75.

Reiter LA. Cyclobutyl-aryloxyarylsulfonylamino hydroxamic acid derivatives. United States Patent US6156798, 2000.

Santos O, McDermott CD, Daniels RG, Appelt K. Rodent pharmacokinetic and anti-tumor efficacy studies with a series of synthetic inhibitors of matrix metalloproteinases. Clin Exp Metastasis 1997; 15: 499–508.

Schnierer S, Kleine T, Gote T, Hillemann A, Knäuper V, Tschesche H. The recombinant catalytic domain of human neutrophil collagenase lacks type I collagen substrate specificity. Biochem Biophys Res Comm 1993; 191: 319–326.

Schröder J, Henke A, Wenzel H, Brandstetter H, Stammler HG, Stammler A, Pfeiffer WD, Tschesche H. Structure-based design and synthesis of potent matrix metalloproteinase inhibitors derived from a thiadiazine scaffold. J Med Chem 2001; 44: 3231–3243.

Schwartz MA, Van Wart HE. Synthetic inhibitors of bacterial and mammalian interstitial collagenases. Prog Med Chem 1992; 29: 271–334.

Shalinsky DR, Brekken J, Zou H, McDermott CD, Forsyth P, Edwards D, Margosiak S, Bender S, Truitt G, Wood A, Varki NM, Appelt K. Broad antitumor and antiangiogenic activities of AG3340, a potent and selective MMP inhibitor undergoing advanced oncology clinical trials. Ann NY Acad Sci 1999; 878: 236–270.

Spurlino JC, Smallwood AM, Carlton DD, Banks TM, Vavra KJ, Johnson JS, Cook ER, Falvo J, Wahl RC, Pulvino TA, et al. 1.56 Å structure of mature truncated human fibroblast collagenase. *Proteins* 1994; **19**: 98–109.

Stams T, Spurlino JC, Smith DL, Wahl RC, Ho TF, Qoronfleh MW, Banks TM, Rubin B. Structure of human neutrophil collagenase reveals large S_1' specificity pocket. Nat Struct Biol 1994; 1: 119–123.

Stetler-Stevenson WG, Krutzsch HC, Wacher MP, Margulies IM, Liotta LA. The activation of human type IV collagenase proenzyme: Sequence identification of the major conversion product following organomercurial activation. J Biol Chem 1989; 264: 1353–1356.

Stetler-Stevenson WG, Talano JA, Gallagher ME, Krutzsch HC, Liotta LA. Inhibition of human type IV collagenase by a highly conserved peptide sequence derived from its prosegment. Am J Med Sci 1991; 302: 163–170.

Steward WP. Marimastat (BB2516): current status of development. Cancer Chemother Pharmacol 1999; 43: S56–60.

Szulzewsky K, Pfeiffer WD, Bulka E, Rossberg H, Schulz B. The crystal-structures of 2-isopropylamino-6-methyl-5-phenyl-6H-1,3,4-thiadiazine and 2-isopropylamino-6-methyl-5-phenyl-6H-1,3,4-selenadiazine. Acta Chem Scand 1993; 47: 302–306.

Tanaka T, Metori K, Mineo S, Matsumoto H, Satoh T. Studies on collagenase inhibitors: II. Inhibitory effects of anthraquinones on bacterial collagenase. J Pharm Soc Jpn 1990; 110: 688–692.

Taraboletti G, Garofalo A, Belotti D, Drudis T, Borsotti P, Scanziani E, Brown PD, Giavazzi R. Inhibition of angiogenesis and murine hemangioma growth by batimastat, a synthetic inhibitor of matrix metalloproteinases. J Natl Cancer Inst 1995; 87: 293–298.

149

Tschesche H, Krumme D. Matrix metalloproteinase inhibitors containing aminomalonic acid derivatives and peptide backbone modified derivatives thereof. World Patent WO0002904, 2000.

Van Wart HE, Birkedal-Hansen H. The cysteine switch: a principle of regulation of metalloproteinase activity with potential applicability to the entire matrix metalloproteinase gene family. Proc Natl Acad Sci (USA) 1990; 87: 5578–5582.

Vassiliou S, Mucha A, Cuniasse P, Georgiadis D, Lucet-Levannier K, Beau F, Kannan R, Murphy G, Knäuper V, Rio MC, Basset P, Yiotakis A, Dive V. Phosphinic pseudo-tripeptides as potent inhibitors of matrix metalloproteinases: a structure-activity study. J Med Chem 1999; 42: 2610–2620.

Vincenti MP, Clark IM, Brinckerhoff CE. Using inhibitors of metallo-proteinases to treat arthritis. Easier said than done? Arthritis Rheum 1994; 37: 1115–1126.

Wallace DA, Bates SR, Walker B, Kay G, White J, Guthrie DJ, Blumson NL, Elmore DT. Competitive inhibition of human skin collagenase by N-benzyloxycarbonyl-L-prolyl-L-alanyl-3-amino-2-oxopropyl-L-leucyl-L-alanylglycine ethyl ester. Biochem J 1986; 239: 797–799.

Wang X, Fu X, Brown PD, Crimmin MJ, Hoffman RM. Matrix metalloproteinase inhibitor BB-94 (batimastat) inhibits human colon tumor growth and spread in a patient-like orthotopic model in nude mice. Cancer Res 1994; 54: 4726–4728.

Watson SA, Morris, TM, Parsons SL, Steele RJ, Brown PD. Therapeutic effect of the matrix metalloproteinase inhibitor, batimastat, in a human colorectal cancer ascites model. Brit J Cancer 1996; 74: 1354–1358.

Woessner JF Jr. Matrix metalloproteinases and their inhibitors in connective tissue remodeling. FASEB J 1991; 5: 2145–2154.

Wu E, Croucher PI, McKie N. Expression of members of the novel membrane linked metalloproteinase family ADAM in cells derived from a range of haematological malignancies. Biochem Biophys Res Comm 1997; 235: 437–442.

Yong VW, Krekoski CA, Forsyth PA, Bell R, Edwards DR. Matrix metalloproteinases and diseases of the CNS. Trends Neurosci 1998; 21: 75–80.

Zook SE, Dagnino R Jr, Deason ME, Bender SL, Melnick MJ. Metalloproteinase inhibitors, pharmaceutical compositions containing them and their pharmaceutical uses, and methods and intermediates useful for their preparation. World Patent WO9720824, 1997.

Chapter 8

TRANSCRIPTIONAL CONTROL OF PROTEASES

H. Allgayer[1], E. Lengyel[2] and D. D. Boyd[3]

[1] *Department Surgery, Klinikum Grosshadern Ludwig-Maximilians University, Munich, D-81377, Germany;* [2] *Department of Obstetrics and Gynecology, Technical University of Munich, Munich 81675, Germany;* [3] *Department of Cancer Biology, M.D. Anderson Cancer Center, Houston, Texas 77303, USA*

1. TRANSCRIPTION FACTORS REGULATING PROTEASE EXPRESSION

There is now ample evidence implicating proteases in tissue remodeling both in physiological (wound repair, mammary involution) and in pathological conditions such as invasive cancer. In these cases, the amount of a protease or proteases are increased leading to sustained extracellular matrix turnover. The increased production of proteases can be ascribed to increased gene transcription and reduced mRNA turnover. In this chapter we will focus on the transcriptional regulation of proteases in cancer and describe some of the *trans* activators that have been shown by various investigators to modulate protease expression. Although we now have extensive knowledge of various *trans*-acting factors, it is unlikely, however, that the control of gene expression by such a limited number of transcription factors can entirely account for the finely-tuned expression of proteases evident in cancer. In this regard, recent studies on gene expression have implicated chromatin-remodeling activities in the regulation of gene expression and these 'activities' may provide an additional level of control of gene expression. The implications of such findings will also be discussed.

1.1. AP-1 family of transcription factors

Activator protein (AP-1) is a sequence-specific transcriptional activator composed of members of the Jun (c-Jun, JunB, JunD) and Fos (c-Fos, Fra-1, Fra-2, and FosB) families of transcription factors. AP-1 was first found as a transcription factor that mediates gene induction by the phorbol ester tumor promoter TPA (12-O-tetradecanoylphorbol-13-acetate), but is also induced by many other stimuli including growth factors, oncogenes, T cell activators,

J.-M. Foidart and R.J. Muschel (eds.), Proteases and Their Inhibitors in Cancer Metastasis, 151–168.

neurotransmitters, and UV irradiation. The AP-1 family member belong to the bZIP group of DNA binding proteins and bind to the TPA response element (TRE: 5'-TGAGTCA-3') in the promoter of many genes. Different AP-1 proteins associate to form a variety of Jun/Jun-homodimers or Jun/Fos-heterodimers that bind to DNA with different affinities and effect (Karin et al, 1997). This myriad of homo- and heterodimers is responsible for the diverse biological effects of distinct AP-1 complexes which ranges from activation to inhibition of gene expression. Two main mechanisms are involved in induction of AP-1 activity. First, at the transcriptional level, AP-1 family members are induced as part of the 'early response' reaction of the cell to stress through several *cis* elements in their promoter. Second, the activity of both preexisting and newly synthesized AP-1 components are modulated through phosphorylation. For example phosphorylation of c-Jun at Ser-73 and Ser-63, located within the transactivation domain increases its ability to activate transcription as either a homodimer or a heterodimer (Deng and Karin, 1995; Karin, 1999).

Members of the metalloproteinase (MMP) family have in general a similar gene organization. They share a common 10-exon structure and contain in their promoter region a TRE and a polyomavirus enhancer activator 3 (PEA-3) consensus site in addition to the typical TATA box (except MMP-2/gelatinase A and MMP-1/stromelysin-3 which have no TATA box) (Westermarck and Kahari, 1999). This common organization suggests a similar regulatory mechanism of gene transcription. A single AP-1 transcriptional binding site is found at approximately −70 base pair (bp) in the promoter region of most inducible MMP genes (Westermarck and Kahari, 1999). As an example, the proximal AP-1 site of the MMP-9 promoter (at −79 bp) is important for its constitutive activity in HT1080 synovial fibrosarcoma cells as shown in transient transfections (Sato and Seiki, 1993). Further, co-transfection of c-Jun and c-Fos expression plasmids stimulated MMP-9 promoter activity in the HT1080 cells (Sato and Seiki, 1993). The proximal AP-1 site of the MMP-9 promoter is not only important for constitutive activity but also for stimulation by the cytokine, TNF-α as well as the induction of MMP-9 by the oncogene H-Ras (Gum et al, 1996). Likewise, analysis of the MMP-1 promoter confirmed the importance of the proximal AP-1 site for constitutive and inducible promoter activity for this MMP gene. For the induction by H-Ras, the distal AP-1 motif at −533 was also required.

Chiu et al (1989) showed that different AP-1 family members exert different effects on the MMP-1 promoter. While c-Jun, as a homodimer, induces MMP-1 and via the proximal AP-1 site, JunB requires the presence of several AP-1 elements in the promoter or the simultaneous expression of c-Fos. White and Brinckerhoff (1995) further analyzed the MMP-1 promoter and presented evidence that mutation of the proximal AP-1 site abrogates basal promoter activity, but remains TPA-inducible. In contrast, mutation of the distal AP-1 site inhibited the inducible expression without much effect on basal MMP-1 promoter activity. Expression of antisense mRNAs for c-Jun also abrogated the induction of MMP-1 gene expression.

1.2. Ets family of transcription factors

Most MMP promoters (with the exception of MMP-2) also contain multiple PEA3 transcription factor binding sites which bind the Ets family of transcription factors. The Ets genes encode a growing family of transcription factors, whose best known members are c-ets-1, c-ets-2, Pu-1 and PEA3. Common to all Ets family members is the so called Ets domain (de Launoit et al, 1997) a region of about 85 amino acids which forms a helix-turn-helix DNA binding domain that binds to the core sequence 5'-GGAA/T-3'. The PEA3 element was identified as an oncogene responsive *cis*-element in the polyoma virus enhancer. A feature of many Ets domain proteins is that they form complexes with transcription factors of unrelated families (e.g. AP-1), thereby strengthening their relatively weak inherent transactivating abilities and, in some instances, their DNA-binding activity. Gutman and Waslyk (1990) were the first to describe a TPA- and oncogene-responsive unit (TORU) in a promoter comprised of PEA3 and AP-1 binding sites. On the interstitial collagenase (MMP-1) promoter, the PEA3 binding site acts synergistically with the AP-1 site to achieve maximum levels of transcription activation by TPA, and non-nuclear oncoproteins. Mutation of either the TRE site or the PEA3 site of MMP-1 reduced the induction of the promoter by TPA greater than 50%. This indicated the functional cooperation of the juxtaposed PEA3 and AP-1 transcription factor binding sites. Similarly, the inducibility of MMP-1 by fibronectin also required the presence of both the AP-1 and PEA3 motifs (Tremble et al, 1995).

A juxtaposed PEA3/AP-1 element also plays a crucial role in the transcriptional regulation of another protease, the serine protease urokinase (Lengyel et al, 1996). The region of the urokinase promoter important for regulation is located approximately 2 kb upstream of the transcriptional start site. Included in this important region is a proximal AP-1 binding site at –1875 and a combined PEA3/AP-1 site at –1965. The regulation through these sites is cell type specific. Thus, Nerlov et al (1991) showed that the PEA3/AP-1 element at –1965 had enhancer activity in HepG2 and HT1080 cells, but not in HeLa cells. Conversely, the proximal AP-1 site at –1875 was most important for basal activity in HeLa cells, but not in the other two cell lines. The reason for the different activities of both sites lies in their differential transcription factor binding properties: The PEA3/AP-1 site at –1965 preferentially binds a heterodimer composed of the ATF transcription factor family member ATF2 and Jun (Jun/ATF-2), whereas the proximal AP-1 site binds preferentially AP-1 family heterodimers (Jun/Fos)

153

(De Cesare et al, 1995). Binding of a Jun/ATF-2 heterodimer activates the PEA3/AP-1 site, however increasing amounts of c-Fos, can titrate c-Jun away from the c-Jun/ATF-2 heterodimer and result in a repression of urokinase promoter activity through the PEA3/AP-1 site (De Cesare et al, 1995). This is a good example that shows that the same transcription factor binding site can work either as an activator or a repressor, depending on the transcription factors binding to it. Presumably, this gives the cell the ability to direct gene expression through activation of a specific subset of transcription factors (Smith and Hager, 1999; Kornberg, 1999; Goodrich et al, 1996).

Watabe et al (1998) analyzed the effect of EGF on both MMP-9 and urokinase expression. Their results showed that stimulation of breast cancer cells by EGF increased the synthesis of both proteases. The induction of urokinase and MMP-9 expression was achieved, in part, by the transcription factors Ets-1 and Ets-2. Interestingly the most invasive breast cancer cell lines also exhibited a high expression of these two Ets family members (Watabe et al, 1998).

The common mechanisms regulating the expression of several proteases through AP-1 transcription factors raises the intriguing possibility that blocking AP-1 or Ets transcriptional activity might inhibit invasion and metastases of cancer cells. Indeed, truncated forms of Jun, lacking most of the transactivation domain act as transdominant negatives, suppressing AP-1 activity in the cell (Brown et al, 1993; Olive et al, 1997). A c-Jun construct in which the N-terminal amino acids are deleted (TAM 67) was found to reduce AP-1 activity on TRE reporter constructs and several TRE-containing promoters in mammalian cells, including the urokinase promoter (Lengyel et al, 1995b). This deletion mutant has also a more general effect on the cell by inhibiting and reversing transformation induced by oncogenes that signal through the Erk MAPK signal transduction pathway (Brown et al, 1993, 1994). Furthermore, down-regulation of AP-1 by 'anti-tumor promoters' such as aspirin and aspirin-like salicylates or retinoic acid inhibits transformation and tumor development. The Ets family is also a potential target for an antitumor therapy. A recent report (Xing et al, 2000) described that overexpression of PEA3 resulted in preferential inhibition of cell growth and tumor development of Her2/neu overexpressing cancer cells.

Taken together, both the Ap-1 and Ets family of transcription factors play a crucial role in regulation of tumor-associated proteases. Given an effective gene delivery systems both transcription factor family members are potentially novel targets for the development of an anti-tumor/invasive therapy.

1.3. Regulation of proteases by AP-2 transcription factors

AP-2 was first isolated from HeLa cells as a 52 kDa transcription factor which binds to a GCCNNNGGC motif. AP-2, or AP-2-related transcription factors, have been implicated in the regulation of expression of a number of protease genes including MMP-2 (Somasundaram et al, 1996; Mertens et al, 1998; Qin et al, 1999), MMP-9 (Munaut et al, 1999), u-PAR (Allgayer et al, 1999a), t-PA (Sumpio et al, 1997; Costa et al, 1998) and potentially MMP-1 (Aho et al, 1997). In most of these cases, AP-2 mediates constitutive gene expression, but in some cases this transcription factor is required for inducible expression (see below).

In several instances, AP-2 interacts with neighboring transcription factors to modulate gene expression. Indeed, there are examples of protease genes which are regulated by combined motifs which allow the binding of AP-2 (or AP-2-related proteins) and other transcription factors. The cis-elements for the different transcription factors can be juxtaposed or overlapping. Often, the Sp family transcription factors are involved as binding partners at combined AP-2 motifs. It may be that the function of these combined motifs is to mediate the different signals from separate signal transduction pathways. One example of this is the regulation of the urokinase-type plasminogen activator receptor (u-PAR) gene, encoding a receptor which promotes extracellular matrix degradation, invasion and metastasis in diverse epithelial carcinomas (Allgayer et al, 1999a, b). Mobility shifting experiments on nuclear extracts of a high u-PAR-expressing colon cancer cell line (RKO) indicated Sp1, Sp3 and a factor similar to, but distinct from, AP-2α bound to a promoter region spanning -152/-135 which contained overlapping, mismatched AP-2-and Sp-1 motifs. Mutations preventing the binding of the AP-2-related factor, but not Sp1 or Sp3, to this region reduced u-PAR promoter activity, indicating that the binding of the AP-2-related factor was required for constitutive promoter activity. Conversely, mutations preventing both AP-2α-like and Sp1/Sp3 binding reduced the u-PAR promoter stimulation by PMA in a low-u-PAR-expressing colon cancer cell line (GEO), indicating that both transcription factor families were mediating PMA-induced u-PAR-promoter activity. Moreover, while transient transfection of SW480 colon cancer cells with a plasmid encoding a constitutively active Src induced u-PAR-promoter activity, mutations preventing Sp1-binding to this promoter region (-152/-135) abolished the induction by this oncogene. These latter findings were supported by the observation that in mobility shift assays increased Sp1 binding to region -152/-135 was evident with nuclear extracts of Src-transfected SW480 cells. Thus, constitutive, PMA-inducible and Src-inducible u-PAR gene expression are differentially mediated through transactivation via a common combined promoter sequence (-152/-135)

155

bound with AP-2α-related factor and Sp1/Sp3. It would appear that the different transcription factors mediate different stimuli leading to altered gene expression. A similar role of the combined AP-2/Sp1 motifs in the differential control of constitutive and inducible gene expression by AP-2 and Sp1 has been reported for the tissue-type plasminogen activator (t-PA) gene in endothelia (Costa et al, 1998). In contrast, while the constitutive expression of another protease, MMP-2, is regulated by the same transcription factors as u-PAR (AP-2, Sp1 and Sp3), experimental evidence indicates that, they act independently (Qin et al, 1999).

Another example of a transcription factor interacting with AP-2 to regulate the expression of a protease gene is YB-1. This single-standed DNA binding transcription factor has been reported to directly interact with AP-2 in the form of AP-2/YB-1 heteromeric complexes at a 40bp-enhancer element (RE-1) of the 5′ flanking region of the MMP-2 gene (Mertens et al, 1998). These complexes generate an extended single-stranded DNA-regions and thus may facilitate the binding of additional proteins. The interaction of AP-2 with YB-1 at the RE-1 element results in a strong synergistic induction of MMP-2 transcription (160 fold) as compared to YB-1 induction alone (3-fold) or AP-2-binding alone which by itself even has a repressive effect on transcription. These examples illustrate how the interaction of AP-2 with other transcription factors can lead to the highly differential regulation of protease gene expression.

There are some studies suggesting that the effect of AP-2 as a transactivator of protease gene expression can be compromised by the E1A oncoprotein. Somasundaram et al (1996) showed that the adenovirus E1A protein physically interacts with AP-2 bound to an enhancer region of the MMP-2 gene and thereby represses MMP-2-gene expression. This suggests a mechanism by which E1A could repress a variety of cellular genes which are regulated by AP-2, including the genes which are involved in promoting tumor-associated proteolysis (for example, MMP-2, MMP-9, u-PAR, c-erbB-2) (Tan et al, 1997). Taken together, it is clear that AP-2 or AP-2-related transcription factors play an essential role in the differential regulation of gene expression of diverse proteases.

1.4. Regulation of proteases by the Sp family transcription factors

The Sp family of transcription factors (including Sp1, Sp2, Sp3 and Sp4), which binds to GC-rich nucleotide sequences, has been implicated in the regulation of a variety of protease genes such as MMP-9 (Farina et al, 1999), MMP-2 (Qin et al, 1999), cathepsin D (Wang et al, 2000), cathepsin B (Yan et al, 2000), MT1-MMP (Lohi et al, 2000), t-PA (Costa et al, 1998; Merchiers et al, 1999), and u-PAR (Allgayer et al, 1999a; Zannetti et al, 2000). Most often, the regulation is achieved by the binding of Sp1 transcription factor to the corresponding cis-element, but for cathepsin B (Yan et al, 2000), MMP-2 (Qin et al, 1999) and u-PAR (Allgayer et al, 1999a), the additional binding of other family members as Sp3 or Sp4 has been reported. The function of the latter in MMP-2 and cathepsin B gene expression is to activate promoter activity. However, regarding the regulation of u-PAR promoter activity, the role of Sp3 binding is not clear yet although current evidence (Allgayer et al, 1999a) indicates that it might be a repressor.

Most often, Sp1 binding mediates basal promoter activity of the protease genes mentioned. However, there are exceptions to this rule. For example, Sp1 was shown to be required for the ability of Src to induce u-PAR expression. (Allgayer et al, 1999b). In addition, there are other examples indicating that Sp1, rather than just maintaining basal levels of transcription, can play distinct roles in inducible gene expression. Thus, for the induction of t-PA gene expression by retinoic acid, Merchiers et al (1999) demonstrated that Sp1 was bound to the CRE element of the t-PA gene.

Again, there are many examples where transactivation of gene expression by Sp1 requires an interaction with other transcription factors. Interactions with the AP-2 transcription factor in the context of the regulation of the genes for MMP-2, t-PA and u-PAR have been described previously. Another very interesting example is the IGF-1-dependent transcriptional activation of the cathepsin D gene in MCF-7 breast cancer cells which is brought about by estrogen receptor/Sp1 binding to GC-rich sites (Wang et al, 2000a). This is a novel finding implicating Sp1 in the ligand-independent, growth-factor activated action of a hormone-receptor, leading to the induction of transcription of a protease gene.

Interestingly, there are data indicating that, in addition to the regulation of protease genes by Sp1, this transcription factor may itself be activated by certain proteases. Edmead et al (1999) reported that the serine protease thrombin activates Sp1 binding as studied by EMSA analysis when using conditions appropriate to prevent the activity of cellular phosphatases. Another study by Zannetti et al (2000) suggests that, in addition to the activation of u-PAR gene transcription in breast cancer by Sp1, the binding of the u-PAR-ligand u-PA results in an induction of Sp1 binding leading to an increased amount of u-PAR protein in MDA-MB-431 breast cancer cells, thus representing a positive regulatory loop.

Taken together, the Sp three-zinc-finger family of transcription factors, and especially of Sp1, has been demonstrated to play distinct roles not only in the constitutive, but also the induced expression of diverse protease genes.

1.5. Regulation of proteases by NFκB

The transcription factor nuclear factor-kappa B (NF-κB), which binds the GGGRNTYYC DNA sequence, has been implicated in the regulation of several proteases including MMP-9 (92kD type IV collagenase). In a highly metastatic H-ras and v-myc transformed rat embryo cell line overexpressing MMP-9, it was demonstrated that NFκB, in addition to Sp1, Ets, AP-1 and a retinoblas-toma-binding element, regulated transcription of this gene (Himelstein et al, 1997). Another study by Farina et al (1999) suggested that NF-κB, together with a GT-box, mediates a switch to MMP-9 expression when neuroblastoma cells undergo spontaneous epithelial to neuroblast conversion. This is paralleled by an enhanced invasive capacity into basement membranes.

There is also evidence for a role of NF-κB in the regulation of the urokinase-type plasminogen activator. In an early study, Novak et al (1991) reported that a DNA element similar to the binding site for NF-κB and located around −1865 was required for the maximal transactivation of the urokinase gene in response to PMA, IL-1 and TNF-α. These studies were extended the following year in pioneering work from Hansen et al (1992). There, it was reported that the NF-κB-like motif in the urokinase promoter was bound with a complex of proteins recognized by anti-c-Rel and anti-p65 but not anti-p50 antibodies. This c-Rel-p65 complex was required for the PMA-dependent induction of uroki-nase gene expression in HepG2 cells. The functional significance of this latter observation was proven subsequently in work from Reuning and co-workers (1995) who convincingly showed that inhibition of NF-κB Rel A activity using antisense oligonucleotides suppressed the synthesis of urokinase but not its inhibitor PAI-1.

NF-κB activity is also involved in the regulation of u-PAR expression. Thus, in a recent study, Wang et al (2000b) implicated NF-κB bound to a non-con-sensus NF-κB motif in the constitutive expression of the u-PAR gene in HCT116 colon cancer cells. Co-transfection with a dominant-negative IκB-Kinase-2 expression vector reduced u-PAR promoter activity up to 75%, demonstrating that this region is required for promoter activity.

2. ROLE OF CHROMATIN IN THE REGULATION OF GENE EXPRESSION

So far, we have seen how protease expression is regulated by various *trans*-acting DNA-binding proteins. However, several lines of evidence suggest that the regulation of transcription is not merely a consequence of the binding of *trans*-acting factors to their recognition motifs. These include the following observations. (1) The regulation of expression of the 50,000–100,000 genes in any human cell cannot be accounted for by the limited number of transcription factors described to date. (2) In many instances, a gene contains consensus binding sites for a particular transcription factor and yet the gene is silent under conditions where the corresponding *trans*-acting factor is activated. For example, the 92 kda type IV collagenase and urokinase genes contains AP-1 and Ets motifs but are transcriptionally silent in tumor cells of colon or breast cancer in which AP-1 and Ets are constitutively active (Pyke et al, 1991, 1993; Nielsen et al, 1996). (3) In several reports, a divergence in promoter activity is observed between studies using transient transfected reporter plasmids (where the reporter is extrachromosomal) and integrated reporter genes. One of the earliest reports in this regard demonstrated that while deletion of the Sp1 binding site in the promoter of the human alpha-globin gene had no effect on reporter activity in transient transfections, stable integration of the deletion reporter plasmid into chromatin of the recipient cells yielded a 90% inhibition (Pondel et al, 1995).

2.1. Packaging of DNA into chromatin

So, if gene expression cannot entirely be accounted for by *trans*-acting factors binding to recognition sequences in the promoter, what other mechanisms exist for the control of gene expression? A discussion of some mechanisms requires knowledge of how DNA is packaged. In the nucleus, DNA is organized into chromatin the latter consisting of about 146 base pairs of sequence wrapped in 1.75 superhelical turns around a histone octamer containing two molecules each of histones H2A, H2B, H3 and H4 (Abe et al, 1999). This unit, referred to as a nucleosome, is repeated approximately every 200 base pairs as a nucleosomal array in chromosomal DNA. The functional consequence of this DNA packaging is considered to be restrictive for transcription factor access. Indeed, biochemical and genetic evidence indicate that nucleosomes are repressive for transcription (Abe et al, 1999).

In the last five years, a great deal of light has been shed on the mechanisms capable of modifying chromatin structure to increase access to transcription factors. These mechanisms can be broadly divided into (a) those functioning as motors to disrupt nucleosomes (ATP-driven chromatin remodeling complexes) and (b) enzymatic machinery that chemically modify histones via acetylation (histone acetyl transferases-HATs) or deacetylation (histone deacetylases-HDACs).

159

2.2. Re-modeling of chromatin alters gene transcription

There are now several reports demonstrating that these two types of chromatin-remodeling activities are involved in the regulation of gene expression. Below are a few examples of how gene expression is altered by either of these activities.

2.2.1. *Histone acetylation/deacetylation*
Previous studies of the integrated, transcriptionally silent, human immunodeficiency virus type 1 (HIV-1) gene has revealed its insensitivity to the transcription factor NF-κB (El Kharroubi et al, 1999). However, this unresponsiveness can be reversed by histone acetylation where the inactive HIV-1 LTR is stimulated by NF-κB (El Kharroubi et al, 1999). These data suggested that a suppressive chromatin structure must be remodeled prior to transcriptional activation by NF-κB. Bearing in mind the rapidly increasing number of histone acetylases and deacetylases reported (Grozinger et al, 1999), some of which are tissue specific, it is tempting to speculate that the control of histone acetylation provides an additional level of regulation of gene expression thereby providing increased specificity.

In a recent study (Michael et al, 2000), the role of chromatin in modulating the transcriptional activity of a DNA-binding factor was reported. Thus, it was shown that the phosphorylation status and hence the transcriptional activity of the cyclic AMP response element binding protein (CREB) was inhibited by nucleosomal arrays on a cAMP-responsive promoter. However, inhibitors of histone deacetylation augmented CREB activity by prolonging its phosphorylation on chromatin (Michael et al, 2000). One can therefore envisage a situation whereby target selectivity for CREB is dictated not only by the presence of cognate DNA-binding sequences in the promoter but also by the chromatin environment which is either permissive or restrictive for CREB phosphorylation and hence activation.

The ability of chromatin to influence the specificity of gene targeting by a specific transcription factor is given further support in a study by Alberts and co-workers. (Xue et al, 1998). These investigators found that while an extra-chromosomal reporter regulated by SRF (serum response factor) was induced by a constitutively active RhoA, upon integration of this reporter into chromosomal DNA, the reporter became unresponsive to RhoA. This block to RhoA, however, could be overcome upon co-stimulation with activators of the JNK pathway (u/v light). Interestingly, the need for such a co-activator could be bypassed by treatment of the cells with histone deacetylase inhibitors and the authors concluded that there was a link between signal-regulated acetylation events and gene transcription. Thus, similar to the above report on CREB,

160

it would appear that again, the binding of a transcription factor (in this case SRF) is insufficient to increase gene transcription and that a co-activation step involving histone modification is required. The study also serves to highlight the fact that the activation of extrachromosomal reporters may, in some instances, be promiscuous.

2.2.2. *ATP-dependent chromatin remodeling*

As mentioned earlier, in addition to the histone-modifying enzymes, chromatin alteration can be achieved by separate activities such as the multisubunit ATPases. These include the Swi-Snf, RSC, NURF (nucleosome-remodeling factor), CHRAC (chromatin accessibility complex) and ACF (ATP-utilizing chromatin assembly and remodeling factor) complexes originally identified in yeast (see (Armstrong and Emerson, 1998; Vignali et al, 2000) for reviews). All are multi-subunit complexes with molecular weights anywhere between 0.5 and 2 Mda. Biochemical studies have demonstrated that these 'motors' can disrupt nucleosomal structures in an ATP-dependent manner, facilitate factor binding (Swi/Snf, NURF, ACF) and transcription from chromatin-assembled genes (NURF, ACF) (see Armstrong and Emerson, 1998 for review). Several observations have suggested that these complexes are functionally and mechanistically distinct (see below for example) and this characteristic may allow for the regulated expression of distinct subsets of genes.

Indeed, there is current evidence to support the concept of such specificity. Thus, in a study by Armstrong and others (Armstrong et al, 1998), it was reported that erythroid Kruppel-like factor (EKLF) required a Swi/Snf-related chromatin remodeling complex to generate a DNaseI hypersenstive, transcriptionally active β-globin promoter on chromatin templates. More importantly, this re-modeling complex demonstrated functional selectivity since it could not activate expression of chromatin-assembled HIV-1 templates with the E box-binding protein TFE-3 (Armstrong et al, 1998). It is worth speculating that such selectivity provides a means of differentially regulating the activation/suppression of genes which have common transcription factor binding sites.

2.2.3. *Functional overlap between the histone acetylating/deacetylating machinery and ATP-dependent chromatin remodeling*

One interesting question is as follows. Does the ATP-dependent class of chromatin-remodeling activities overlap with the histone-modifying enzymes with respect to target genes? This issue was addressed in a study using yeast (Biggar and Crabtree, 1999) and determining the effect of knocking out the genes encoding these chromatin-remodeling activities. The authors concluded that three general classes of genes based on their requirements for Swi-Snf

(ATP-dependent remodeling complex) and Gcn5 (a histone acetyl transferase) could be distinguished. Expression of one class of genes, which included *Ho* and *SUC2*, depended on both activities. A second category including *PGK1* and *ACT1* depended on either activity. A third group, which included *TCM1*, was affected minimally in terms of its expression. Thus, at least in this system, there is both functional overlap and independence of both chromatin-remodeling activities with respect to target genes.

2.2.4. *Evidence for a role of chromatin in the regulation of protease function*
Studies on the role of chromatin in the regulation of protease expression studies are few. However, the findings from transgenic studies, when compared with data generated by transient transfections, suggest a role for chromatin in the regulation of expression of the 92 kDa type IV collagenase gene. In transgenic mice harboring a MMP-9 promoter LacZ reporter, a region of the promoter (–522/+19) was found to be critical for developmental regulation *in vivo*. In contrast, this region was dispensable in transient transfections (Mohan et al, 1998) utilizing MMP-9 promoter sequences fused to a reporter gene. In a separate study also focusing on MMP-9 expression, a sequence residing between –2722 and –7745 was shown to be required for its expression in osteoclasts and migrating keratinocytes (Munaut et al, 1999). Again, these data contrast with transient transfection assays where 670 base pairs of flanking sequence has been shown to be necessary and sufficient for 'driving' constitutive- and inducible-expression of this collagenase (Sato and Seiki, 1993; Sato et al, 1993; Gum et al, 1996).

These differences probably reflect the altered environments of the transiently transfected and transgenic constructs. For transgenic systems, the reporter construct is integrated into the mouse DNA, and therefore appropriately chromatinized, and probably also organized into nucleosomal particles. In contrast, the extrachromosomal reporter plasmids used in transient transfections are poorly chromatinized and are not organized into nucleosomal particles by virtue of their circular geometry. Thus, it may be inferred that the different promoter requirements demonstrated by the two different methods reflect the influence of chromatin structure and possibly nucleosome positioning on MMP-9 expression in transgenic mice. Certainly, further studies will be necessary to confirm the influence of chromatin on MMP-9 expression *in vivo*.

Although studies on *in vivo* regulation of protease expression are scarce, one study has been published on the role of chromatin remodeling in the regulation of urokinase expression by phorbol ester. In this investigation, biochemical approaches were employed to study phorbol ester stimulated urokinase expression *in vivo* (Ibanez-Tallon et al, 1999). The authors reported that the enhancer previously identified by *in vitro* techniques and which lies about

2 kb upstream of the transcriptional start site, became hypersensitive to DNaseI upon induction of urokinase transcription by treatment with phorbol ester. All *cis* elements of the enhancer were occupied *in vivo* upon phorbol ester stimulation. Further, there was no evidence of nucleosomal boundaries *in vivo* in close proximity to the enhancer either before or after phorbol ester stimulation. The authors concluded that phorbol ester induced the binding of transcription factors to the urokinase enhancer without chromatin remodeling of this region. While the data presented support this contention, since a functional analysis was not undertaken, the role of elements outside (upstream or downstream) of the region of the urokinase promoter investigated in this study was not addressed. For example, it is possible that elements further upstream are also required for the induction for urokinase expression. Indeed, the authors did document DNaseI hypersenstive sites at −4500 upon stimulation with phorbol ester but the role of this region (presumably bound with *trans* -activators) remains to be determined. Future functional experiments utilizing a transgenic system or cultured cells harboring a stably integrated urokinase promoter-reporter construct will be required to answer this question.

2.2.5. *Alterations of chromatin-remodeling activity in cancer*
If chromatin remodeling activities are important for regulating gene expression, is there any evidence that these activities are altered in cancer? A study by Versteege and co-workers (Versteege et al, 1998) is important in this regard. These workers reported that deletion of region 11.2 on the long arm of chromosome 22 is a recurrent characteristic of malignant rhabdoid tumors. In a panel of 13 cell lines, they found 6 homozygous deletions. Interestingly, this region contains the chromatin remodeling SNF5/INI1 and analysis of this sequence indicated frameshift or nonsense mutations in another 6 cell lines. Thus, the authors concluded that this 'loss of function' was suggestive for a role for SNF5/INI1 to oncogenesis.

Another intriguing link between chromatin-remodeling activities and cancer comes from a report by Xue and co-workers (Xue et al, 1998). These investigators described a novel human complex (NURD) which contained not only ATP-dependent nucleosome disrupting activity but also histone deacetylase activity which is usually associated with transcriptional repression. Interestingly, deacetylation was found to be stimulated by ATP on nucleosomal templates suggesting that nucleosome disruption gives the deacetylase access to its substrates. Importantly, one subunit of NURD turned out to be identical to MTA1, a 703 amino acid, 80 kDa metastasis-associate protein whose expression is 4 fold higher in metastatic breast cancer compared with non-metastatic disease (Toh et al, 1994). Interestingly, we have recently determined that MTAl represses MMP-9 expression by binding directly to the promoter (Yan et al,

2003). While these findings provide a potential link between chromatin remodeling and the metastatic disease process, caution should be exercised in making such an interpretation since a causal role of MTA1 in the metastatic process has not yet been established.

3. CONCLUSIONS

We now have a good knowledge of the *trans* -acting factors and *cis* elements involved in the regulation of protease expression in cancer. However, there are still issues which remain unanswered. For example, in many cancers, protease expression is not in the tumor cells but in the surrounding stromal cells. How then can this be explained if a variety of *trans* acting factors such as AP-1, NF-κB are constitutively active in the cancer cells. Future studies will have to address this question. It may very well be that the chromatin environment and epigenetic factors, such as methylation shown to regulate urokinase expression (Xing and Rabbani, 1999), play a crucial role in the regulation of gene expression and works in concert with the know trans acting factors to exert control of gene expression.

REFERENCES

Abe J, Urano T, Konno H, Erhan Y, Tanaka T, Nishino N, Takada A, Nakamura S. Larger and more invasive colorectal carcinoma contains larger amounts of plasminogen activator inhibitor type 1 and its relative ratio over urokinase receptor correlates well with tumor size. Cancer 1999; 86: 2602–2611.

Allgayer H, Wang H, Wang Y, Heiss MM, Bauer R, Nyormoi O, Boyd DD. Transactivation of the urokinase-type plasminogen activator receptor gene through a novel promoter motif bound with an activator protein-2α-related factor. J Biol Chem 1999a; 274: 4702–4714.

Allgayer H, Wang H, Gallick GE, Crabtree A, Mazar A, Jones T, Kraker AJ, Boyd DD. Transcriptional induction of the urokinase receptor gene by a constitutively active Src. Requirement of an upstream motif (-152/-135) bound with Sp1. J Biol Chem 1999b; 274: 18428–18445.

Armstrong JA, Bieker JJ, Emerson WA. A SWI/SNF-related chromatin remodeling complex E-RC1, is required for tissue-specific transcriptional regulation of EKLF in vitro. Cell 1998; 95: 93–104.

Armstrong JA, Emerson BM. Transcription of chromatin: these are complex times. Current Opinion in Genetics and Development 1998; 8: 165–172.

Aho S, Rouda S, Kennedy SH, Qin H, Tan EM. Regulation of human interstitial collagenase (matrix metalloproteinase 1) promoter activity by fibroblast growth factor. Eur J Biochem 1997; 247: 503–510.

Biggar SR, Crabtree GR. Continuous and widespread roles for the Swi-Snf complex in transcription. EMBO J 1999; 18: 2254–2264.

Brown PH, Alani R, Preis LH, Szabo E, Birrer MJ. Suppression of oncogene-induced transformation by a deletion mutant of c-jun. Oncogene 1993; 8: 877–886.

Brown PH, Chen TK, Birrer MJ. Mechanism of action of a dominant-negative mutant of c-Jun. Oncogene 1994; 9: 791–799.

Chiu R, Angel P, Karin M. Jun-B differs in its biological properties from, and is a negative regulator of, c-Jun. Cell 1989; 59: 979–986.

Costa M, Shen Y, Maurer F, Medcalf RL. Transcriptional regulation of the tissue-type plasminogen activator gene in human endothelial cells: identification of nuclear factors that recognise functional elements in the tissue-type plasminogen activator gene promoter. Eur J Biochem 1998; 258: 123–131.

Deng T, Karin M. c-Fos transcriptional activity stimulated by H-ras-activated protein kinase distinct from JNK and ERK. Nature 1995; 371: 171–175.

De Cesare D, Vallone D, Caracciolo A, Sassone-Corsi P, Nerlov C, Verde P. Heterodimerization of c-jun with ATF-2 and c-fos is required for positive and negative regulation of the human urokinase enhancer. Oncogene 1995; 11: 365–376.

de Launoit Y, Baert J, Chotteau A, Monte D, Defossez PA, Coutte L, et al. Structure-function relationships of the PEA3 group of ets-related transcription factors. Biochemical and Molecular Medicine 1997; 61: 127–135.

Edmead C, Kanthou C, Benzakour O. Thrombin activates transcription factors Sp1, NfkappaB, and CREB: importance of the use of phosphatase inhibitors in nuclear protein extraction for the assessment of transcription factor DNA-binding activities. Anal Biochem 1999; 275: 180–186.

El Kharroubi A, Piras G, Zensen R, Martin MA. Transcriptional activation of the integrated chromatin-associated human immunodeficiency virus type 1 promoter. Mol Cell Biol 1999; 18: 2535–2544.

Farina AR, Tacconelli A, Vacca A, Maroder M, Gulino A, Mackay AR. Transcriptional up-regulation of matrix-metalloproteinase-9 expression during spontaneous epithelial to neuroblast phenotype conversion by SK-N-SH neuroblastoma cells, involved in enhanced invasivity, depends upon GT-box and nuclear factor kappaB elements. Cell Growth Differ 1999; 10: 353–367.

Fini ME, Bartlett JD, Matsubara M, Rinehart WB, Mody MK, Rainville M. The rabbit gene for 92-kDa matrix metalloproteinase. Role of AP1 and AP2 in cell type-specific transcription. J Biol Chem 1994; 269: 28620–28628.

Goodrich JA, Cutler G, Tjian R. Contacts in context: Promoter specificity and macromolecular interactions in transcription. Cell 1996; 84: 825–830.

Grozinger CM, Hassig CA, Schreiber SL. Three proteins define a class of human histone deacetylases related to yeast Hda1p. Proc Natl Acad Sci (USA) 1999; 96: 4868–4873.

Gum R, Lengyel E, Juarez J, Chen JH, Sato H, Seiki M, et al. Stimulation of 92-kDA gelatinase B promoter activity by ras is mitogen-activated protein kinase kinase 1-independent and requires multiple transcription factor binding sites including closely spaced PEA3/ets and AP-1 sequences. J Biol Chem 1996; 271: 10672–10680.

Gutman A, Wasylyk B. The collagenase gene promoter contains a TPA and oncogene-responsive unit encompassing the PEA3 and AP-1 binding sites. EMBO J 1990; 9: 2241–2246.

Hansen SK, Nerlov C, Zabel U, Verde P, Johnsen M, Baeuerle PA, Blasi F. A novel complex between the p65 subunit of NF-kB and c-Rel binds to a DNA element involved in the phorbol ester induction of the human urokinase gene. EMBO J 1992; 11: 205–213.

Himelstein BP, Lee EJ, Sato H, Seiki M, Muschel RJ. Transcriptional activation of the metrix metalloproteinase-9 gene in an H-ras and v-myc transformed rat embryo cell line. Oncogene 1997; 14: 1995–1998.

165

Michael LF, Hiroshi A, Shulman AI, Kraus WL, Montminy M. The phosphorylation status of a cyclic AMP-responsive activator is modulated via a chromatin-dependent mechanism. Mol Cell Biol 2000; 20: 1596–1603.

Ibanez-Tallon I, Caretti G, Blasi F, Crippa MP. In vivo analysis of the state of the human uPA enhancer following stimulation by TPA. Oncogene 1999; 18: 2836–2845.

Karin M, Liu ZG, Zandi E. AP-1 function and regulation. Curr Opin Cell Biol 1997; 9: 240–246.

Karin M. The regulation of AP-1 activity by mitogen-activated protein kinases. J Biol Chem 1995; 270: 16483–16486.

Kornberg R. Eukaryotic transcriptional control. Trends Biochem Sci 1999; 9: 46–49.

Lengyel E, Gum R, Stepp E, Juarez J, Wang H, Boyd D. Regulation of urokinase-type plasminogen activator expression by an ERK1-dependent signaling pathway in a squamous cell carcinoma cell line. J Cell Biochem 1996; 61: 430–438.

Lengyel E, Stepp E, Gum R, Boyd D. Involvement of a mitogen-activated protein kinase signaling pathway in the regulation of urokinase promoter activity by c-Ha-ras. J Biol Chem 1995a; 270: 23007–23012.

Lengyel E, Singh B, Gum R, Nerlov C, Sabichi A, Birrer MJ, et al. Regulation of urokinase-type plasminogen activator expression by the v-mos oncogene. Oncogene 1995b; 11: 2639–2648.

Lohi J, Lehti K, Valtanen H, Parks WC, Keski-Oja J. Structural analysis and promoter characterization of membrane-type matrix metalloproteinase-1 (MT1-MMP). Gene 2000; 242: 75–86.

Merchiers P, Bulens F, De Vriese A, Collen D, Belayew A. Involvement of Sp1 in basal and retinoic acid induced transcription of the human tisue-type plasminogen activator gene. FEBS Lett 1999; 456: 149–154.

Mertens PR, Alfonso-Jaume MA, Steinmann K, Lovett DH. A synergistic interaction of transcription factors AP-2 and YB-1 regulates gelatinase A enhancer-dependent transcription. J Biol Chem 1998; 273: 32957–32965.

Mohan R, Rinehart WB, Bargagna-Mohan P, Fini ME. Gelatinase B/lacZ transgenic mice, a model for mapping gelatinase B expression during developmental and injury-related tissue remodeling. J Biol Chem 1998; 273: 25903–25914.

Munaut C, Salonurmi T, Kontusaari S, Reponen P, Morita T, Foidart JM, Tryggvason K. The murine matrix metalloproteinase 9 gene. J Biol Chem 1999; 274: 5588–5596.

Nerlov C, Rorth P, Blasi F, Johnsen M. Essential AP-1 and PEA3 binding elements in the human urokinase enhancer display cell type-specific activity. Oncogene 1991; 6: 1583–1593.

Nielsen BS, Timshel S, Kjeldsen L, Sehested M, Pyke C, Borregaard N, Dano K. 92 kDa type IV collagenase (MMP-9) is expressed in neutrophils and macrophages but not in malignant epithelial cells in human colon cancer. Int J Cancer 1996; 65: 57–62.

Novak U, Cocks G, Hamilton J. A labile repressor acts through the NFkB-like binding sites of the human urokinase gene. Nucleic Acids Research 1991; 19: 3389–3393.

Olive M, Krylov D, Echlin DR, Gardner K, Taparowsky E, Vinson C. A dominant negative to activation protein-1 (AP-1) that abolishes DNA binding and inhibits oncogenesis. J Biol Chem 1997; 272: 18586–18594.

Pondel MD, Murphy S, Pearson L, Craddock C, Proudfoot NJ. Sp1 functions in a chromatin-dependent manner to augment human α-globin promoter activity. Proc Natl Acad Sci (USA) 1995; 92: 7237–7241.

Pyke C, Kristensen P, Ralfkiaer E, Grondahl-Hansen J, Eirksen J, Blasi F, Dano K. Urokinase-type plasminogen activator is expressed in stromal cells and its receptor in cancer cells at invasive foci in human colon adenocarcinomas. Amer J Pathol 1991; 138: 1059–1067.

Pyke C, Ralfkiaer E, Tryggvason K, Dano K. Messenger RNA for two type IV collagenases is located in stromal cells in human colon cancer. Amer J Pathol 1993; 142: 359–365.

Qin H, Sun Y, Benveniste EN. The transcription factors Sp1, Sp3, and AP-2 are required for constitutive matrix metalloproteinase-2 gene expression in astroglioma cells. J Biol Chem 1999; 274: 29130–29137.

Reuning U, Wilhelm O, Nishiguchi T, Guerrini L, Blasi F, Graeff H, Schmitt M. Inhibition of NF-kB-rel A expression by antisense oligodeoxynucleotides suppresses synthesis of urokinase-type plasminogen activator (uPA) but not its inhibitor PAI-1. Nucleic Acids Research 1995; 23: 3887–3893.

Sato H, Seiki M. Regulatory mechanism of 92 kDa type IV collagenase gene expression which is associated with invasiveness of tumor cells. Oncogene 1993; 8: 395–405.

Sato H, Kita M, Seiki M. v-src activates the expression of 92-kDa type IV collagenase through the AP-1 site and the GT Box homologous to retinoblastoma control elements. J Biol Chem 1993; 268: 23460–23468.

Smith CL, Hager GL. Transcriptional regulation of mammalian genes in vivo. J Biol Chem 1997; 272: 27493–27496.

Somasundaram K, Jayaraman G, Williams T, Moran E, Frisch S, Thimmapaya B. Repression of a matrix metalloprotease gene by E1A correlates with its ability to bind to cell type-specific transcription factor AP-2. Proc Natl Acad Sci (USA) 1996; 93: 3088–3093.

Sumpio BE, Chang R, Xu WY, Wang X, Du W. Regulation of t-PA in endothelial cells exposed to cyclic strain: role of CRE, AP-2, and SSRE binding sites. Am J Physiol 1997; 273: C1441–C1448.

Tan M, Yao J, Yu D. Overexpression of the c-erbB-2 gene enhanced intrinsic metastasis potential in human breast cancer cells without increasing their transformation abilities. Cancer Res 1997; 57: 1199–1205

Toh Y, Pencil SD, Nicolson GL. A novel candidate metastasis-associated gene, mta1, differentially expressed in highly metastatic mammary adenocarcinoma cell lines. cDNA cloning, expression and protein analysis. J Biol Chem 1994; 269: 22958–22963.

Tremble P, Damsky CH, Werb Z. Components of the nuclear signaling cascade that regulate collagenase gene expression in response to integrin-derived signals. J Cell Biol 1995; 129: 1707–1720.

Vignali M, Hassan AH, Neely KE, Workman JL. ATP-dependent chromatin-remodeling complexes. Mol Cell Biol 2000; 20: 1899–1910.

Versteege I, Sevenet N, Lange J, Rousseau-Merck M-F, Ambros P, Handgretinger R, Aurias A, Delattre O. Truncating mutations of hSNF5/INI1 in aggressive paediatric cancer. Nature 1998; 394: 203–206.

Walter M, Hugel A, Huang H, Cavenee WK, Wiestler OD, Pietsch T, et al. Expression of the Ets-1 transcription factor in human astrocytomas is associated with Fms-like tyrosine kinase-1 (Flt-1)/vascular endothelial growth factor receptor-1 synthesis and neoangiogenesis. Cancer Res 1999; 59: 5608–5614.

Wang F, Duan R, Chirgwin J, Safe SH. Transcriptional activation of cathepsin D gene expression by growth factors. J Mol Endocrinol 2000a; 24: 193–202.

Wang Y, Dang J, Wang H, Allgayer H, Murrell GA, Boyd D. Identification of a novel nuclear factor-kappaB sequence involved in expression of urokinase-type plasminogen activator receptor. Eur J Biochem 2000b; 267: 3248–3254.

Watabe T, Yoshida K, Shindoh M, Kaya M, Fujikawa K, Sato H, et al. The Ets-1 and Ets-2 transcription factors activate the promoters for invasion-associated urokinase and collagenase genes in response to epidermal growth factor. Int J Cancer 1998; 77: 128–137.

Westermarck J, Kähäri V-M. Regulation of matrix metalloproteinase expression in tumor invasion. FASEB J 1999; 13: 781–792.

White L, Brinckerhoff CE. Two AP-1 elements in the collagenase (MMP-1) promoter have dif-

167

ferential effects on transcription and bind JunD, c-Fos, and Fra-2. Matrix Biol 1995; 14: 715–725.

Xing RH, Rabbani SA. Transcriptional regulation of urokinase (uPA) gene expression in breast cancer cells: role of DNA methylation. Int J Cancer 1999; 81: 443–450.

Xing X, Wang S, Xia W, Zou Y, Shao R, Kwong KY, et al. The Ets protein PEA3 suppresses Her2/neu overexpression and inhibits tumorigenesis. Nature Med 2000; 6: 189–195.

Yan S, Berquin IM, Troen BR, Sloane BF. Transcription of human cathepsin B is mediated by Sp family factors in glioma. DNA Cell Biol 2000; 19: 79–91.

Zannetti A, Del Vecchio S, Carriero MV, Fonti R, Franco P, D'Aiuto G, Stoppelli MP, Salvatore M. Co-ordinate up-regulation of Sp1 DNA-binding activity and urokinase-receptor expression in breast carcinoma. Cancer Res 2000; 60: 1546–1551.

Xue Y, Wong J, Moreno GT, Young MK, Cote J, Wang W. NURD, a novel complex with both ATP-dependent chromatin-remodeling and histone deacetylase activities. Molecular Cell 1998; 2: 851–861.

Yan C, Wang H, Toh Y, Boyd DD. Repression of 92 kDa type IV collagenase expression by MTA1 is mediated through direct interactions with the promoter via a mechanism which is both dependent and independent of histone deacetylation. J Biol Chem 2003; in press.

168

Chapter 9

TISSUE INHIBITORS OF METALLOPROTEINASES IN CANCER

Yves A. DeClerck

Division of Hematology-Oncology, Departments of Pediatrics and Biochemistry and Molecular Biology, Childrens Hospital Los Angeles, USC Keck School of Medicine, Los Angeles, CA 90027, USA

Abstract

Our understanding of the biological function of tissue inhibitors of metalloproteinases (TIMP) has significantly evolved from an initial focus on the extracellular matrix (ECM) to a much broader function that includes a regulatory role on cell growth, survival and transformation. The bases for this larger role of TIMPs are several. 1. The group of proteins proteolytically altered by matrix metalloproteinases (MMPs) that TIMPs control, includes many non-ECM proteins. 2. TIMPs not only target MMPs but also non-matrix metalloproteinases involved in growth factors and cytokines activation and processing. 3. TIMPs have a direct effect on cell growth and survival independent of their anti-MMP activity. It is therefore not surprising that the effects of TIMPs in cancer are complex and include tumor suppressor as well as tumor promoting activities. In this chapter the complexity of the biological activities of TIMPs is reviewed, and how it brings light to some paradoxical effects of TIMPs reported in cancer is discussed. The lesson from the review of these data is that our perspective on cancer must include the role of the extracellular environment in which TIMPs are integral contributors.

1. STRUCTURE OF TIMP

Four members of the TIMP family have been so far described in many species, including human. These 4 inhibitors have in common many structural features but also differ in several aspects, which are responsible for important differences in their role (Table 1). TIMPs are secreted proteins with a molecular weight ranging between 21 kDa and 28 kDa. A unique feature of the primary structure common to the four TIMPs is the presence of 12 Cys residues all involved in disulfide bonds. The positions of these disulfide bonds are such that they create 2 domains (N-terminal and C-terminal) of 3 overlapping bonds. While there is a significant degree of homology in the N-terminal domain among the TIMPs, more divergence is seen in their C-terminal domain. This is consistent with the fact that the N-terminal domain of TIMPs is responsible for their common function on MMP inhibition, whereas the C-terminal domain is

J.-M. Foidart and R.J. Muschel (eds.), Proteases and Their Inhibitors in Cancer Metastasis, 169–194.
© 2002 *Kluwer Academic Publishers. Printed in the Netherlands.*

Table 1. Characteristics of tissue inhibitors of matrix metalloproteinases.

Characteristic	TIMP-1	TIMP-2	TIMP-3	TIMP-4
Mol. weight (kDa)	28	21	24	22
Chromosome (human)	x	17q25	22q13.1	3p25
mRNA (kb)	0.9	1.2, 1.7, 3.5	2.4, 2.8, 4.5	1.4
Glycosylation	Yes	No	No	No
Amino acids	184	194	188	195
Binding	Pro-MMP-9, cell surface	Pro-MMP-2, cell surface	ECM	Pro-MMP-2

involved in properties more specific to each TIMP. The tertiary structure of TIMP-2 has been partially elucidated by X-ray crystallography to 2.1 Ångstrom resolution (Tuuttila et al, 1998). The structure of the N-terminal domain (residues1 to 110) revealed a beta-barrel-like structure similar to the oligonucleotide/ oligosaccharide-binding fold found in DNA-binding proteins. The structure of the C-terminal domain (residues 111 to 194) consisted of a beta hairpin plus beta-loop-beta motif. The crystal structure of a TIMP-1/MMP-3 complex and a TIMP-2/MT1-MMP and TIMP-2/MMP-3 complex have pointed to specific residue sequences located in the N-terminal domain that are involved in binding to the active (zinc pocket) domain of MMPs (Muskett et al, 1998; Fernandez-Catalan et al, 1998; Gomis-Rüth et al, 1997). In the case of TIMP-1, a first sequence involves Cys^1-Thr^2-Cys^3-Ala^4 and a second sequence is made of Ser^{68}-Val^{69}. In the case of TIMP-2, binding sequences include residues 1 to 11, 27 to 41, 68 to 73, 87 to 90 and 97 to 104. The C-terminal domain of TIMPs is more variable and contains sequences that bind to the hemopexin domain of several MMPs, in particular MMP-9 for TIMP-1 and MMP-2 for TIMP-2 and TIMP-4 (Goldberg et al, 1992; Bigg et al, 1997; Overall et al, 1999). In the case of TIMP-3, the C-terminal domain is responsible for its unique ability to bind to the ECM (Langton et al, 1998). The C-terminal domain of TIMP-2 also plays a role in its high affinity binding to the cell surface (Ko et al, 1997).

2. REGULATION OF TIMP EXPRESSION AND ACTIVITY

It has long been considered that the major regulatory mechanism controlling TIMP activity was at the level of transcription. However more recently, attention has been paid to potentially important post-transcriptional mechanisms of regulation.

2.1. Transcriptional regulation of TIMP expression

The transcriptional regulation of TIMPs has been extensively studied over the past years and these studies have revealed significant differences among the different TIMPs. TIMP-1 and TIMP-3 are transcriptionally regulated by a variety of growth factors and cytokines that are also involved in the regulation of MMPs. Some of these factors, such as transforming growth factor beta-1, up-regulate TIMP-1 and TIMP-3 expression and down-regulate MMP expression, and therefore have a coordinated effect that decreases the degradation of the ECM (Edwards et al, 1996; Su et al, 1996). Other factors such as interleukin-1, interleukin-6, oncostatin M or tumor necrosis alpha (TNF-alpha) have a less predictable effect on the ECM because they simultaneously increase or decrease the expression of TIMPs and MMPs (Kossakowska et al, 1999; Botelho et al, 1998; Gatsios et al, 1996; Bugno et al, 1999). Most cytokines and growth factors do not affect the expression of TIMP-2, and therefore this inhibitor has been considered to have a housekeeping function. However we have recently demonstrated that TIMP-2 is up-regulated by cAMP in a delayed response that involves a cooperative activity between two transcription factors NF-Y and Sp1 which are also involved in the transcriptional regulation of several ECM proteins such as fibronectin and collagen I. Up-regulation of TIMP-2 by cAMP does not affect MMP-2 and MMP-9 and therefore switches the balance toward MMP inhibition (Zhong et al, 2000). These differences in TIMP transcriptional regulation have their basis on the presence of specific DNA binding motifs in their respective promoters. Among those is the AP-1/PEA-3 motif present in TIMP-1 and TIMP-3, and also in the promoters of many MMPs. The promoters of TIMP-2 and TIMP-3 also contain a CpG island, which is methylated. However it is only in TIMP-3 that methylation of the promoter suppresses gene expression (Pennie et al, 1999; Kang et al, 2000; Bachman et al, 1999). The TIMP-3 promoter is also cell cycle regulated and contains a p53 binding motif, but it is unclear whether the expression of TIMP-3 is specifically regulated by p53 (Wick et al, 1995; Bian et al, 1996a; Loging and Reisman, 1999). In the case of TIMP-2, TIMP-3 and TIMP-4, several mRNAs that differ by their polyadenylation signal sites have been reported but these differences do not affect their stability (Sun et al, 1995; Hammani et al, 1996). Much less is known on the nature of specific signaling pathways that regulate the transcriptional expression of TIMPs. The Jak/Stat pathway is involved in mediating the transcriptional up-regulation of TIMP-1 by gp130 family of receptor proteins that transmit signals from interleukin-6 and oncostatin M (Korzus et al, 1997) and a cAMP dependent pathway is involved in TIMP-2 regulation (Zhong et al, 2000). The mitogen-activated protein kinase pathway is involved in the up-regulation of TIMP-3 by oncostatin M (Li and Zafarullah, 1998).

2.2. Temporor-spatial expression of TIMPs

Studies in the mouse have indicated that TIMPs differ in their temporo-spatial expression during development and in adult tissues. For example the abundant and selective expression of TIMP-1 in the bone suggests a more specific role in bone development (Nomura et al, 1989). In contrast, TIMP-2 is highly expressed in the reproductive system, the lung, the skin and the heart (Blavier and DeClerck, 1997), TIMP-3 in the kidney, the heart, the lung and the ovary (Zeng et al, 1998; Leco et al, 1994) and TIMP-4 is abundant in the heart and the muscle (Leco et al, 1997). In the murine placenta, TIMP-1 is not expressed but spongiotrophoblastic cells at the invasive edge of the placenta abundantly express both TIMP-2 and TIMP-3 (Blavier and DeClerck, 1997).

2.3. Post-transcriptional regulation of TIMP activity

Much less is known of the factors that regulate TIMP at a post-transcriptional level. Glycosylation is a post-translational modification that occurs during the biosynthesis of TIMP-1. However it does not appear to affect the inhibitory activity or the biological half-life of the protein (Caterina et al, 1998; Murphy et al, 1991). Recently a novel post-translation regulatory mechanism for TIMP-2 has been suggested by the demonstration that secreted TIMP-2 is internalized and degraded intracellularly by a MT1-MMP-dependent mechanism (Maquoi et al, 2000). Extracellular proteolytic degradation of TIMP could also occur by proteases such as cathepsin B (Kostoulas et al, 1999). The study of the mechanisms involved in the regulation of TIMPs at a post-transcriptional level deserves further investigation.

3. FUNCTIONS OF TIMPs

For many years, TIMPs have been considered as having a single regulatory function toward the inhibition of the proteolytic activity of MMPs in the extra-cellular milieu and the preservation of the ECM. The ability of TIMPs to inhibit proteolysis mediated by MMPs not only affects insoluble proteins that form the complex composition of the ECM but also soluble non-ECM proteins. Furthermore it has now become apparent that TIMPs are multifunctional proteins and that their spectrum of activity extends beyond the inhibition of MMP activity (Table 2). Four major functions for TIMPs have been recognized.

Table 2. Functions of tissue inhibitors of matrix metalloproteinases.

Function	TIMP-1	TIMP-2	TIMP-3	TIMP-4
Inhibition of MMPs	Yes	Yes	Yes	Yes
Inhibition of ADAMs	Yes	No	Yes	No
	Yes	Yes	Yes	Unknown
Activation of proMMPs	Inhibits	Stimulates proMMP-2 activation	Unknown	Unknown
Cell growth	Stimulates	Stimulates	Suppresses	No effect
Apoptosis	Suppresses	Protects/stimulates	Enhances	No effect

3.1. TIMPs inhibit the degradation of ECM proteins

The primary function of TIMPs is to control the activity of active MMPs in the extracellular milieu. This function is based on the ability of the N-terminal domain of TIMP to form high affinity (Kd in the nM range) complexes with the active form of all MMPs. There is no significant difference among the TIMPs in their ability to inhibit most MMPs *in vitro* and very little specificity exists among the TIMPs in regard to MMP inhibition (Murphy and Willenbrock, 1995). Because MMPs have a broad spectrum of proteolytic activity for all major components of the ECM, TIMPs exert a broad inhibitory activity on all the components of the ECM. It is generally agreed that the effect of TIMPs on the ECM is to decrease its turnover and overexpression of TIMP with increased deposition of ECM proteins and tissue fibrosis has been well documented in many physiological and pathological processes such as implantation, embryogenesis, organogenesis, wound healing, angiogenesis, osteoarthritis and cancer. Because the ECM plays an important role in regulating critical cellular functions such as growth, survival and differentiation, TIMPs indirectly affect cell behavior (Werb, 1997; Lukashev and Werb, 1998). For example, degradation of the basement membrane during involution of the mammary gland is a result of subtle changes in MMP-3 and TIMP-1 expression and is required for the induction of apoptosis in mammary epithelial cells (Boudreau et al, 1995). This indirect effect of TIMPs on cell behavior plays an important role in cancer, as will become apparent later.

3.2. TIMPs inhibit the processing of non-ECM proteins

It has now become apparent that MMPs are also involved in the proteolytic processing of proteins others than those of the ECM. Those include growth

173

factor binding proteins, growth factor and cytokines and their receptors, adhesion molecules and precursor proteins of biologically active peptides. It is anticipated that the list of these novel targets for MMP mediated proteolysis will continue to grow. Several MMPs can proteolytically cleave the insulin-like growth factor binding protein 3 (IGFBP-3) (Manes et al, 1999; Fowlkes et al, 1997) and MMP-3 degrades perlecan, a proteoglycan that sequesters basic fibroblast growth factor (Whitelock et al, 1996). MMP-3 can also activate HB-EGF by cleaving its precursor proHB-HGF and this activity is inhibited by the synthetic MMP inhibitor batimastat which consequently inhibits EGF receptor transactivation (Suzuki et al, 1997; Prenzel et al, 1999). MMP-7, which is expressed by Paneth cells in the intestinal mucosa, is responsible for the pro-teolytic activation of defensin, a peptide with anti-bacterial activity (Wilson et al, 1999). It has also been suggested that MMP-3 cleaves the extracellular domain of E-cadherin in mammary epithelial cells triggering an epithelium to mesenchyme conversion and a malignant behavior in immunocompromised mice (Lochter et al, 1997; Christofori and Semb, 1999). Several MMPs can also pro-teolytically cleave precursors of anti-angiogenic factors such as plasminogen and collagen XVIII to generate angiostatin and endostatin respectively (O'Reilly et al, 1999; Wen et al, 1999; Patterson and Sang, 1997; Dong et al, 1997; Lijnen et al, 1998). The effect of inhibition of the proteolytic cleavage of these sub-strates by TIMPs is still poorly understood but it is anticipated that it will affect growth regulatory processes, inflammatory reactions and angiogenesis among others. Another mechanism by which TIMPs affect the proteolytic processing of non-ECM proteins has been recently recognized. TIMPs can inhibit the pro-teolytic activity of non-matrix metalloproteinases such as the ADAMs (A Disintegrin And Metalloproteinase) and other metalloproteases involved in the shedding of cell membrane associated proteins. Some members of the ADAM family of membrane associated metalloproteinases are proteolytically active and are involved in the activation of growth factors and cytokines. For example, the TNF-alpha converting enzyme (TACE or ADAM 17) which releases soluble TNF-alpha is inhibited by TIMP-3 (Black et al, 1997; Amour et al, 1998). TIMP-2 but not TIMP-1 also inhibits the shedding of TNF-alpha receptor in colon carcinoma cells (Lombard et al, 1998) and TIMP-3 inhibits the shedding of L-selectin from leukocytes (Borland et al, 1999). The activity of TIMPs on these proteases has become an area of active investigation.

3.3. TIMPs control the activation of MMPs

TIMPs exert a second level of control over MMP activity in the extracellular milieu by controlling the activation of proMMPs. Activation of proMMPs is a complex process that differs among the MMPs but typically involves a two step proteolytic cleavage of the prodomain (Nagase, 1997). A first step includes a proteolytic cleavage by a serine protease (such as plasmin or furin) and a second step consists of an MMP-dependent cleavage that involves either an auto-proteolytic cleavage or a cleavage mediated by another MMP. This second step is inhibited by TIMPs (DeClerck et al, 1991a; Ward et al, 1991). However, in other situations TIMPs can promote rather that inhibit MMP activation. This is well illustrated in the case of TIMP-2, which can form trimolecular complexes with MT1-MMP and proMMP-2 at the cell surface. In these complexes, TIMP-2 acts as an adapter molecule of which N-terminal domain binds to the active domain of a first molecule of MT1-MMP anchored to the cell surface and which C-terminal domain binds to the hemopexin domain of proMMP-2. As a result, proMMP-2 is brought to the cell surface where it is activated by a second molecule of MT1-MMP (Strongin et al, 1995). Binding of TIMP-2 to MT1-MMP also prevents the autocatalytic inactivation of cell surface associated MT1-MMP, thus further promoting proMMP-2 activation (Hernandez-Barrantes et al, 2000). Whether TIMP-2 acts as an enhancer or inhibitor of proMMP-2 activation depends on a delicate stoichiometric balance between MT1-MMP, TIMP-2 and proMMP-2 (Butler et al, 1998). A clear illustration of the role of TIMP-2 in proMMP-2 activation has been recently provided *in timp-2* deficient mice which cannot activate proMMP-2 (Wang et al, 2000).

3.4. TIMPs affect cell growth and survival

Since the original report in 1985 that TIMP-1 was identical to an erythroid potentiating activity factor (Docherty et al, 1985), it has been suggested that TIMPs could act as growth stimulatory factors through an interaction with TIMP-specific cell surface receptors. There have been numerous reports indicating that TIMP-1 and TIMP-2 bind with high affinity to the surface of many normal and malignant cells and stimulate cell growth *in vitro* (Hayakawa et al, 1992; Hayakawa et al, 1994; Corcoran and Stetler-Stevenson, 1995). In support for the existence of a potential receptor for TIMPs, is the observation that TIMP-1 can stimulate adenylate cyclase and the cAMP dependent activation of protein kinase and that TIMP-2 increases tyrosine phosphorylation and MAP kinase activity (Yamashita et al, 1996; Corcoran and Stetler-Stevenson, 1995). A few cell surface associated TIMP binding proteins have been described such as MT1-MMP or possibly $\alpha_v\beta_3$ integrin which binds MMP-2 at the cell surface (Brooks et al, 1996), however TIMP specific receptors have yet to be identified and characterized. In contrast to TIMP-1 and TIMP-2, TIMP-3 has been identified as an epidermal growth factor-regulated growth suppressor (Andreú et al, 1998). TIMPs can also affect cell apoptosis. TIMP-1 but not TIMP-2 can suppress programmed cell death induced by CD95 (Fas ligand) or by heat shock, serum deprivation and gamma-radiation in malignant Burkitt cells (Guedez et al, 1998a). TIMP-1 can also inhibit apoptosis in human breast epithelial cells induced by Adriamycin or X-ray irradiation (Li et al, 1999) and inhibit apoptosis and induce differentiation in germinal B center B cells (Guedez et al, 1998b). A decrease in NF(B activity and an up-regulation of Bcl-X$_L$ by TIMP-1 has been reported (Guedez et al, 1998a). In contrast TIMP-3 has been shown to enhance programmed cell death (Baker et al, 1999; Ahonen et al, 1998). The mechanisms by which TIMP-1 or TIMP-3 affect apoptosis are presently unknown. However the observation that these effects can be abrogated by anti-TIMPs blocking antibodies and can be reproduced by exogenous TIMPs suggests that it involves an extracellular function of TIMPs. In the case of TIMP-1, suppression of apoptosis in B cells could not be reproduced by synthetic MMP inhibitors suggesting a novel activity independent of an anti-MMP activity (Baker et al, 1999). An interaction with sheddases that affect cytokine activity such as TNF-alpha and a direct receptor mediated mechanism affecting signal transduction pathways involved in apoptosis are possibilities that should be considered.

3.5. Nuclear function of TIMPs?

It has also been suggested that TIMPs could have a function in the cell nucleus. Investigators have reported that TIMP-1 accumulates in the nucleus of gingival fibroblasts in a cell cycle dependent manner (Zhao et al, 1998) and that TIMP-1 bound to the surface of MCF-7 cells is transported to the nucleus (Ritter et al, 1999). The selective presence of TIMP-1 in the nucleus and the structural analogy between the N-terminal domain of TIMPs and oligonucleotide/oligosaccharides binding proteins might suggest that TIMPs could play an intranuclear role in regulating gene transcription. It is however unknown whether TIMPs bind to specific DNA sequences or DNA/protein complexes and this aspect will require further investigation.

In summary, it is now clear that the biological roles of TIMPs are much more complex than it was initially anticipated and consist of more than the single regulation of the amount of ECM protein proteolytically modified in connective tissues. The relevance of these observations is becoming apparent as one examines the effect and role of TIMPs in cancer (Figure 1).

4. ROLE OF TIMPs IN CANCER PROGRESSION

The importance of the degradation of the ECM during tumor invasion and metastasis has been recognized for many years and the role of matrix degrading

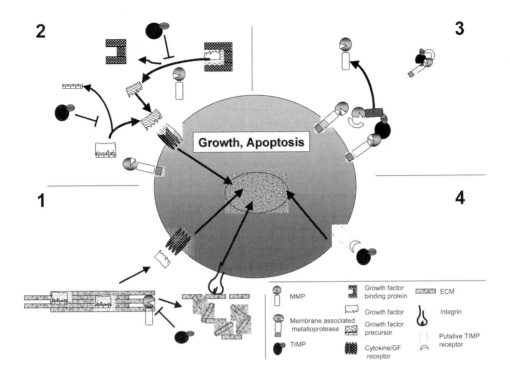

Figure 1. TIMPs affect cell growth and apoptosis in multiple ways. 1. TIMPs inhibit the degradation of the ECM by MMPs. As a result, matrix bound growth factors are released and become more available to interact with membrane bound receptors (a). Inhibition of the degradation of the ECM by TIMPs prevents novel interaction between integrin and a proteolyzed ECM that influences cell survival (b). 2. TIMPs inhibit membrane bound metalloproteinases and soluble MMPs that process growth factors, growth receptors and growth factor binding proteins. As a result, the interaction between growth factors and their receptors is altered. 3. TIMPs control the activation of MMPs. TIMPs can either inhibit proMMP activation (a) by preventing the auto-catalytic cleavage of the prodomain (a) or – as illustrated for TIMP-2 – stimulate proMMP-2 activation (b). 4. TIMPs can directly affect cell growth and apoptosis by interacting with a putative cell surface receptor.

proteases abundantly present in tumor tissue in this process has been much emphasized. As TIMPs were discovered and characterized as MMP specific natural inhibitors, it was hypothesized that a shift in the MMP/TIMP balance in favor of the proteases as a result of a direct increase in protease expression, a decrease in inhibitor expression or a combination of both changes, was a key step in tumor progression toward invasion, metastasis and angiogenesis. As the role of TIMPs in cancer began to be investigated *in vitro* and *in vivo*, the simplistic nature of this concept became apparent when tumor suppressor as well as tumor promoting activities for TIMPs were reported.

4.1. Tumor suppressor activity of TIMPs

4.1.1. *Experimental evidence*

There is pharmacological and genetic evidence supporting a tumor suppressor activity of TIMPs.

Pharmacological evidence. We have previously demonstrated that exogenous rTIMP-1 and rTIMP-2 inhibit the degradation of ECM proteins by MMP-expressing rodent and human tumor cells in culture and that inhibition of ECM degradation by rTIMPs prevents the invasion of the ECM (Alvarez et al, 1990; DeClerck et al, 1991b; Montgomery et al, 1993). Our laboratory and those of others have also shown that administration of rTIMP-1 and rTIMP-2 in mice inhibits lung colonization of B16 melanoma and transformed rat embryo cells injected into the tail vein (Schultz et al, 1988; Alvarez et al, 1990). This approach has not yet been tested for TIMP-3 and TIMP-4.

Genetic evidence. Modulation of TIMP expression in tumor cells and in mice by genetic manipulation has been an invaluable method to examine how alteration of the MMP/TIMP balance affects tumor progression and to discriminate between the contribution of tumor cells and host cells in this aspect. The first evidence supporting a tumor suppressor activity of TIMPs was obtained from antisense experiments in which down-regulation of TIMP-1 in Swiss 3T3 fibroblasts was shown to confer to these cells a tumorigenic and metastatic phenotype (Khokha et al, 1989). Overexpression of TIMP-1, TIMP-2, TIMP-3 and TIMP-4 in several rodent and human tumor cell lines by cDNA transfection has been accomplished by many groups of investigators who have shown that transfected cells overexpressing TIMPs consistently have an impaired ability to degrade the ECM and to invade *in vitro* (Koop et al, 1994; Khokha, 1994; DeClerck et al, 1992; Montgomery et al, 1994; Valente et al, 1998; Bian et al, 1996b; Wang et al, 1997). However in animals, their behavior has been less consistent. Somewhat unexpectedly, little or no effect of TIMP-1 and TIMP-2 overexpression was seen on distant metastasis whereas a definitive effect on the growth of primary tumors was demonstrated (Yoneda et al, 1997; DeClerck et al, 1992; Koop et al, 1994). This observation pointed to a role for TIMPs in controlling the growth of primary tumors through a series of mechanisms discussed later in this chapter. In tumor tissues, stromal cells substantially contribute to TIMP expression and high levels of TIMP expression by stromal cells at the invasive front of cancer has been considered as a mechanism of host defense against tumor invasion. The contribution of host cells to TIMP expression in cancer has been examined in transgenic mice in whom expression was either stimulated in a tissue specific manner or abolished by gene knockout.

Some of these experiments have indicated that host derived TIMPs play an important role in cancer control but not necessarily, as initially anticipated, on invasion and metastasis. For example, in transgenic mice in whom MMP-3 is overexpressed in the mammary gland, there is an increased incidence of mammary tumors which can be abrogated by either local administration of TIMP-1 or by crossing these mice with TIMP-1 over-expressing transgenic mice (Sternlicht et al, 2000; Sternlicht et al, 1999). In mice overexpressing TIMP-1 in the liver, TIMP-1 blocks the development of Tag-induced hepatocellular carcinoma (Martin et al, 1996). In contrast, in TIMP-1 deficient mice, absence of TIMP-1 expression in the host does not affect the formation of experimental metastasis in the lungs (Soloway et al, 1996). These data thus suggest that TIMP-1 expressed by host cells control early steps of tumor progression including transformation and primary growth, and has no effect on later stages of progression such as metastasis. The role of other TIMPs in this aspect has not yet been explored.

4.1.2. *Mechanisms of action*
It was initially anticipated that the primary target for the anti-cancer activity of TIMPs would be the latest steps of cancer progression such as invasion and metastasis. The above described experiments however suggest that a main target for the activity of TIMPs in cancer are the earliest steps of tumor formation and primary tumor growth. At least five mechanisms of action supporting an inhibitory activity of TIMPs on tumor growth can be identified. Some of these mechanisms involve an anti-metalloproteinase function and the ECM, others appear independent from an anti-proteolytic activity of TIMPs. A first mechanism is on angiogenesis. TIMPs inhibit angiogenesis because of a direct inhibitory effect on endothelial cell proliferation and migration and because they also inhibit the activity of MMPs required for local invasion of the ECM by endothelial cells upon stimulation by angiogenic factors (Murphy et al, 1993; Johnson et al, 1994; Anand-Apte et al, 1997). TIMP-1 and TIMP-2 have been purified from cartilage extracts with anti-angiogenic activity and TIMP-3 inhibits the motility and proliferation of endothelial cells grown in collagen gels or implanted in the chorioallantoic membrane (Moses et al, 1990; Anand-Apte et al, 1997). A second mechanism supporting a growth inhibitory effect on tumor cell growth is the control of the bioavailability of growth factors. This effect has been elegantly demonstrated for TIMP-1. In mice overexpressing TIMP-1 in the liver, there is a decrease in IGFBP-3 degradation and a concomitant decrease in IGFII release and bioavailability. These changes are responsible for the lower incidence of hepatocellular carcinoma tumors that develop in the liver of these mice upon induction by the large Tag (Martin et al, 1999). A third mechanism, which has been in particular studied by our group, is the ECM.

It is now well recognized that the ECM plays a key role in controlling cell behavior (Lukashev and Werb, 1998). Thus, it is anticipated that by preventing the degradation of the ECM, TIMPs allow the ECM to maintain control on essential functions such as growth, migration, survival and differentiation. However it was uncertain whether anchorage independent tumor cells would remain sensitive to regulation by the ECM. Such a regulatory effect has been demonstrated by us in human melanoma cells. We had previously shown that in these cells, the administration of exogenous rTIMP-2 and overexpression of TIMP-2 achieved by cDNA transfection inhibited the growth of melanoma cells on intact fibrillar collagen but not on non-fibrillar (denatured) collagen (Montgomery et al, 1994). We have now demonstrated that inhibition of growth is the result of a specific block at the G1/S checkpoint and is associated with elevated levels of p27 and a concomitant decrease in cyclin E associated CDK-2 activity. This block in cell cycle progression is lifted upon degradation of fibrillar collagen by MMP-1 or in the absence of TIMP-2 (Henriet et al, 2000). A fourth mechanism of action is an effect on apoptosis. An apoptosis inducing activity has been in particular suggested in the case of TIMP-3, which when overexpressed in tumor cells inhibits invasion and triggers apoptosis (Baker et al, 1999; Ahonen et al, 1998). In the case of TIMP-1, a protective rather than a stimulatory effect on apoptosis has been reported as discussed later. A fifth mechanism supporting an inhibitory effect of TIMPs on tumor progression consists of the effects of TIMPs on the activity of ADAMs or other proteases that process and activate growth factors and cytokines and their receptors at the cell surface (Gallea-Robache et al, 1997; Arribas et al, 1996). For example TIMP-2 and TIMP-3 as well as synthetic inhibitors of MMPs but not TIMP-1 inhibit TNF-alpha receptor shedding in colon carcinoma cells increasing therefore the response of these cells to TNF (Lombard et al, 1998). Inhibition of TNF-alpha shedding by TIMP-3 also restores the TNF-alpha p55 signaling pathway and apoptosis (Bian et al, 1996b; Smith et al, 1997). Another example is the HER2/neu tyrosine kinase receptor, which undergoes cleavage of its extracellular domain by MMPs. Shedding of the extracellular domain of HER2/neu is inhibited in breast cancer cells by TIMP-1 and not by TIMP-2 (Codony-Servat et al, 1999). CD44, the receptor for hyaluronic acid expressed by many metastatic tumor cells is cleaved by a membrane associated MMP and cleavage is inhibited by TIMP-1 as well as synthetic inhibitors of MMPs. Inhibition of CD44 cleavage by TIMP-1 impairs tumor cell migration (Okamoto et al, 1999).

4.2. Tumor promoting activity of TIMPs

There has been a series of observations suggesting that TIMPs could also stimulate tumor development and progression. Such evidence comes from animal experiments as well as from the analysis of the expression of TIMPs and MMPs in human tumors.

4.2.1. *Experimental evidence*

Animal studies. Some experiments in mice suggest that TIMP-1 may accelerate the incidence of tumors. TIMP-1 overexpression in tumorigenic cells can either increase or decrease lung colonization (Soloway et al, 1996). In *min* null mice that have a higher incidence of intestinal tumors, forced TIMP-1 expression had either no effect on tumor formation or augmented tumor multiplicity whereas synthetic inhibitors of MMPs inhibited tumor formation (Goss et al, 1998).

Analysis of TIMP expression in human tumors. Analysis of TIMP expression in human tumor specimens has been the subject of a large number of publications. These studies have consistently reported the expression of TIMPs by both tumor cells and stromal cells and more specifically in regions adjacent to the invasive edge of the tumors. However most studies have shown that TIMPs – in particular TIMP-1 and TIMP-2 – are indicators of poorer rather than better survival (see below), suggesting therefore a potentially negative effect of TIMPs in cancer. A limitation in these studies is the absence of information on the effect of the expression of TIMPs on the proteolytic activity present in tumor tissues and how TIMPs affect the nature and structure of the ECM. The interpretation of these data is therefore not simple. Overexpression of TIMPs at the tumor-stroma interface could be interpreted as the result of a defensive reaction from the host to prevent local invasion and metastasis in more aggressive forms of cancer. Alternatively, it could be seen as providing a direct advantage to tumor cells and several mechanisms of action of TIMPs in support of this latter hypothesis exist.

4.2.2. *Mechanisms of action supporting a tumor promoter activity of TIMPs*
At least five mechanisms of action that support a tumor promoter activity can be considered. First among those is the growth promoting activity of TIMP-1 and TIMP-2. Initially identified as having an activity on the growth of erythroid precursor cells, TIMP-1 and TIMP-2 were later reported to stimulate the growth of a variety of malignant cells *in vitro* (Hayakawa et al, 1992; Hayakawa et al,

1994). The existence of a TIMP/TIMP cell surface receptor interaction could theoretically account for differences observed in the effect of TIMPs in cancer progression. For example the presence of a TIMP-1 receptor in colon cancer cells and not in melanoma cells could explain why higher TIMP-1 levels correlate with more aggressive colon cancers and not in melanoma (Lu et al, 1991; MacDougall et al, 1999). Whether the growth stimulatory effect of TIMPs, which has so far only been reported *in vitro*, has any pathophysiological relevance in tumor progression remains unclear. A second mechanism in support of a stimulatory role of TIMPs on tumor progression is the effect of TIMPs on programmed cell death. TIMP-1 inhibits apoptosis in B cells and this effect could explain the association between high levels of TIMP-1 and poorer prognosis in B lymphoma (Guedez et al, 1998a). In the case of TIMP-3, as previously mentioned, an inducing rather than protective effect on apoptosis has been reported and in the case of TIMP-2, a protective effect on apoptosis in melanoma (Valente et al, 1998) and a promoting effect on T lymphocytes (Lim et al, 1999) have been reported. A third mechanism of action is a positive effect of TIMP on the activation of proMMP. This effect has been well characterized and studied in the case of TIMP-2 which is required for the activation of proMMP-2 at the cell surface by MT1-MMP. It is likely that in response to an increase in proMMP-2 and MT1-MMP expression in tumor cells during invasion, a corresponding increase in TIMP-2 is needed to maintain optimal activation of the proenzyme and to prevent autocatalytic degradation of MT1-MMP (Hernandez-Barrantes et al, 2000). A fourth mechanism of action is on angiogenesis where TIMPs have a complex activity that includes a positive and a negative regulation (Sang, 1998). Inhibition of the MMP-mediated proteolytic cleavage of plasminogen and collagen XVIII by TIMPs may prevent the generation of anti-angiogenic factors such as angiostatin and endostatin and will therefore positively affect angiogenesis. A fifth mechanism is the anti-sheddase activity of TIMPs previously discussed. Inhibition of growth factors/cytokines and their receptors cleavage by TIMP could have a positive as well as a negative effect on cancer. A better knowledge of the effect of growth factor and cytokine shedding on cancer is needed to further appreciate the importance of this mechanism of action of TIMPs.

5. CAN TIMPS CONTRIBUTE TO CANCER PROGNOSIS?

5.1. Analysis of TIMP and MMP/TIMP levels in tumor tissues

The analysis of TIMP and MMP/TIMP tissue levels in a large variety of cancer types has been accomplished using methods such as Northern blot analysis, quantitative RT-PCR, *in situ* hybridization, semi-quantitative immunohisto-chemistry and semi-quantitative zymography (Brummer et al, 1999; Thomas et al, 2000; Sugiura et al, 1998). These analyses have often generated conflicting data. In the majority of the cases, overexpression of TIMP-1 and TIMP-2, in particular in association with elevated levels of MMPs is associated with a poorer rather than a better prognosis. In colon cancer, TIMP-1 tissue levels are higher in more invasive stages (Lu et al, 1991) and the same observation was made in non-Hodgkin's lymphoma (Kossakowska et al, 1992). Similar data were reported in the case of TIMP-2 in which elevated levels in bladder and breast cancer predicts an unfavorable clinical outcome (Grignon et al, 1996; Visscher et al, 1994). These observations have been recently confirmed in breast cancer patients by another group of investigators (Remacle et al, 2000; McCarthy et al, 1999). Higher tissue levels of TIMP-1 or TIMP-2 have also been reported in more advanced non-small cell lung cancer (Fong et al, 1996), melanoma (Airola et al, 1999), ovarian carcinoma (Kikkawa et al, 1997), and acute myelogenous leukemia (Janowska-Wieczorek et al, 1999). Considering the very large number of MMPs that could be involved in cancer, the diverse effect of TIMPs and the lack of sensitive methods to examine the proteolytic activity in tumor tissue, it is uncertain whether these time-consuming and costly analyses will have any clinical value.

5.2. Analysis of TIMP and MMP/TIMP levels in serum

TIMP-1 and TIMP-2 as well as MMPs and TIMP-MMP complexes can also be measured by immunological methods in many biological fluids including the serum. This analysis has therefore been regarded as a simpler and potentially cost-effective method to predict either clinical outcome or the reoccurrence of occult metastases and to provide a sensitive marker to monitor response to anti-cancer treatment (Zucker et al, 1999). In gastric cancer, preoperative plasma levels of TIMP-1 were reported to be an independent and most powerful prognosticator for (poor) survival in patients (Yoshikawa et al, 2000). In colon cancer patients, significantly higher plasma levels of TIMP-1 than in healthy individuals were reported and the highest levels were found in patients with more advanced cancer (Holten-Andersen et al, 1999). In patients with lung cancer, TIMP-1 serum levels were found to be higher than in controls whereas TIMP-2 and MMP-2/TIMP-2 complex levels were lower than in the control population (Ylisirnio et al, 2000). However in colon cancer, only the serum levels of TIMP-1 were found significantly higher in Dukes' D stages compared with Dukes' A but these levels did not predict survival (Oberg et al, 2000). Altogether these studies suggest that among the TIMPs, the measurement of TIMP-1 may have a value in cancer prognosis. Whether other measurements of MMPs/TIMPs would have any value in predicting response to treatment or survival is unclear.

6. DO TIMPs HAVE ANY ROLE IN THE THERAPY OF CANCER?

Inhibition of MMP activity in tumors has been considered to be a potentially important and novel target for cancer treatment. Supported by a large number of encouraging *in vitro* data and preclinical studies suggesting the efficacy and low toxicity of several synthetic inhibitors of MMPs, many clinical trials with these inhibitors have recently been initiated in a large variety of cancer types (Wojtowicz-Praga et al, 1998; Tierney et al, 1999; Bramhall, 1997). Several of these trials have however been discontinued because of either a lack of effect or because of adverse effects. The recent realization that metalloproteinases targeted by these inhibitors have a much broader spectrum of activity than initially anticipated is providing some explanation for the unexpected effects of MMP inhibitors in cancer. A better understanding of the complex effect of MMPs will be needed to reevaluate the therapeutic value of MMP inhibitors in cancer and other diseases. Thus, a similar cautious statement should apply to the potential use of TIMPs in therapy in particular considering that the activity of these natural inhibitors on cancer cells could be even more complex. Nevertheless, two potential avenues for the therapeutic administration of TIMPs in cancer have been considered and tested *in vitro* and in pre-clinical models in mice.

6.1. Pharmacological administration of TIMPs in mice

A major limiting factor in the pharmacological administration of TIMPs in animals has been the relatively short serum half life of the protein (2 to 5 min) and the amount of proteins required to achieve an anti-tumor activity in mouse (4 mg/kg). These observations have made the cost effective use of recombinant TIMPs unlikely. A second limiting factor – shared with many other biologically active agents that are non cytotoxic – is the need for a chronic administration. As an alternative to some of these limitations, investigators have attempted to modify TIMP to improve its pharmacological properties. For example, peggylation of TIMP-2 increases its half-life from 4.5 min to 2.5 h without altering its antiproteolytic activity. Mutation of a single amino acid in the region Cys^1-Cys^3, Ser^{68}-Cys^{72} or Ser^{31}-Ile^{41} of TIMP-2 affects its affinity for several MMPs and therefore such protein engineering might be useful in generating TIMPs with a more specific activity (Butler et al, 1999). Information obtained from the tertiary structure of TIMP/MMP complexes may also lead to the generation of TIMP-like peptides that may have better pharmacological properties. However early data have shown that the interaction between TIMP and MMP involves more than one domain so that the generation of small TIMP-like peptides may not be feasible (Nagase et al, 1999). Until now, TIMPs have not been considered as potentially useful proteins in the treatment of cancer.

6.2. Gene therapy

The fact that TIMPs are natural inhibitors of MMPs, and the demonstration that when overexpressed in tumor cells by genetic manipulation they inhibit the growth of primary tumors, have led to postulate that overexpression of TIMPs by gene therapy could have a role in cancer treatment. The use of TIMPs in gene therapy has a potentially important advantage over the use of other tumor suppressor genes such as pRb or p53, which have been among the top candidates for such an approach. Because TIMPs primarily act in the extracellular milieu, expression of TIMPs in every single tumor cell by either direct transfection or by bystander effect should not be needed because expression in a limited number of tumor cells could be sufficient to produce enough TIMPs to inhibit MMP activity in the vicinity of tumor cells. This possibility was tested in our group who showed that overexpression of TIMP-2 could be achieved by retroviral mediated gene transfer in primary tumors in mice with an efficiency of approximately 10%. Expression of TIMP-2 by tumor cells was sufficient to increase the amount of ECM present at the tumor edge, to limit local invasion into the muscle and to inhibit primary growth (Imren et al, 1996). Since this report, other gene delivery models have been tested *in vitro* by several groups of investigators, including temperature sensitive herpes simplex virus based vectors and adenovirus and adeno-associated virus based vectors (Hoshi et al, 2000; Indraccolo et al, 1999). These vectors could be used for *in vivo* intramuscular delivery of TIMP cDNA containing plasmids and systemic expression of TIMP or alternatively for local gene delivery to tumor tissues. A major limiting factor of this latter approach however has been the present lack of tumor specific vectors.

7. CONCLUSION

Our understanding of the mechanisms of action of TIMPs in cancer has significantly changed from a relatively simple concept that the essential function of TIMPs is the maintenance of the homeostasis of the ECM to the understanding that TIMPs can affect tumor cell growth, transformation and survival. The complex nature of the biological activity of TIMPs resides in the large number of ECM and non-ECM proteins whose proteolytic processing is affected by matrix and non-matrix metalloproteinases that TIMPs control. Another level of complexity is the fact that TIMPs directly interact with cells. It is clear that in regard to these extended activities, each TIMP is different. It is therefore not surprising that it has been difficult to predict the effect of over-expression of a particular TIMP in a specific cancer. An important lesson we learn from the analysis of the effects of TIMPs in cancer is that the extracellular milieu plays an important role in controlling the behavior of malignant cells. Our view on cancer can no longer be restricted to a genetic concept and must be broadened to include the regulatory function of the ECM in which TIMPs play an important part.

REFERENCES

Ahonen M, Baker AH, Kähäri VM. Adenovirus-mediated gene delivery of tissue inhibitor of metalloproteinases-3 inhibits invasion and induces apoptosis in melanoma cells. Cancer Res 1998; 58: 2310–2315.

Airola K, Karonen T, Vaalamo M, Lehti K, Lohi J, Kariniemi AL, Keski-Oja J, Saarialho-Kere UK. Expression of collagenases-1 and -3 and their inhibitors TIMP-1 and -3 correlates with the level of invasion in malignant melanomas. Br J Cancer 1999; 80: 733–743.

Alvarez OA, Carmichael DF, DeClerck YA. Inhibition of collagenolytic activity and metastasis of tumor cells by a recombinant human tissue inhibitor of metalloproteinases. J Natl Cancer Inst 1990; 82: 589–595.

Amour A, Slocombe PM, Webster A, Butler M, Knight CG, Smith BJ, Stephens PE, Shelle C, Hutton M, Knäuper V, Docherty AJP, Murphy G. TNF-α converting enzyme (TACE) is inhibited by TIMP-3. FEBS Lett 1998; 435: 39–44.

Anand-Apte B, Pepper MS, Voest E, Montesano R, Olsen B, Murphy G, Apte SS, Zetter B. Inhibition of angiogenesis by tissue inhibitor of metalloproteinase-3. Invest Ophthalmol Vis Sci 1997; 38: 817–823.

Andreú T, Beckers T, Thoenes E, Hilgard P, Von Melchner H. Gene trapping identifies inhibitors of oncogenic transformation – The tissue inhibitor of metalloproteinases-3 (TIMP3) and collagen type I (2 (COL1A2) are epidermal growth factor-regulated growth repressors. J Biol Chem 1998; 273: 13848–13854.

Arribas J, Coodly L, Vollmer P, Kishimoto TK, Rose-John S, Massague J. Diverse cell surface protein ectodomains are shed by a system sensitive to metalloprotease inhibitors. J Biol Chem 1996; 271: 11376–11382.

Bachman KE, Herman JG, Corn PG, Merlo A, Costello JF, Cavenee WK, Baylin SB, Graff JR. Methylation-associated silencing of the tissue inhibitor of metalloproteinase-3 gene suggest a suppressor role in kidney, brain, and other human cancers. Cancer Res 1999; 59: 798–802.

Baker AH, George SJ, Zaltsman AB, Murphy G, Newby AC. Inhibition of invasion and induction of apoptotic cell death of cancer cell lines by overexpression of TIMP-3. Br J Cancer 1999; 79: 1347–1355.

Bian JH, Jacobs C, Wang YL, Sun Y. Characterization of a putative p53 binding site in the promoter of the mouse tissue inhibitor of metalloproteinases-3 (TIMP-3) gene: TIMP-3 is not a p53 target gene. Carcinogenesis 1996a; 17: 2559–2562.

Bian J, Wang Y, Smith MR, Kim H, Jacobs C, Jackman J, Kung HF, Colburn NH, Sun Y. Suppression of in vivo tumor growth and induction of suspension cell death by tissue inhibitor of metalloproteinases (TIMP)-3. Carcinogenesis 1996b; 17: 1805–1811.

Bigg HF, Shi YE, Liu YLE, Steffensen B, Overall CM. Specific, high affinity binding of tissue inhibitor of metalloproteinases-4 (TIMP4) to the COOH-terminal hemopexin-like domain of human gelatinase A – TIMP-4 binds progelatinase A and the COOH-terminal domain in a similar manner to TIMP-2. J Biol Chem 1997; 272: 15496–15500.

Black RA, Rauch CT, Kozlosky CJ, Peschon JJ, Slack JL, Wolfson MF, Castner BJ, Stocking KL, Reddy P, Srinivasan S, Nelson N, Boiani N, Schooley KA, Gerhart M, Davis R, Fitzner JN, Johnson RS, Paxton RJ, March CJ, Cerretti DP. A metalloproteinase disintegrin that releases tumour-necrosis factor-α from cells. Nature 1997; 385: 729–733.

Blavier L, DeClerck YA. Tissue inhibitor of metalloproteinases-2 is expressed in the interstitial matrix in adult mouse organs and during embryonic development. Mol Biol Cell 1997; 8: 1513–1527.

Borland G, Murphy G, Ager A. Tissue inhibitor of metalloproteinases-3 inhibits shedding of L-selectin from leukocytes. J Biol Chem 1999; 274: 2810–2815.

Botelho FM, Edwards DR, Richards CD. Oncostatin M stimulates c-fos to bind a transcription-ally responsive AP-1 element within the tissue inhibitor of metalloproteinase-1 promoter. J Biol Chem 1998; 273: 5211–5218.

Boudreau N, Sympson CJ, Werb Z, Bissell MJ. Suppression of ICE and apoptosis in mammary epithelial cells by extracellular matrix. Science 1995; 267: 891–893.

Bramhall SR. The matrix metalloproteinases and their inhibitors in pancreatic cancer. Int J Pancreatol 1997; 21: 1–12.

Brooks PC, Stromblad S, Sanders LC, von Schalscha TL, Aimes RT, Stetler-Stevenson WG, Quigley JP, Cheresh DA. Localization of matrix metalloproteinase MMP-2 to the surface of invasive cells by interaction with integrin alpha v beta 3. Cell 1996; 85: 683–693.

Brummer O, Athar S, Riethdorf L, Loning T, Herbst H. Matrix-metalloproteinases 1, 2, and 3 and their tissue inhibitors 1 and 2 in benign and malignant breast lesions: an in situ hybridiza-tion study. Virchows Arch 1999; 435: 566–573.

Bugno M, Witek B, Bereta J, Bereta M, Edwards DR, Kordula T. Reprogramming of TIMP-1 and TIMP-3 expression profiles in brain microvascular endothelial cells and astrocytes in response to proinflammatory cytokines. FEBS Lett 1999; 448: 9–14.

Butler GS, Butler MJ, Atkinson SJ, Will H, Tamura T, Van Westrum SS, Crabbe T, Clements J, D'Ortho MP, Murphy G. The TIMP2 membrane type 1 metalloproteinase 'receptor' regu-lates the concentration and efficient activation of progelatinase A – A kinetic study. J Biol Chem 1998; 273: 871–880.

Butler GS, Hutton M, Wattam BA, Williamson RA, Knäuper V, Willenbrock F, Murphy G. The specificity of TIMP-2 for matrix metalloproteinases can be modified by single amino acid mutations. J Biol Chem 1999; 274: 20391–20396.

Caterina NCM, Windsor LJ Bodden MK, Yermovsky AE, Taylor KB, Birkedal Hansen H, Engler JA. Glycosylation and NH₂-terminal domain mutants of the tissue inhibitor of metallopro-teinases-1 (TIMP-1). Biochim Biophys Acta Protein Struct Mol Enzymol 1998; 1388: 21–34.

Christofori G, Semb H. The role of the cell-adhesion molecule E-cadherin as a tumour-suppressor gene. Trends Biochem Sci 1999; 24: 73–76.

Codony-Servat J, Albanell J, Lopez-Talavera JC, Arribas J, Baselga J. Cleavage of the HER2 ectodomain is a pervanadate-activable process that is inhibited by the tissue inhibitor of met-alloproteases-1 in breast cancer cells. Cancer Res 1999; 59: 1196–1201.

Corcoran ML, Stetler-Stevenson WG. Tissue inhibitor of metalloproteinase-2 stimulates fibrob-last proliferation via a cAMP-dependent mechanism. J Biol Chem 1995; 270: 13453–13459.

187

DeClerck YA, Perez N, Shimada H, Boone TC, Langley KE, Taylor SM. Inhibition of invasion and metastasis in cells transfected with an inhibitor of metalloproteinases. Cancer Res 1992; 52: 701–708.

DeClerck YA, Yean TD, Lu HS, Ting J, Langley KE. Inhibition of autoproteolytic activation of interstitial procollagenase by recombinant metalloproteinase inhibitor MI/TIMP-2. J Biol Chem 1991a; 266: 3893–3899.

DeClerck YA, Yean TD, Chan D, Shimada H, Langley KE. Inhibition of tumor invasion of smooth muscle cell layers by recombinant human metalloproteinase inhibitor. Cancer Res 1991b; 51: 2151–2157.

Docherty AJ, Lyons A, Smith BJ, Wright EM, Stephens PE, Harris TJ, Murphy G, Reynolds JJ. Sequence of human tissue inhibitor of metalloproteinases and its identify to erythroid-potentiating activity. Nature 1985; 318: 66–69.

Dong Z, Kumar R, Yang X, Fidler IJ. Macrophage-derived metalloelastase is responsible for the generation of angiostatin in Lewis lung carcinoma. Cell 1997; 88: 801–810.

Edwards DR, Leco KJ, Beaudry PP, Atadja PW, Veillette C, Riabowol KT. Differential effects of transforming growth factor-beta 1 on the expression of matrix metalloproteinases and tissue inhibitors of metalloproteinases in young and old human fibroblasts. Exp Gerontol 1996; 31: 207–223.

Fernandez-Catalan C, Bode W, Huber R, Turk D, Calvete JJ, Lichte A, Tschesche H, Maskos K. Crystal structure of the complex formed by the membrane type 1-matrix metalloproteinase with the tissue inhibitor of metalloproteinases-2, the soluble progelatinase A receptor. EMBO J 1998; 17: 5238–5248.

Fong KM, Kida Y, Zimmerman PV, Smith PJ. TIMP1 and adverse prognosis in non-small cell lung cancer. Clin Cancer Res 1996; 2: 1369–1372.

Fowlkes JL, Thrailkill KM, Serra DM, Nagase H. Insulin-like growth factor binding protein (IGFBP) substrate zymography – A new tool to identify and characterize IGFBP-degrading proteinases. Endocrine 1997; 7: 33–36.

Gallea-Robache S, Morand V, Millet S, Bruneau JM, Bhatnagar N, Chouaib S, Roman-Roman S. A metalloproteinase inhibitor blocks the shedding of soluble cytokine receptors and processing of transmembrane cytokine precursors in human monocytic cells. Cytokine 1997; 9: 340–346.

Gatsios P, Haubeck HD, Van de Leur E, Frisch W, Apte SS, Greiling H, Heinrich PC, Graeve L. Oncostatin M differentially regulates tissue inhibitors of metalloproteinases TIMP-1 and TIMP-3 gene expression in human synovial lining cells. Eur J Biochem 1996; 241: 56–63.

Goldberg GI, Strongin A, Collier IE, Genrich LT, Marmer BL. Interaction of 92-kDa type IV collagenase with the tissue inhibitor of metalloproteinases prevents dimerization, complex formation with interstitial collagenase, and activation of the proenzyme with stromelysin. J Biol Chem 1992; 267: 4583–4591.

Gomis-Rüth FX, Maskos K, Betz M, Bergner A, Huber R, Suzuki K, Yoshida N, Nagase H, Brew K, Bourenkov GP, Bartunik H, Bode W. Mechanism of inhibition of the human matrix metalloproteinase stromelysin-1 by TIMP-1. Nature 1997; 389: 77–81.

Goss KJH, Brown PD, Matrisian LM. Differing effects of endogenous and synthetic inhibitors of metalloproteinases on intestinal tumorigenesis. Int J Cancer 1998; 78: 629–635.

Grignon DJ, Sakr W, Toth M, Ravery V, Angulo J, Shamsa F, Pontes JE, Crissman JC, Fridman R. High levels of tissue inhibitor of metalloproteinase-2 (TIMP-2) expression are associated with poor outcome in invasive bladder cancer. Cancer Res 1996; 56: 1654–1659.

Guedez L, Courtemanch L, Stetler-Stevenson M. Tissue inhibitor of metalloproteinase (TIMP)-1 induces differentiation and an antiapoptotic phenotype in germinal center B cells. Blood 1998b; 92: 1342–1349.

Guedez L, Stetler-Stevenson WG, Wolff L, Wang J, Fukushima P, Mansoor A, Stetler-Stevenson M. In vitro suppression of programmed cell death of B cells by tissue inhibitor of metalloproteinases-1. J Clin Invest 1998a; 102: 2002–2010.

Hammani K, Blakis A, Morsette D, Bowcock AM, Schmutte C, Henriet P, DeClerck YA. Structure and characterization of the human tissue inhibitor of metalloproteinases-2 (TIMP-2) gene. J Biol Chem 1996; 271: 25498–25505.

Hayakawa T, Yamashita K, Ohuchi E, Shinagawa A. Cell growth-promoting activity of tissue inhibitor of metalloproteinases-2 (TIMP-2). J Cell Sci 1994; 107: 2373–2379.

Hayakawa T, Yamashita K, Tanzawa K, Uchijima E, Iwata K. Growth-promoting activity of tissue inhibitor of metalloproteinases-1 (TIMP-1) for a wide range of cells. A possible new growth factor in serum. FEBS Lett 1992; 298: 29–32.

Henriet P, Zhong ZD, Brooks PC, Weinberg KI, DeClerck YA. Contact with fibrillar collagen inhibits melanoma cell proliferation by up-regulating p27KIP1. Proc Natl Acad Sci (USA) 2000; 97: 10026–10031.

Hernandez-Barrantes S, Toth M, Bernardo MM, Yurkova M, Gervasi DC, Raz Y, Sang QA, Fridman R. Binding of active (57 kDa) membrane type 1-matrix metalloproteinase (MT1-MMP) to tissue inhibitor of metalloproteinase (TIMP)-2 regulates MT1-MMP processing and pro-MMP-2 activation. J Biol Chem 2000; 275: 12080–12089.

Holten-Andersen MN, Murphy G, Nielsen HJ, Pedersen AN, Christensen IJ, Hoyer-Hansen G, Brunner N, Stephens RW. Quantitation of TIMP-1 in plasma of healthy blood donors and patients with advanced cancer. Br J Cancer 1999; 80: 495–503.

Hoshi M, Harada A, Kawase T, Uyemura K, Yazaki T. Antitumoral effects of defective herpes simplex virus-mediated transfer of tissue inhibitor of metalloproteinases-2 gene in malignant glioma U87 in vitro: consequences for anti-cancer gene therapy. Cancer Gene Ther 2000; 7: 799–805.

Imren S, Kohn, DB, Shimada H, Blavier L, DeClerck YA. Overexpression of tissue inhibitor of metalloproteinases-2 in vivo by retroviral mediated gene transfer inhibits tumor growth and invasion. Cancer Res 1996; 56: 2891–2895.

Indraccolo S, Minuzzo S, Gola E, Habeler W, Carrozzino F, Noonan D, Albini A, Santi L, Amadori A, Chieco-Bianchi L. Generation of expression plasmids for angiostatin, endostatin and TIMP-2 for cancer gene therapy. Int J Biol Markers 1999; 14: 251–256.

Janowska-Wieczorek A, Marquez LA, Matsuzaki A, Hashmi HR, Larratt LM, Boshkov LM, Turner AR, Zhang MC, Edwards DR. Expression of matrix metalloproteinases (MMP-2 and -9) and tissue inhibitors of metalloproteinases (TIMP-1 and -2) in acute myelogenous leukaemia blasts: comparison with normal bone marrow cells. Br J Haematol 1999; 105: 402–411.

Johnson MD, Kim HR, Chesler L, Tsao Wu G, Bouck N, Polverini PJ. Inhibition of angiogenesis by tissue inhibitor of metalloproteinase. J Cell Physiol 1994; 160: 194–202.

Kang SH, Choi HH, Kim SG, Jong HS, Kim NK, Kim SJ, Bang YJ. Transcriptional inactivation of the tissue inhibitor of metalloproteinase-3 gene by dna hypermethylation of the 5'-CpG island in human gastric cancer cell lines. Int J Cancer 2000; 86: 632–635.

Khokha R. Suppression of the tumorigenic and metastatic abilities of murine B16-F10 melanoma cells in vivo by the overexpression of the tissue inhibitor of the metalloproteinases-1. J Natl Cancer Inst 1994; 86: 299–304.

Khokha R, Waterhouse P, Yagel S, Lala PK, Overall CM, Norton G, Denhardt DT. Antisense RNA-induced reduction in murine TIMP levels confers oncogenicity on Swiss 3T3 cells. Science 1989; 243: 947–950.

Kikkawa F, Tamakoshi K, Nawa A, Shibata K, Yamagata S, Yamagata T, Suganuma N. Positive correlation between inhibitors of matrix metalloproteinase 1 and matrix metalloproteinases in malignant ovarian tumor tissues. Cancer Lett 1997: 120: 109–115.

Ko YC, Langley, KE, Mendiaz, EA, Parker VP, Taylor SM, DeClerck YA. The C-terminal domain of tissue inhibitor of metalloproteinases-2 is required for cell binding but not for antimetalloproteinase activity. Biochem Biophys Res Commun 1997; 236: 100–105.

Koop S, Khokha R, Schmidt EE, MacDonald IC, Morris VL, Chambers AF, Groom AC. Overexpression of metalloproteinase inhibitor in B16-F10 cells does not affect extravasation but reduces tumor growth. Cancer Res 1994; 54: 4791–4797.

Korzus E, Nagase H, Rydell R, Travis J. The mitogen-activated protein kinase and JAK-STAT signaling pathways are required for an oncostatin M-responsive element-mediated activation of matrix metalloproteinase 1 gene expression. J Biol Chem 1997; 272: 1188–1196.

Kossakowska AE, Edwards DR, Prusinkiewicz C, Zhang MC, Guo DL, Urbanski SJ, Grogan T, Marquez LA, Janowska-Wieczorek A. Interleukin-6 regulation of matrix metalloproteinase (MMP-2 and MMP-9) and tissue inhibitor of metalloproteinase (TIMP-1) expression in malignant non-Hodgkin's lymphomas. Blood 1999; 94: 2080–2089.

Kossakowska AE, Urbanski SJ, Huchcroft SA, Edwards, DR. Relationship between the clinical aggressiveness of large cell immuno-blastic lymphomas and expression of 92 kDa gelatinase (type IV collagenase) and tissue inhibitor of metalloproteinases-1 (TIMP-1) RNAs. Oncol Res 1992; 4: 233–240.

Kostoulas G, Lang A, Nagase H, Baici A. Stimulation of angiogenesis through cathepsin B inactivation of the tissue inhibitors of matrix metalloproteinases. FEBS Lett 1999; 455: 286–290.

Langton KP, Barker MD, McKie N. Localization of the functional domains of human tissue inhibitor of metalloproteinases-3 and the effects of a Sorsby's fundus dystrophy mutation. J Biol Chem 1998; 273: 16778–16781.

Leco KJ, Apte SS, Taniguchi GT, Hawkes SP, Khokha R, Schultz GA, Edwards DR. Murine tissue inhibitor of metalloproteinases-4 (Timp-4): cDNA isolation and expression in adult mouse tissues. FEBS Lett 1997; 401: 213–217.

Leco KJ, Khokha R, Pavloff N, Hawkes SP, Edwards DR. Tissue inhibitor of metalloproteinases-3 (TIMP-3) is an extracellular matrix-associated protein with a distinctive pattern of expression in mouse cells and tissues. J Biol Chem 1994; 269: 9352–9360.

Li G, Fridman R, Kim HR. Tissue inhibitor of metalloproteinase-1 inhibits apoptosis of human breast epithelial cells. Cancer Res 1999; 59: 6267–6275.

Li WQ, Zafarullah M. Oncostatin M up-regulates tissue inhibitor of metalloproteinases-3 gene expression in articular chondrocytes via de novo transcription, protein synthesis, and tyrosine kinase- and mitogen-activated protein kinase-dependent mechanisms. J Immunol 1998; 161: 5000–5007.

Lijnen HR, Ugwu F, Bini A, Collen D. Generation of an angiostatin-like fragment from plasminogen by stromelysin-1 (MMP-3). Biochemistry 1998; 37: 4699–4702.

Lim MS, Guedez L, Stetler-Stevenson WG, Stetler-Stevenson M. Tissue inhibitor of metalloproteinase-2 induces apoptosis in human T lymphocytes. Ann NY Acad Sci 1999; 878: 522–523.

Lochter A, Galosy S, Muschler J, Freedman N, Werb Z, Bissell MJ. Matrix metalloproteinase stromelysin-1 triggers a cascade of molecular alterations that leads to stable epithelial-to-mesenchymal conversion and a premalignant phenotype in mammary epithelial cells. J Cell Biol 1997; 139: 1861–1872.

Loging WT, Reisman D. Inhibition of the putative tumor suppressor gene TIMP-3 by tumor-derived p53 mutants and wild type p53. Oncogene 1999; 18: 7608–7615.

Lombard MA, Wallace TL, Kubicek MF, Petzold GL, Mitchell MA, Hendges SK, Wilks JW.

190

Synthetic matrix metalloproteinase inhibitors and tissue inhibitor of metalloproteinase (TIMP)-2, but not TIMP-1, inhibit shedding of tumor necrosis factor-α receptors in a human colon adenocarcinoma (Colo 205) cell line. Cancer Res 1998; 58: 4001–4007.

Lu XQ, Levy M, Weinstein IB, Santella RM. Immunological quantitation of levels of tissue inhibitor of metalloproteinase-1 in human colon cancer. Cancer Res 1991; 51: 6231–6235.

Lukashev ME, Werb Z. ECM signalling: orchestrating cell behaviour and misbehaviour. Trends Cell Biol 1998; 8: 437–441.

MacDougall JR, Bani MR, Lin Y, Muschel RJ, Kerbel RS. 'Proteolytic switching': opposite patterns of regulation of gelatinase B and its inhibitor TIMP-1 during human melanoma progression and consequences of gelatinase B overexpression. Br J Cancer 1999; 80: 504–512.

Manes S, Llorente M, Lacalle RA, Gomez-Mouton C, Kremer L, Mira E, Martinez A. The matrix metalloproteinase-9 regulates the insulin-like growth factor-triggered autocrine response in DU-145 carcinoma cells. J Biol Chem 1999; 274: 6935–6945.

Maquoi E, Frankenne F, Baramova E, Munaut C, Sounni NE, Remacle A, Noel A, Murphy G, Foidart JM. Membrane type 1 matrix metalloproteinase-associated degradation of tissue inhibitor of metalloproteinase 2 in human tumor cell lines. J Biol Chem 2000; 275: 11368–11378.

Martin DC, Fowlkes JL, Babic B, Khokha R. Insulin-like growth factor II signaling in neoplastic proliferation is blocked by transgenic expression of the metalloproteinase inhibitor TIMP-1. J Cell Biol 1999; 146: 881–892.

Martin DC, Ruther U, Sanchez Sweatman OH, Orr FW, Khokha R. Inhibition of SV40 T antigen-induced hepatocellular carcinoma in TIMP-1 transgenic mice. Oncogene 1996; 13: 569–576.

McCarthy K, Maguire T, McGreal G, McDermott E, O'Higgins N, Duffy MJ. High levels of tissue inhibitor of metalloproteinase-1 predict poor outcome in patients with breast cancer. Int J Cancer 1999; 84: 44–48.

Montgomery AM, DeClerck YA, Langley KE, Reisfeld, RA, Mueller BM. Melanoma-mediated dissolution of extracellular matrix: contribution of urokinase-dependent and metalloproteinase-dependent proteolytic pathways. Cancer Res 1993; 53: 693–700.

Montgomery AM, Mueller BM, Reisfeld RA, Taylor SM, DeClerck YA. Effect of tissue inhibitor of the matrix metalloproteinases-2 expression on the growth and spontaneous metastasis of a human melanoma cell line. Cancer Res 1994; 54: 5467–5473.

Moses MA, Sudhalter J, Langer R. Identification of an inhibitor of neovascularization from cartilage. Science 1990; 248: 1408–1410.

Murphy AN, Unsworth, EJ, Stetler Stevenson WG. Tissue inhibitor of metalloproteinases-2 inhibits bFGF-induced human microvascular endothelial cell proliferation. J Cell Physiol 1993; 157: 351–358.

Murphy G, Houbrechts A, Cockett MI, Williamson RA, O Shea M, Docherty AJ. The N-terminal domain of tissue inhibitor of metalloproteinases retains metalloproteinase inhibitory activity. Biochemistry 1991; 30: 8097–8102.

Murphy G, Willenbrock F. Tissue inhibitors of matrix metalloendopeptidases. Methods Enzymol 1995; 248: 496–510.

Muskett FW, Frenkiel TA, Feeney J, Freedman RB, Carr MD, Williamson RA. High resolution structure of the N-terminal domain of tissue inhibitor of metalloproteinases-2 and characterization of its interaction site with matrix metalloproteinase-3. J Biol Chem 1998; 273: 21736–21743.

Nagase H. Activation mechanisms of matrix metalloproteinases. Biol Chem Hoppe Seyler 1997; 378: 151–160.

Nagase H, Meng Q, Malinovskii V, Huang W, Chung L, Bode W, Maskos K, Brew K. Engineering of selective TIMPs. Ann NY Acad Sci 1999; 878: 1–11.

191

Nomura S, Hogan BL, Wills AJ, Heath JK, Edwards DR. Developmental expression of tissue inhibitor of metalloproteinase (TIMP) RNA. Development 1989; 105: 575–583.

O'Reilly MS, Wiederschain D, Stetler-Stevenson WG, Folkman J, Moses MA. Regulation of angiostatin production by matrix metalloproteinase-2 in a model of concomitant resistance. J Biol Chem 1999; 274: 29568–29571.

Oberg A, Hoyhtya M, Tavelin B, Stenling R, Lindmark G. Limited value of preoperative serum analyses of matrix metalloproteinases (MMP-2, MMP-9) and tissue inhibitors of matrix metalloproteinases (TIMP-1, TIMP-2) in colorectal cancer. Anticancer Res 2000; 20: 1085–1091.

Okamoto I, Kawano Y, Tsuiki H, Sasaki J, Nakao M, Matsumoto M, Suga M, Ando M, Nakajima M, Saya H. CD44 cleavage induced by a membrane-associated metalloprotease plays a critical role in tumor cell migration. Oncogene 1999; 18: 1435–1446.

Overall CM, King AE, Sam DK, Ong AD, Lau TTY, Wallon UM, DeClerck YA, Atherstone J. Identification of the tissue inhibitor of metalloproteinases-2 (TIMP-2) binding site on the hemopexin carboxyl domain of human gelatinase a by site-directed mutagenesis – The hierarchical role in binding TIMP-2 of the unique cationic clusters of hemopexin modules III and IV. J Biol Chem 1999; 274: 4421–4429.

Patterson BC, Sang QA. Angiostatin-converting enzyme activities of human matrilysin (MMP-7) and gelatinase B/type IV collagenase (MMP-9). J Biol Chem 1997; 272: 28823–28825.

Pennie WD, Hegamyer GA, Young MR, Colburn NH. Specific methylation events contribute to the transcriptional repression of the mouse tissue inhibitor of metalloproteinases-3 gene in neoplastic cells. Cell Growth Differ 1999; 10: 279–286.

Prenzel N, Zwick E, Daub H, Leserer M, Abraham R, Wallasch C, Ullrich A. EGF receptor transactivation by G-protein-coupled receptors requires metalloproteinase cleavage of proHB-EGF. Nature 1999; 402: 884–888.

Remacle A, McCarthy K, Noel A, Maguire T, McDermott E, O'Higgins N, Foidart JM, Duffy MJ. High levels of TIMP-2 correlate with adverse prognosis in breast cancer. Int J Cancer 2000; 89: 118–121.

Ritter LM, Garfield SH, Thorgeirsson UP. Tissue inhibitor of metalloproteinases-1 (TIMP-1) binds to the cell surface and translocates to the nucleus of human MCF-7 breast carcinoma cells. Biochem Biophys Res Commun 1999; 257: 494–499.

Sang QX. Complex role of matrix metalloproteinases in angiogenesis. Cell Res 1998; 8: 171–177.

Schultz RM, Silberman S, Persky B, Bajkowski AS, Carmichael DF. Inhibition by human recombinant tissue inhibitor of metalloproteinases of human amnion invasion and lung colonization by murine B16-F10 melanoma cells. Cancer Res 1988; 48: 5539–5545.

Smith MR, Kung H, Durum SK, Colburn NH, Sun Y. TIMP-3 induces cell death by stabilizing TNF-alpha receptors on the surface of human colon carcinoma cells. Cytokine 1997; 9: 770–780.

Soloway PD, Alexander CM, Werb Z, Jaenisch R. Targeted mutagenesis of Timp-1 reveals that lung tumor invasion is influenced by Timp-1 genotype of the tumor but not by that of the host. Oncogene 1996; 13: 2307–2314.

Sternlicht MD, Bissell MJ, Werb Z. The matrix metalloproteinase stromelysin-1 acts as a natural mammary tumor promoter. Oncogene 2000; 19: 1102–1113.

Sternlicht MD, Lochter A, Sympson CJ, Huey B, Rougier JP, Gray JW, Pinkel D, Bissell MJ, Werb Z. The stromal proteinase MMP3/stromelysin-1 promotes mammary carcinogenesis. Cell 1999; 98: 137–146.

Strongin AY, Collier, I, Bannikov G, Marmer BL, Grant GA, Goldberg GI. Mechanism of cell surface activation of 72-kDa type IV collagenase.Isolation of the activated form of the membrane metalloprotease. J Biol Chem 1995; 270: 5331–5338.

Su SM, Dehnade F, Zafarullah M. Regulation of tissue inhibitor of metalloproteinases-3 gene expression by transforming growth factor-α and dexamethasone in bovine and human articular chondrocytes. DNA Cell Biol 1996; 15: 1039–1048.

Sugiura Y, Shimada H, Seeger RC, Laug WE, DeClerck YA. Matrix metalloproteinases-2 and -9 are expressed in human neuroblastoma: contribution of stromal cells to their production and correlation with metastasis. Cancer Res 1998; 58: 2209–2216.

Sun Y, Hegamyer G, Kim H, Sithanandam K, Li H, Watts R, Colburn NH. Molecular cloning of mouse tissue inhibitor of metalloproteinases-3 and its promoter. Specific lack of expression in neoplastic JB6 cells may reflect altered gene methylation. J Biol Chem 1995; 270: 19312–19319.

Suzuki M, Raab G, Moses MA, Fernandez CA, Klagsbrun M. Matrix metalloproteinase-3 releases active heparin-binding EGF- like growth factor by cleavage at a specific juxtamembrane site. J Biol Chem 1997; 272: 31730–31737.

Thomas P, Khokha R, Shepherd FA, Feld R, Tsao MS. Differential expression of matrix metalloproteinases and their inhibitors in non-small cell lung cancer. J Pathol 2000; 190: 150–156.

Tierney GM, Griffin NR, Stuart RC, Kasem H, Lynch KP, Lury JT, Brown PD, Millar AW, Steele RJC, Parsons SL. A pilot study of the safety and effects of the matrix metalloproteinase inhibitor marimastat in gastric cancer. Eur J Cancer [A] 1999; 35: 563–568.

Tuuttila A, Morgunova E, Bergmann U, Lindqvist Y, Maskos K, Fernandez-Catalan C, Bode W, Tryggvason K, Schneider G. Three-dimensional structure of human tissue inhibitor of metalloproteinases-2 at 2.1 Å resolution. J Mol Biol 1998; 284: 1133–1140.

Valente P, Fassina G, Melchiori A, Masiello L, Cilli M, Vacca A, Onisto M, Santi L, Stetler-Stevenson WG, Albini A. TIMP-2 over-expression reduces invasion and angiogenesis and protects B16-F10 melanoma cells from apoptosis. Int J Cancer 1998; 75: 246–253.

Visscher DW, Hoyhtyea M, Ottosen SK, Liang CM, Sarkar FH, Crissman JD, Fridman R. Enhanced expression of tissue inhibitor of metalloproteinase-2 (TIMP-2) in the stroma of breast carcinomas correlates with tumor recurrence. Int J Cancer 1994; 59: 339–344.

Wang MS, Liu YLE, Greene J, Sheng SJ, Fuchs A, Rosen EM, Shi YE. Inhibition of tumor growth and metastasis of human breast cancer cells transfected with tissue inhibitor of metalloproteinase 4. Oncogene 1997; 14: 2767–2774.

Wang Z, Juttermann R, Soloway PD. TIMP-2 is required for efficient activation of proMMP-2 in vivo. J Biol Chem 2000.

Ward RV, Atkinson SJ, Slocombe PM, Docherty AJ, Reynolds JJ, Murphy G. Tissue inhibitor of metalloproteinases-2 inhibits the activation of 72 kDa progelatinase by fibroblast membranes. Biochim Biophys Acta 1991; 1079: 242–246.

Wen W, Moses, MA, Wiederschain D, Arbiser JL, Folkman J. The generation of endostatin is mediated by elastase. Cancer Res 1999; 59: 6052–6056.

Werb Z. ECM and cell surface proteolysis: regulating cellular ecology. Cell 1997; 91: 439–442.

Whitelock JM, Murdoch AD, Iozzo RV, Underwood PA. The degradation of human endothelial cell-derived perlecan and release of bound basic fibroblast growth factor by stromelysin, collagenase, plasmin, and heparanases. J Biol Chem 1996; 271: 10079–10086.

Wick M, Hareonen R, Mumberg D, Burger C, Olsen BR, Budarf ML, Apte SS, Muller R. Structure of the human TIMP-3 gene and its cell cycle-regulated promoter. Biochem J 1995; 311: 549–554.

Wilson CL, Ouellette AJ, Satchell DP, Ayabe T, López-Boado YS, Stratman JL, Hultgren SJ, Matrisian LM, Parks WC. Regulation of intestinal-defensin activation by the metalloproteinase matrilysin in innate host defense. Science 1999; 286: 113–117.

Wojtowicz-Praga S, Torri J, Johnson M, Steen V, Marshall J, Ness E, Dickson R, Sale M,

Rasmussen HS, Chiodo TA, Hawkins MJ. Phase I trial of marimastat, a novel matrix metalloproteinase inhibitor, administered orally to patients with advanced lung cancer. J Clin Oncol 1998; 16: 2150–2156.

Yamashita K, Suzuki M, Iwata H, Koike T, Hamaguchi M, Shinagawa A, Noguchi T, Hayakawa T. Tyrosine phosphorylation is crucial for growth signaling by tissue inhibitors of metalloproteinases (TIMP-1 and TIMP-2). FEBS Lett 1996; 396: 103–107.

Ylisirnio S, Hoyhtya M, Turpeenniemi-Hujanen T. Serum matrix metalloproteinases -2, -9 and tissue inhibitors of metalloproteinases -1, -2 in lung cancer – TIMP-1 as a prognostic marker. Anticancer Res 2000; 20: 1311–1316.

Yoneda T, Sasaki A, Dunstan C, Williams PJ, Bauss F, DeClerck YA, Mundy GR. Inhibition of osteolytic bone metastasis of breast cancer by combined treatment with the bisphosphonate ibandronate and tissue inhibitor of the matrix metalloproteinase-2. J Clin Invest 1997; 99: 2509–2517.

Yoshikawa T, Tsuburaya A, Kobayashi O, Sairenji M, Motohashi H, Yanoma S, Noguchi Y. Prognostic value of tissue inhibitor of matrix metalloproteinase-1 in plasma of patients with gastric cancer. Cancer Lett 2000; 151: 81–86.

Zeng Y, Rosborough RC, Li YJ, Gupta AR, Bennett J. Temporal and spatial regulation of gene expression mediated by the promoter for the human tissue inhibitor of metalloproteinases- 3 (TIMP-3)-encoding gene. Dev Dyn 1998; 211: 228–237.

Zhao WQ, Li H, Yamashita K, Guo XK, Hoshino T, Yoshida S, Shinya T, Hayakawa T. Cell cycle-associated accumulation of tissue inhibitor of metalloproteinases-1 (TIMP-1) in the nuclei of human gingival fibroblasts. J Cell Sci 1998; 111: 1147–1153.

Zhong ZD, Hammani K, Bae WS, DeClerck YA. NF-Y and Sp1 cooperate for the transcriptional activation and cAMP response of human tissue inhibitor of metalloproteinases-2. J Biol Chem 2000; 275: 18602–18610.

Zucker S, Hymowitz M, Conner C, Zarrabi HM, Hurewitz AN, Matrisian L, Boyd D, Nicolson G, Montana S. Measurement of matrix metalloproteinases and tissue inhibitors of metalloproteinases in blood and tissues – Clinical and experimental applications. Ann NY Acad Sci 1999; 878: 212–227.

Chapter 10

CLINICAL ASPECTS OF MATRIX METALLOPROTEINASES

Béatrice Nawrocki-Raby, Christine Clavel, Myriam Polette and Philippe Birembaut
I.N.S.E.R.M. U. 514, I.F.R. 53, and Laboratoire Pol Bouin, C.H.U. of REIMS, France

Abstract

Tumor metastasis is ultimately responsible for most cancer deaths. Tumor invasion and metastasis represent a multistep process including basement membrane disruption, stromal infiltration, angiogenesis, intravasation and extravasation and invasion of target organs by tumor cells. All these events require degradation and remodeling of the extracellular matrix (ECM) by various proteolytic enzymes. Among these enzymes, matrix metalloproteinases (MMPs) play a key role at various levels. These enzymes are associated with degradation of a broad spectrum of ECM components. MMPs are also implicated in the remodeling the ECM by creating and maintaining a microenvironment that facilitates angiogenesis and growth of tumors. Thus, in the last years, the exploration of MMPs expression has led to a large bunch of studies on their biological activities and their clinical implications.

1. THE MMP FAMILY

The MMP family consists of 4 principal subclasses which include the collagenases, the gelatinases (type IV collagenases), the stromelysins, and the Membrane-Type MMPs (MT-MMPs) (Nagase and Woessner, 1999). These enzymes are secreted and are membrane-bound in a latent, proenzyme form and require activation to digest ECM components. The activation process consists in a proteolytic cleavage of a propeptide domain at the N-terminus of the MMP molecule which can be accomplished by proteolytic enzymes including plasmin and other MMPs. For example, most of the MT-MMPs participate in the activation of pro-MMP-2. After this activation, most MMPs are able to degrade a broad spectrum of ECM components, allowing tumor cells to penetrate the stroma. The interstitial collagenases (MMP-1, MMP-8, MMP 13 and MMP-18) cleave a specific peptide bond in triple helical fibrillar collagens I, II and III. The two gelatinases A (MMP-2) and B (MMP-9) target denatured collagen, gelatin and the type IV collagen present in basement membranes. The stromelysins have the broadest spectrum of substrates, cleaving proteoglycans, gelatin, laminin, fibronectin. This subfamily includes stromelysin 1 (MMP-3),

J.-M. Foidart and R.J. Muschel (eds.), Proteases and Their Inhibitors in Cancer Metastasis, 195–204.
© 2002 *Kluwer Academic Publishers. Printed in the Netherlands.*

stromelysin 2 (MMP-10), stromelysin 3 (MMP-11) and matrilysin (MMP-7). The last group encompasses five membrane-bound MMPs (MT1 to MT5-MMPs). There is a good evidence that one of their principal functions is to localize and activate secreted MMPs, particularly MMP-2 and MMP-13. However the role of MMPs is not limited to the ECM degradation. Indeed, recent studies implicate these enzymes in the activation of growth factors and/or their receptors, in the degradation of enzyme inhibitors, in the degradation of cell-matrix attachments, cell adhesion complexes and in the production of ECM products of degradation promoting angiogenesis and tumor invasion (Mc Cawley and Matrisian, 2000). Of particular interest is the case of MMP-11 (stromelysin-3). At the present time, no known ECM component has been reported degraded by this enzyme. Nevertheless it has been shown that this MMP-11 functions *in vivo* as a protease by remodeling ECM and probably by inducing it to release the necessary microenvironmental factors for tumor growth (Noël et al, 2000). This represents a new important role of MMPs and a new approach for understanding cancer progression.

MMP activity is regulated at multiple levels. At the transcriptional level, most of the MMP genes are responsive to a wide variety of growth factors, cytokines, hormones and oncogenes. Tissue inhibitors of MMPs (TIMPs) block enzymatic activity. At the present time, four members of the TIMP family are known, capable of binding and inhibiting the activity of all the members of the MMP family. However, TIMPs display differences in tissue distribution and differ in their capacity to form complexes with the inactive form of MMP and thereby in their ability to control MMP activation and activity. Interestingly, TIMP-2 is also involved in the activation process of MMP-2 as it binds to MT1-MMP and pro-MMP-2 at cell surface, resulting in proteolytic activation of the pro-MMP-2 by adjacent activated MT1-MMP (Strongin et al, 1995). TIMP-1 and TIMP-2 also display some growth factors properties (Bertaux et al, 1991; Stetler- Stevenson et al, 1992).Thus the regulation of MMPs activity cannot be reduced to a simple balance between MMPs and inhibitors.

2. DETECTION OF MMPs IN TUMORS

In the literature, various methodologies have been used for the detection of MMP expression in tumors. Numerous *in vivo* studies have reported the local-ization and production of these enzymes within tumor and stromal cells using immunohistochemistry and *in situ* hybridization. The expression of steady state level of mRNAs encoding MMPs in tumor tissues has been tested and quanti-fied by Northern Blot and/or RT-PCR. In another way, zymographic detection for MMPs and reverse zymographic detection of TIMPs, western blot analyses and ELISA from tumor extracts have given indication of enzymatic activities, activations and potential inhibitions of MMPs. Moreover, MMPs in blood have been used as diagnostic markers of invasion and metastasis. Each of these approaches has given different, sometimes contradictory, but complementary informations, with possible clinical applications.

The first observation of the role of MMPs *in vivo* in human tumoral pathology was made by Barsky et al (1983) who detected a type IV collagenase in tumor cells of breast carcinomas. Since then, numerous works have focused on the study of MMP expression in almost all tumors. The expression of MMPs in carcinomas is an early event. MMPs such as MMP-2, MMP-11 and MT1-MMP, are expressed *in vivo* in preinvasive lesions such as intraductal carcinomas of the breast and in bronchial squamous preinvasive lesions (Galateau-Salle et al, 2000; Polette et al, 1993). Although initially it was assumed that the tumor cells were the major source of MMPs expression, there was growing evidence that most MMPs were produced by host stromal cells. If MMP-7 (matrilysin) is commonly expressed in the epithelial compartment of adenocarcinomas, MMP-2, MT1-MMP, MMP-9, MMP-1, MMP-3, MMP-11 and MMP-13 which are the principal MMPs detected in cancers, are largely synthesized by fibroblasts, myofibroblasts and inflammatory cells of the stroma, as shown by *in situ* hybridization studies. The concept of stromal cell expression of MMPs has been particularly well established by the demonstration of MMP-11 (stromelysin 3) associated with breast cancer (Basset et al, 1990). Since this fundamental study, numerous papers have reported the same observations (Nelson et al, 2000). Moreover, some tumor cells in carcinomas may also undergo an epithelial-to-mesenchymal transition, with the apparition of vimentin in their cytoplasm (Gilles and Thompson, 1996). They acquire the fully metastatic phenotype and produce these MMPs. This concept has been well described in *in vitro* models. These tumor cells could represent *in vivo*, a limited population of metastatic cancer cells which would not require the contribution of stromal MMPs to be able to disseminate (Martinella-Catusse et al, 1999). At last, MMPs play a direct role in the neoangiogenesis observed in most tumors. Indeed, MMP-2 and MMP-9 have been detected *in vivo* in endothelial cells of the neovasculature of breast tumors (Heppner et al, 1996; Polette et al, 1993). All these observations underline the role of MMPs in the various steps of tumor progression.

The concept of cooperation between tumor and stromal cells for tumor progression is now well accepted. Multiple diffusible growth factors regulating MMPs expression are produced by tumor cells. For example, it has been reported that breast cancer cell lines MCF-7 and 8701-BC produced several growth factors such as TGFα and TGFβ which are known to modulate the production of MMPs (Bates et al, 1988; Knabbe et al, 1987; Noël et al, 1994;

Polette et al, 1997) have also observed an enhancement of MMP-2 and MT1-MMP in human fibroblasts in response to breast adenocarcinoma cell lines. This paracrine regulation concept has largely been well developed by Biswas et al (1995) leading to the characterization and cloning of EMMPRIN (Extracellular Matrix MetalloPRoteinase INducer). This factor produced by tumor cells increases the expression of MMP-1, MMP-2 and MMP-3 by stromal fibroblasts. EMMPRIN expression has been demonstrated *in vivo* in tumor cells in breast and lung carcinomas. Its detection in some endothelial cells and fibroblasts by immunohistochemistry seems to indicate that EMMPRIN binds selectively to a receptor on these cells (Caudroy et al, 1999). Moreover, it has been recently demonstrated that EMMPRIN can bind to MMP-1 (Guo et al, 2000). The degradation of stromal ECM may also produce additional MMP-inducing factors, such as fibronectin or elastin fragments which have been shown to initiate MMP expression (Brassart et al, 1998; Werb et al, 1989). In another way, fibroblasts in close contact to tumor clusters overexpress mRNAs encoding type I collagen in breast carcinomas. Type I collagen increases the steady-state MT1-MMP mRNA levels resulting in a local activation of MMP-2 (Gilles et al, 1997). At last, a tumor cell surface-associated binding site for MMP-2 (Emonard et al, 1992) and a cell surface binding for TIMP-2 (Emmert-Buck et al, 1995) have been described in breast carcinoma cell lines MCF-7 and MDA-MB231. These binding sites could play a role for the binding of MMP-2 produced by stromal cells, at the cell surface of tumor cells. The $\alpha_v\beta_3$ integrin might also serve to recruit activated MMP-2 to the tumor cell membrane (Brooks et al, 1996). Taken together, these data emphasize a complex cooperation between stromal and tumor cells in the production and activation of MMPs.

3. CLINICAL APPLICATIONS

From all these data showing the large MMP expression *in vivo* in tumors, numerous studies have been conducted to use MMP expression as a diagnostic or prognostic marker. MMP-11 has been particularly associated with malignant lesions (Basset et al, 1990). Indeed this MMP is specifically detected in most carcinomas whereas their benign counterparts do not express this enzyme. However, this stromal MMP has also been detected in wound healing in epithelial bronchial cells exhibiting an epithelial to mesenchymal transition (Buisson et al, 1996). Moreover, in the light of the activation mechanism of MMP-2, it is not surprising that the coexpression of MMP-2 and its principal activator MT1-MMP is more frequently reported in cancers than in the adjacent benign lesions and/or normal tissues. *In situ* hybridization studies clearly show that the same stromal cells produce both enzymes in breast carcinomas, but generally with a more restricted pattern of distribution for MT1-MMP than for MMP-2. These observations may be paralleled to the findings that the ratio of activated to total MMP-2 levels increases in advanced, metastatic diseases in breast carcinomas (Brown et al, 1993; Davies et al, 1993). In a general way, malignant tumors tend to express a wider variety of MMPs than benign lesions and/or normal tissues. For example, MMP-7 is the only MMP detected in benign polyps, whereas colon adenocarcinomas express MMP-1, MMP-2, MMP-3, MMP-7 and MMP-11 (Newell et al, 1994). In bronchopulmonary carcinomas, MMP expression frequencies also increased as compared with the adjacent lung tissue, with particularly the coexpression of MMP-2 and its activator MT1-MMP in cancers (Nawrocki et al, 1997). Thus, there is a positive correlation between tumor aggressiveness and the expression of multiple MMP family members.

There is a good correlation between the stage progression of most tumors and their level of MMP expression. In lung carcinomas, Northern blot analysis has shown that MMP mRNA levels increased progressively with malignant phenotype, lack of differentiation and TNM stages of the tumors (Nawrocki et al, 1997). Several groups have identified an association between the MMP-11 expression levels, lymph node metastasis and/or a shorter disease-free survival in patients with invasive ductal carcinoma of the mammary gland (Ahmad et al, 1998; Chenard et al, 1996; Tetu et al, 1998). The increased gene expression of this MMP-11 is also associated with local invasiveness in head and neck squamous cell carcinomas (Muller et al, 1993). In colon carcinomas, immuno-histochemical detection of interstitial collagenase has been found associated with a poor prognosis independent of Dukes' stage (Murray et al, 1996). MMP-1 detection levels are associated with poor prognosis in esophageal cancer (Murray et al, 1998). MMP-7 expression detected by immunohistochemistry has also been suggested of prognostic value in squamous cell esophageal carcinomas (Yamamoto et al, 1999). Patients with no MMP-7 expression had a better disease-free and overall survival. Moreover, the demonstration of mRNAs encoding this MMP by RT-PCR has been considered as a reliable marker of occult lymph node metastasis in colon cancer patients (Ichikawa et al, 1998). In melanomas, the expression of MMP-9 is associated with the conversion from radial growth phase to vertical growth phase and subsequent metastasis (MacDougall et al, 1995), whereas MMP-2 expression increases with increasing tumor grade (Vaisanen et al, 1996). In prostate carcinomas, tissue expression of activated MMP-2 has been also found associated with Gleason score and poor prognosis. The highest levels of MMP-2 were observed in prostatic carcinomas with the highest Gleason scores and lymph node metastases (Stearns and Stearns, 1996). By contrast, Remacle et al (1998) using ELISA and gelatin zymography, have reported that, in breast carcinomas, the levels of MMP-2, MMP-3 and MMP-9 correlated inversely with numbers of nodal metastases. In their series, neither MMP-2 nor MMP-9 levels were significantly related to patient outcome. Nevertheless, taken together, these observations generally plead for a frequent increased expression of some MMPs, principally MMP-2, its activator MT1-MMP, MMP-11 and MMP-7, associated with a high aggressiveness of tumors.

The balance between MMPs and their inhibitors (TIMPs) has been seen important during tumor invasion and progression. Most data from model systems have suggested that high levels of these inhibitors prevent metastasis. Indeed, we have demonstrated in lung carcinomas a decrease of TIMPs expression very early during tumor progression, underlining a progressive disruption of the MMP/TIMP balance leading to an excess of several MMPs acting in concert *in vivo* (Nawrocki et al, 1997). Paradoxally, in human breast cancers, high levels of TIMP-2 quantified by ELISA correlate with both shortened disease-free interval and overall survival (Remacle et al, 2000). TIMP-2 levels correlated significantly with those of TIMP-1 in these tumors. In the same way, enhanced expression of TIMP-2 in the stroma of breast carcinomas correlated with tumor recurrence (Visscher et al, 1994). Increased expression of TIMPs 1, 2 or 3 in highly malignant tumors of the gastrointestinal tract (Newell et al, 1994), of the bladder (Grignon et al, 1996), of the lung (Karameris et al, 1997) has been also demonstrated. These apparent discrepant observations according to the inhibiting role of TIMP-2 may reflect the promoting role of TIMP-2 in the activation process of MMP-2. Moreover TIMPs may also promote tumor cell proliferation at some stage of tumor progression (Gomez et al, 1997). Whatever is the balance between MMPs and TIMPs in terms of activity, an overexpression of both MMPs and TIMPs seems to occur in most cancers.

Since tissue alterations are often reflected in body fluids, MMPs in blood have been recommended as diagnostic markers of the invasive and metastatic behavior of carcinomas.Thus, MMP-9 has been reported increased in the plasma of patients with colon cancer and breast cancer but MMP-9 concentrations were not significantly increased in patients with metastatic disease as compared to those with non-metastatic cancer (Zucker et al, 1993). Plasma MMP-9/TIMP-1 complexes were also significantly increased in patients with gastrointestinal and gynecologic cancers, but not in patients with breast cancer. In stage IV gastrointestinal carcinomas, the patient survival was shorter in the group with increased MMP-9 and MMP-9/TIMP-1 complexes than those with normal plasma levels (Zucker et al, 1995). Gohji et al (1996) have also reported that the circulating MMP-2/TIMP-2 ratio was significantly higher in patients with recurrence of urothelial cancer than in patients without recurrence. Serum levels of MMP-2 were found to be significantly higher in men with prostate cancer than in those with benign prostate hyperplasia or with no disease (Gohji et al, 1998). Nevertheless, these preliminary results have not been confirmed by other authors (Jung et al, 1998). Similarly plasma TIMP-1 is associated with prostate cancer but not with benign lesions or normal prostate tissue (Baker et al, 1994; Jung et al, 1997). The variable results obtained with this approach may be partly due to technical problems (serum or plasma measurements, difference of assays). Nevertheless, the generally increased levels of MMPs found in cancers again emphasize the role of these enzymes in tumor progression.

4. CONCLUSION

The key role of MMPs in tumor invasion and metastasis is now well established in a clinical point of view. It has led to the development of new therapeutic agents, the MMP inhibitors, which are largely tested in phases I to III clinical trials with some successes. These components act at the different stages of tumor progression, from the stromal invasion to the intravasation and neoangiogenesis. Nevertheless, if MMPs are largely involved in the ECM remodeling of cancers, the important physiological role of these enzymes in the maintenance of the normal ECM should not be underestimated.

REFERENCES

Ahmad A, Hanby A, Dublin E, Poulson R, Smith P, Barnes R, Anglard P, Hart I. Stromelysin 3: an independent prognostic factor for relapse-free survival in breast cancer represents a tumor-induced host response. Am J Pathol 1998; 152: 721–728.

Baker T, Tickle S, Wasan H, Docherty A, Isenberg D, Waxman J. Serum metalloproteinases and their inhibitor. Markers for malignant potential. Br J Cancer 1994; 70: 506–512.

Barsky SH, Togo S, Garbisa S, Liotta LA. Type IV collagenase immunoreactivity in invasive breast carcinoma. Lancet 1983; 1: 296–297.

Basset P, Bellocq JP, Wolf C, Stoll I, Hutin P, Limacher JM, Podahjcer OL, Chenard MP, Rio MC, Chambon P. A novel metalloproteinase gene specifically expressed in stromal cells of breast carcinomas. Nature 1990; 348: 699–704.

Bates SE, Davidson NE, Valverius EM, Freter CE, Dickson RB, Tam J.P, Kudlow JE, Lippman ME, Salomon DS. Expression of transforming growth factor-α and its messenger ribonucleic acid in human breast cancer: its regulation by oestrogen and its possible functional significance. Mol Endocrinol 1988; 2: 543–555.

Bertaux B, Hornebeck W, Eisen AZ, Dubertret L. Growth stimulation of human keratinocytes by tissue inhibitor of metalloproteinases. J Invest Dermatol 1991; 97: 679–685.

Biswas C, Zhang Y, Decastro R, Guo H, Nakamura T, Kataoka H. The human tumor cell-derived stimulatory factor (renamed EMMPRIN) is a member of the immunoglobulin superfamily. Cancer Res 1995; 55: 434–439.

Brassart B, Randoux A, Hornebeck W, Emonard H. Regulation of matrix metalloproteinase-2 (gelatinase A, MMP-2), membrane-type matrix metalloproteinase-1 (MT1-MMP) and tissue inhibitor of metalloproteinases-2 (TIMP-2) expression by elastin-derived peptides in human HT-1080 fibrosarcoma cell line. Clin Exp Metastasis 1998; 16: 489–500.

201

Brooks PC, Stomblad S, Sanders LC, von Schalscha TL, Aimes RT, Stetler-Stevenson WG, Quigley JP, Cheresh DA. Localization of matrix metalloproteinase MMP-2 to the surface of invasive cells by interaction with integrin alpha V beta 3. Cell 1996; 85: 683–693.

Brown PD, Bloxidge RE, Anderson E, Howell A. Expression of activated gelatinase in human invasive breast carcinoma. Clin Exp Metast 1993; 11: 183–189.

Buisson AC, Gilles C, Polette M, Zahm JM, Birembaut P, Tournier JM. Wound repair induced expression of stromelysins is associated to the acquisition of a mesenchymal phenotype in human respiratory epithelial cells. Lab Invest 1996; 74: 658–669.

Caudroy S, Polette M, Tournier JM, Burlet H, Toole B, Zucker S, Birembaut P. Expression of the Extracellular matrix metalloproteinase inducer (EMMPRIN) and the matrix metalloproteinase-2 in bronchopulmonary and breast lesions. J Histochem Cytochem 1999; 47: 1575–1580.

Chenard MP, O'Siorain L, Shering S, Rouyer N, Lutz Y, Wolf C, Basset P, Bellocq JP, Duffy MJ. High levels of stromelysin-3 correlate with poor prognosis in patients with breast carcinoma. Int J Cancer 1996; 69: 448–451.

Davies B, Miles DW, Happerfield LC, Naylor MS, Bobrow LG, Rubens RD, Balkwill FR. Activity of type IV collagenases in benign and malignant breast diseases. Br J Cancer 1993; 67: 126–131.

Emmert-Buck MR, Emonard HP, Corcoran M, Krutzsch HC, Foidart JM, Stetler-Stevenson WG. Cell surface binding of TIMP-2 and pro-MMP-2/TIMP-2 complex. FEBS Lett 1995; 364: 28–32.

Emonard H, Remacle A, Noël A, Grimaud JA, Stetler-Stevenson WG, Foidart JM. Tumor cell surface associated binding site for the Mr 72,000 type IV collagenase. Cancer Res 1992; 52: 845–848.

Galateau-Salle F, Luna RE, Horiba K, Sheppard MN, Hayashi T, Fleming MV, Colby TV, Bennett W, Harris CC, Stetler-Stevenson WG, Liotta L, Ferrans VJ, Travis WD. Matrix metalloproteinases and tissue inhibitors of metalloproteinases in bronchial squamous preinvasive lesions. Hum Pathol 2000; 31: 296–305.

Gilles C, Thompson EW. The epithelial to mesenchymal transition and metastatic progresion in carcinoma. Breast J 1996; 2: 83–96.

Gilles C, Polette M, Seiki M, Birembaut P, Thompson EW. Implication of collagen type I-induced membrane-type 1-matrix metalloproteinase expression and matrix metalloproteinase-2 activation in the metastatic progression of breast carcinoma. Lab Invest 1997; 76: 651–660.

Gohji K, Fujimoto N, Fuji A, Komiyama T, Okawa J, Nakajima M. Prognostic significance of circulating matrix metalloproteinase-2 to tissue inhibitor of metalloproteinase-2 ratio in recurrence of urothelial cancer after complete resection. Cancer Res 1996; 56: 3196–9198.

Gohji K, Fujimoto N, Hara I, Fujii A, Gotoh A, Okada H, Arakawa S, Kitazawa S, Miyake H, Kamidono S, Nakajima M. Serum matrix metalloproteinase-2 and its density in men with prostate cancer as a new predictor of disease extension. Int J Cancer 1998; 79: 96–101.

Gomez DE, Alonso DF, Yoshiji H, Thorgeirsson UP. Tissue inhibitors of metalloproteinases: structure, regulation and biological functions. Eur J Cell Biol 1997; 74: 111–122.

Grignon DJ, Sakr W, Toth M, Ravery V, Angulo J, Shamsa F, Pontes JE, Crissman JC, Fridman R. High levels of tissue inhibitor of metalloproteinases-2 (TIMP-2) expression are associated with poor outcome in invasive bladder cancer. Cancer Res 1996; 56: 1654–1659.

Guo H, Li R, Zucker S, Toole BP. EMMPRIN (CD147), an inducer of Matrix Metalloproteinase synthesis, also binds to interstitial collagenase to the tumor cell surface. Cancer Res 2000; 60: 888–891.

Heppner KJ, Matrisian LM, Jensen RA, Rodgers WH. Expression of most matrix metalloproteinase family members in breast cancer represents a tumor-induced host response. Am J Pathol 1996; 149: 273–282.

Ichikawa Y, Ishikawa T, Momiyama N, Yamaguchi S, Masui H, Hasegawa S, Chishima T, Takimoto A, Kitamura H, Akitaya T, Hosokawa T, Mitsuhashi M, Shimada H. Detection of regional lymph node metastases in colon cancer by using RT-PCR for matrix metallo-proteinase-7, matrilysin. Clin Exp Metastasis 1998; 16: 3–8.

Jung K, Nowak L, Lein M, Priem F, Schnorr D, Loening S. Matrix metalloproteinases 1 and 3, tissue inhibitor of metalloproteinase-1 and the complex of metalloproteinase-1/tissue inhibitor in plasma of patients with prostate cancer. Int J Cancer 1997; 74: 220–223.

Jung K, Laube C, Lein M, Türk I, Lichtinghagen R, Rudolph B, Schnorr D, Loening S. Matrix metalloproteinase-2 in blood does not indicate the progression of prostate cancer. Int J Cancer 1998; 78: 392–393.

Karameris A, Panagou P, Tsilalis T, Bouros D. Association of expression of metalloproteinases and their inhibitors with the metastatic potential of squamous cell lung carcinomas. Am J Respir Crit Care Med 1997; 156: 1930–1936.

Knabbe C, Lippman ME, Wakefield LM, Flanders KC, Kasid A, Derynck R, Dickson RB. Evidence that transforming growth factor-α is a hormonally regulated negative growth factor in human breast cancer cells. Cell 1987; 48: 417–428.

McCawley LJ, Matrisian LM. Matrix metalloproteinases: multifunctional contributors to tumor progression. Mol Med Today 2000; 6: 149–156.

MacDougall JR, Bani MR, Lin Y, Rak Y, Kerbel RS. The 92 kDa gelatinase B is expressed by advanced stage melanoma cells: suppression by somatic cell hybridization with early stage melanoma cell. Cancer Res 1995; 55: 4174–4181.

Martinella-Catusse C, Nawrocki B, Gilles C, Birembaut P, Polette M. Matrix-metalloproteinases in bronchopulmonary carcinomas. Histol Histopathol 1999; 14: 839–843.

Muller D, Wolf C, Abecassis J, Millon R, Engelmann A, Bronner G, Chambon P, Basset P. Increased stromelysin-3 is associated with local invasiveness in head and neck squamous cell carcinomas. Cancer Res 1993; 53: 165–169.

Murray GI, Duncan ME, O'Neil P, Melvin WT, Fothergill JE. Matrix metalloproteinase-I is associated with poor prognosis in colorectal cancer. Nat Med 1996; 2: 461–462.

Murray GI, Duncan ME, O'Neil P, McKay JA, Melvin WT, Fothergill JE. Matrix metallo-proteinase-I is associated with poor prognosis in eosophageal cancer. J Pathol 1998; 185: 256–261.

Nagase H, Woessner JF Jr. Matrix metalloproteinases. J Biol Chem 1999; 274: 21491–21494.

Nawrocki B, Polette M, Marchand V, Monteau M, Gillery P, Tournier JM, Birembaut P. Expression of matrix metalloproteinases and their inhibitors in human bronchopulmonary carcinomas: quantificative and morpohological analyses. Int J Cancer 1997; 72: 556–564.

Nelson AR, Fingleton B, Rothenberg ML, Matrisian LM. Matrix metalloproteinases: biologic activity and clinical implications. J Clin Oncol 2000; 18: 1135–1149.

Newell KJ, Witty JP, Rodgers W, Matrisian LM. Expression and localization of matrix-degrading metalloproteinases during colorectal carcinogenesis. Mol Carcinog 1994; 10: 199–206.

Noël A, Boulay A, Kebers F, Kannan R, Hajitou A, Calberg-Bacq CM, Basset P, Rio MC, Foidart JM. Demonstration in vivo that stromelysin-3 functions through its proteolytic activity. Oncogene 2000; 19: 1605–1612.

Noël A, Polette M, Lewalle JM, Munaut C, Emonard H, Birembaut P, Foidart JM. Coordinate enhancement of gelatinase A mRNA and activity levels in human fibroblasts in response to breast adenocarcinoma cells. Int J Cancer 1994; 56: 331–336.

Polette M, Clavel C, Cockett M, Girod de Bentzmann S, Murphy G, Birembaut P. Detection and localization of mRNAs encoding matrix metalloproteinases and their tissue inhibitor in human breast pathology. Invas Metast 1993; 13: 31–37.

Polette M, Gilles C, Marchand V, Seiki M, Tournier JM, Birembaut P. Induction of membrane-type matrix metalloproteinase (MT1-MMP) expression in human fibroblasts by breast adenocarcinoma cells. Clin Exp Metastasis 1997; 15: 157–163.

Remacle A, Noël A, Duggan C, McDermott E, O'Higgins N, Foidart JM, Duffy MJ. Assay of matrix metalloproteinases types 1, 2, 3 and 9 in breast cancer. Br J Cancer 1998; 77: 926–931.

Remacle A, McCarthy K, Noël A, Maguire T, McDermott E, O'Higgins N, Foidart JM, Duffy MJ. High levels of TIMP-2 correlate with adverse prognosis in breast cancer. Int J Cancer 2000; 89: 118–121.

Stearns MM, Stearns M. Immunohistochemical studies of activated matrix metalloproteinase-2 (MMP-2a) expression in human prostate cancer. Oncol Res 1996; 8: 63–67.

Stetler-Stevenson WG, Bersch N, Golde DW. Tissue inhibitor of metalloproteinases-2 (TIMP-2) has erythroid-potentiating activity. FEBS Lett 1992; 296: 231–234.

Strongin AY, Collier I, Bannikov G, Marmer BL, Grant GA, Goldberg GI. Mechanism of cell surface ectivation of the 72 kD type IV collagenase: isolation of the activated form of the membrane metalloproteinase. J Biol Chem 1995; 270: 5331–5338.

Tetu B, Brisson J, Lapointe H, Bernard P. Prognostic significance of stromelysin 3, gelatinase A and urokinase expression in breast cancer. Hum Pathol 1998; 29: 979–985.

Vaisanen A, Tuominen H, Kallioinen M, Turpeenniemi-Hujanen T. Matrix metalloproteinase-2 (72 kD type IV collagenase) expression occurs in the early stage of human melanocytic tumour progression and may have prognostic value. J Pathol 1996; 180: 283–289.

Visscher DW, Hoyhtya M, Ottosem SK, Liang CM, Sarkar FH, Crissman JD, Fridman R. Enhanced expression of tissue inhibitor of metalloproteinase-2 (TIMP-2) in the stroma of breast carcinomas correlates with tumor recurrence. Int J Cancer 1994; 59: 339–344.

Werb Z, Tremble PM, Behrendtsen D, Crowley E, Damsky CH. Signal transduction through the fibronectin receptor induces collagenase and stromelysin gene expression. J Cell Biol 1989; 109: 877–889.

Yamamoto H, Adachi Y, Itoh F, Iku S, Matsuno K, Kusano M, Arimura Y, Endo T, Hinoda Y, Hosokawa M, Imai K. Association of matrilysin expression with recurrence and poor prognosis in human esophageal squamous cell carcinoma. Cancer Res 1999; 59: 3313–3316.

Zucker S, Lysik RM, Zarrabi MH, Moll U. Mr 92,000 type IV collagenase is increased in plasma of patients with colon cancer and breast cancer. Cancer Res 1993; 53: 140–146.

Zucker S, Lysik RM, Dimassimo BI, Zarrabi MH, Moll UM, Grimson R, Tickle SP, Docherty AJ. Plasma assay of gelatinase B/tissue inhibitor of metalloproteinase complexes in cancer. Cancer 1995; 76: 700–708.

Chapter 11

TISSUE MODELS TO STUDY TUMOR-STROMA INTERACTIONS

N. E. Fusenig, M. Skobe, S. Vosseler, M. Hansen, W. Lederle, K. Airola,
P. Tomakidi, H.-J. Stark, H. Steinbauer, N. Mirancea, P. Boukamp and
D. Breitkreutz
German Cancer Research Center (DKFZ), Division of Differentiation and Carcinogenesis,
Im Neuenheimer Feld 280, D-69120 Heidelberg, Germany

1. INTRODUCTION

Cancer develops as a progressive multi-step process in which cells pass through consecutive genetic alterations gradually acquiring phenotypic changes enabling the transformed cells to grow to malignant tumors. Whereas our understanding of the genetic alterations causing cell transformation has greatly improved during the last two decades, the characteristic phenotypic changes which enable a cancer cell to grow to a tumor are still less apparent. This is mainly due to the fact that these studies are restricted to the tissue level, a much more complicated situation than the conventional cell culture models. *In vivo*, the tumor is a complex ecosystem comprising the genetically altered neoplastic cells and the tumor stroma, a framework of connective tissue cells with extracellular matrix (ECM) and the embedded vasculature. Although changes in the cellularity and ECM composition of the tumor stroma had been noticed, this connective tissue component of epithelial malignancies have long been considered mainly as a passive supporting and nourishing system for the cancer cells. Concomitantly with the increasing interest in tumor angiogenesis and the recognition of its essential role for tumor progression and as a new target for tumor therapy, a new view of the significance of the stromal compartment in tumor biology emerged. There is increasing evidence of the importance of the microenvironment for tumor development and progression indicating that the genetic alterations in the tumor cells themselves are not sufficient to generate a tumor but that a permissive stromal environment is needed as well. As compared to the connective tissue of normal organs, both composition of the ECM and the functional state of the stromal cells are altered in tumors and these alterations seem to be crucial for tumor growth, invasion, and metastasis (Morikawa et al, 1988; Fidler, 1990). The stroma of malignant tumors often

J.-M. Foidart and R.J. Muschel (eds.), Proteases and Their Inhibitors in Cancer Metastasis, 205–223.

closely resembles granulation tissue such as found in healing wounds (Dvorak, 1986). It is assumed that the various features of a granulation-tissue-like-stroma may favour or even induce tumor invasion (Pauli and Knudson, 1988; Dingemans et al, 1993). Growth-promoting effects of activated stromal cells on tumor cells have been reported (Cornil et al, 1991; Gregoire et al, 1995) indicating persistent functional alterations in fibroblasts (Olumi et al, 1999; Turner et al, 1997). Furthermore, many reports have emphasized the importance of tumor-stroma interactions in the regulation of matrix-degrading proteases which are considered essential players in the process of cancer invasion and metastasis (for review see Noël et al, 1997).

All these reports stress the importance of the stromal compartment in malignant tumors and strongly indicate that continuous interaction between tumor and stromal cells (resulting in their reciprocal regulation and modulation) are prerequisite for carcinoma development and progression. Because of the complex composition of the tumor stroma, *in vitro* models developed so far are not able to faithfully mimic the interactions occurring *in vivo* and thus reflect only a small facet of the *in vivo* reality. On the other hand, *in vivo* studies on established neoplasms, either autochthonous or transplanted tumors, are often difficult to interpret concerning the functional role of the stroma due to the intermingled close association of tumor and stroma elements. Furthermore, the analysis of tumor-stroma interactions and their role in tumor development requires experimental *in vivo* systems reflecting different tumor stages and corresponding environmental conditions.

We have elaborated such an *in vivo* model which apparently fulfills all those requirements for the study of tumor-stroma interactions of squamous cell carcinomas (SCC) including the dynamics of angiogenesis, induction and maintenance. This *surface transplantation model* has been developed initially to study interactions between normal epithelial and stromal cells and their regulatory mechanisms on growth and differentiation (Fusenig, 1992). Based on this *in vivo* model, simplified organotypic coculture systems have been established mimicking structure and function of a native tissue such as epidermis (for review see Fusenig, 1994). Although comparable *in vitro* models for tumor invasion have not yet been achieved, some principles of tumor-stroma interaction could be investigated in these assays (Borchers et al, 1994, 1997).

2. SURFACE TRANSPLANTATION SYSTEM FOR NORMAL EPITHELIAL TISSUE RECONSTRUCTION

To elaborate mechanisms of epidermal regeneration, we have established a transplantation technique allowing the complete restoration of skin epithelium under the influence of the connective tissue environment, however, without direct contact between the epithelial and stromal cells, as schematically shown in Figure 1 (Fusenig et al, 1983; Fusenig, 1994). In this model, keratinocytes (of mouse or human origin) are cultured for one day on a 1–2 mm thick collagen (type I) gel mounted between two concentric teflon rings (CRD, Noser and Limat, 1987). When a confluent monolayer has formed, the culture assembly is covered by a silicone transplantation chamber and transplanted *in toto* onto the back muscle fascia of mice (syngeneic, allogeneic or nude) and held in place by the surrounding mouse skin fixed by wound clips (Fusenig, 1994).

By this technique, standardized grafts are obtained with a controlled number of epithelial cells firmly attached to the collagen gel yielding highly reproducible 'take-rates' and optimal survival of the transplanted cells. Although separated from the host stroma by the collagen matrix, the grafted cells rapidly develop into highly proliferative stratified epithelia which, after one to two

Surface transplantation model for normal and transformed epithelia

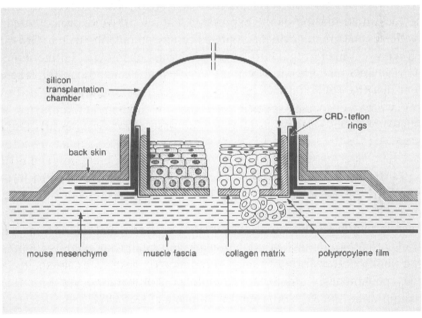

Figure 1. Schematic cross-section of the surface transplantation assay on collagen gels placed on the back muscle fascia of mice. Intact epithelial monolayers are transplanted attached to the collagen gel (type I), mounted in concentric teflon rings (Combi Ring Dish, CRD), and covered with a hat-shaped silicone transplantation chamber. Transplanted tumor cells proliferate to form a multilayered epithelium, while the collagen gel is replaced by a well-vascularized granulation tissue. Normal and premalignant cells form surface epithelia (*left side*), while malignant cells infiltrate the newly formed host stroma (*right side*).

207

weeks, have grown to form epidermis-like tissues with all typical characteristics (Breitkreutz et al, 1997, and further references therein). Complete regeneration of a regularly organized and differentiated epidermis, including a structured basement membrane, occurs within two weeks, while the epithelium is still separated from the host stromal tissue by the collagen gel. Later on, this gel is gradually replaced by a highly vascularized granulation tissue, which eventually gets in close contact to the epithelium. Thus, this model mimics principle stages of epidermal tissue regeneration and differentiation, functions which are regulated by diffusible factors provided by the host connective tissue.

This model of tissue reconstruction could be mimicked *in vitro* by organotypic cocultures of keratinocytes growing on fibroblast-populated collagen gels yielding a rather normal epidermis including a structured basement membrane (Smola et al, 1998; Stark et al, 1999). With this model we were able to further elaborate the mechanism of a rather complex double paracrine pathway of epithelial-mesenchymal interactions regulating keratinocyte proliferation and differentiation (Smola et al, 1993; Maas-Szabowski et al, 1999, 2000; Szabowski et al, 2000). Through release of interleukin-1 (IL-1) keratinocytes upregulate in the cocultured fibroblasts the expression and release of keratinocyte growth factor (KGF) and granulocyte macrophage colony-stimulating factor (GM-CSF), which represent major regulators of the epidermal phenotype. Furthermore, by this *in vitro* assay and the corresponding *in vivo* transplantation model, it became evident that the epithelial-mesenchymal interactions operating via diffusible factors were not species-specific, because the human keratinocytes were stimulated by mouse as well as human fibroblasts (Szabowski et al, 2000).

3. EPITHELIAL-MESENCHYMAL INTERACTIONS IN DIFFERENT STAGES OF KERATINOCYTE TRANSFORMATION

In order to determine alterations in epithelial-mesenchymal interactions during the transformation process in premalignant and malignant stages of epithelial cells, a family of transformed human keratinocyte lines was established. Based on the spontaneously immortalized human skin keratinocyte line HaCaT (Boukamp et al, 1988), benign and malignant clones have been derived following H-ras oncogene transfection (Boukamp et al, 1990) and a metastasizing variant obtained after repeated passaging as tumor transplant in nude mice (Fusenig and Boukamp, 1998; Mueller et al, submitted).

3.1. Immortal nontumorigenic HaCaT cells

Immortal nontumorigenic HaCaT cells being genetically altered but functionally rather normal, represent a very early but stable stage in the keratinocyte transformation process (Boukamp et al, 1988, 1997). In surface transplants, HaCaT cells still respond to mesenchymal signals comparable to normal keratinocytes and form a rather normal epidermis with all major differentiation markers and a regularly structured basement membrane. However, full differentiation is delayed and proliferation activity maintained at a higher level as compared to normal keratinocyte transplants (Breitkreutz et al, 1997, 1998). Furthermore, collagen replacement by mouse granulation tissue occurs more rapidly, so that usually after two weeks mesenchymal cells are already in close vicinity to the epithelium. Thus, these immortal keratinocytes have largely maintained their normal function and their responsiveness to mesenchymal signals, although distinct differences to normal keratinocytes were obvious.

These became even more pronounced in the *in vitro* tissue model of organotypic cocultures of HaCaT cells with normal fibroblasts embedded in collagen gels. Under these conditions, proliferation and differentiation were further delayed and, astonishingly, even more dependent on fibroblasts. Thus, higher fibroblast cell numbers were required than for normal keratinocytes and even after three weeks normal epidermal architecture and keratinization were not fully achieved (Schoop et al, 1999). Preliminary results indicate that both the release of IL-1 by HaCaT cells and their response to KGF and GM-CSF (but not to TGF-α) are significantly decreased. Taken together, these less optimal *in vitro* growth condition deficiencies in the regulation of epithelial-mesenchymal interactions were more obvious than *in vivo*, where other compensatory mechanisms may be effective.

3.2. Benign and malignant HaCaT-*ras* clones

Benign and malignant HaCaT-*ras* clones exhibited significant transformation-stage-dependent alterations in their interactions with stromal cells *in vivo*. First, they maintained their proliferative potential after subcutaneous injection in nude mice giving rise to slowly enlarging benign encapsulated cystic tumors and rapidly enlarging invasive carcinomas, respectively. On the other hand, HaCaT cells, though immortalized *in vitro*, rapidly lost their proliferative potential when injected subcutaneously into nude mice, both at low and high passage levels (Boukamp et al, 1990, 1997). Thus, the tumorigenic clones had gained the potential for continued proliferation at ectopic sites *in vivo*, though at different degrees depending on the stage of transformation. Their different tumorigenic potential was even more evident in surface transplants, where benign clones formed

209

slightly dysplastic keratinizing epithelia, while malignant cells developed into invasive, although well differentiating carcinomas (Boukamp et al, 1990; Breitkreutz et al, 1991) (Figure 2). These differences in growth behaviour were reflected in drastically altered interactions with the host stroma at the individual tumor stages. In contrast to HaCaT transplants, a strong stromal reaction was noticed within the first week in tumor transplants below the collagen gel visible as increased cell density and strong angiogenesis. The start and strength of this reaction clearly correlated with the stage of transformation, being later and weakest in transplants of benign and earliest and strongest in those of metastatic cells. With time, this stromal reaction expanded with host cells and vessels penetrating into the collagen gel which was progressively replaced by granulation tissue. At this stage, both benign and malignant cells had formed thick epithelia with more or less pronounced differentiating layers depending on the degree of transformation but did not exhibit invasive growth behaviour. In malignant transplants, invasion started as soon as the newly formed granulation tissue had replaced the collagen gel and had reached the tumor cells. This was the first indication of an essential inductive or permissive role of the stroma for tumor invasion. In contrast, transplants of benign cells did never invade, though in contact with stroma, but formed well delineated slightly dysplastic keratinizing epithelia. Moreover, proliferation was reduced and proliferating cells were mainly localized in the basal layer exclusively, adjacent to a fully developed basement membrane comparable to normal keratinocyte transplants (Skobe et al, 1997; Tomakidi et al, 1999) (Figure 2). Transplants of malignant cells still exhibited distinct stretches of basement membrane, as long as they stayed separated from the stroma by the collagen gel, but lost these features when stromal elements approached the epithelium (Tomakidi et al, 1999). Nevertheless, immunostaining for most basement membrane components was

Epithelial-Mesenchymal Interactions in Surface Transplants

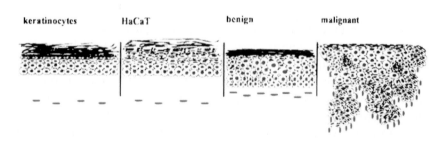

Figure 2. Schematic cross-sections through 3-week-old transplants of different stages of keratinocyte transformation indicating epithelial morphology, stromal replacement of the collagen gel, as well as vessel density and orientation.

maintained around the infiltrating epithelia, though sometimes discontinuous indicating a rapid turnover. Accordingly, integrins localized in the basal layer of the normal epidermis which are generally overexpressed in benign and malignant transplants at one week were largely normalized in benign epithelia when stromal vicinity was reached, while upregulation persisted in invasive malignant tissues.

Also differentiation epithelial markers were differentially clearly discriminating benign and malignant epithelial transplants. Distinct cytokeratins (K19, 4, 13, 8, 18), not expressed in normal epidermis, were produced at a similar level in benign and malignant HaCaT-*ras* clones in cell culture (Breitkreutz et al, 1993) and in early transplants as long as they were separated from stroma by the collagen gel (one week). With increasing vicinity to the newly developed host granulation tissue, these markers were downregulated in benign but persisted in malignant transplants (Tomakidi et al, submitted). In addition, malignant transplants exhibited *de novo* expression of vimentin, the mesenchymal intermediate filament protein, mostly in peripheral cells of invading tumor areas. These differential alterations occurring in benign and malignant transplants clearly indicate distinct regulatory mechanisms exerted by the stroma. Thus, with decreasing distance between tumor epithelia and stromal elements, this control became increasingly evident as normalizing effect in benign but not in malignant cells. Presumably, regular signal transduction mechanisms are still operative in benign cells but have been compromised in malignant cells. On the other hand, the granulation tissue induced by malignant cells (i.e. tumor stroma) may have lost these controlling functions and/or instead acquired different regulatory capacities favouring malignant tumor growth, i.e., leading to invasion and metastasis.

4. TRANSFORMATION STAGE-DEPENDENT KINETICS OF STROMAL ACTIVATION AND ANGIOGENESIS

4.1. The surface transplantation model on collagen matrix

The surface transplantation model on collagen matrixwas particularly advantageous for displaying early stages of tumor-stroma interactions. Remarkably, the major initial consequences of tumor-stroma interactions were observed in the stromal compartment by the onset and intensity of granulation tissue formation and induction of angiogenesis below the collagen gel. Although tumor cells rapidly proliferated forming multilayered epithelia on top of the gel, invasive growth, the hallmark of malignancy, did not manifest before the vascularized granulation tissue had replaced the gel and approached the tumor cells.

Thus, a close association and interaction between tumor and stromal tissue was obviously prerequisite for tumor invasion. This sequential course of stromal activation and tumor invasion indicated that rapid interactions between tumor and host cells occurred upon transplantation resulting first in activation of stromal tissue. However, this early sequence of events became only apparent by this particular transplantation technique, where a collagen gel was interposed between tumor cells and stromal elements. Clearly, this matrix-inserted transplantation assay has several crucial advantages: 1) The collagen matrix provides an appropriate substratum for attachment of tumor cells and their transfer to the *in vivo* environment as an intact confluent cell layer. As a consequence, a nearly full take-rate of the transplanted tumor cells is accomplished resulting in a rapid initiation of their cell proliferation. This way, a major loss of the transplanted tumor cells is prevented and also a delay of initial attachment which is usually the case when cells are injected as cell suspension into ectopic or orthotopic sites (e.g. Stanbridge et al, 1975; Fidler, 1990). 2) As consequence, only a rather low number of transplanted cells (2×10^5) is required. This as well as the virtual absence of degenerating cells immediately after transplantation on the other (both adding up to a low burden of immunogenic material) may be a major reason for the lack of an immediate serious immune reaction when normal or tumor cells are transplanted to allogeneic recipients (Fusenig et al, 1980, 1983) and heterozygous transgenic animals (Bajou et al, 1998).

3) The inserted collagen gel serves as temporal 'barrier' preventing immediate contact between grafted tumor cells and host cells. Nevertheless, the interposed biocompatible and permeable matrix, however, does not block interactions between grafted and host cells via diffusible factors. As a consequence, transplanted cells will rapidly assume proliferation and form multilayered tissues. On the other hand, tumor cells produce inducible factors which give rise to a granulation tissue formation and angiogenesis on the host side. 4) Most importantly, the early steps of this host stroma response to the tumor signals, i.e. the induction of a vascularized granulation tissue becomes inspectable during a time window defined by the speed of replacement of the collagen gel by the newly formed stroma. Although tumor-stroma interactions and invasion are similarly developed when carcinoma cells are transplanted as cell suspension onto the muscle fascia using the silicon transplantation chamber without CRD, they are not as clearly discernible (Fusenig et al, 1983; Hornung et al, 1987). Under those conditions, when immediate contact between tumor cells and stromal tissue is not prevented, the evolution and progression of the tumor-stroma including its vascularization could not be studied in detail. Thus, the interposed collagen gel, although delaying the onset of tumor invasion, apparently did not seriously hinder the reciprocal interactions between both compartments, at least not those mediated by diffusible factors could be demonstrated by the

application of stromal activating factors. When these factors were applied prior to transplantation onto the upper side of the collagen gel, a rapid formation of granulation tissue was induced at the opposite (stromal) side of the gel which was of comparable strength to that seen in transplants of tumor cells (Skobe, 1996).

4.2. Differential dynamics of stromal activation by benign and malignant cells

Differential dynamics of stromal activation by benign and malignant cells have become apparent as novel characteristics of tumor-stroma interactions due to these particular conditions of the transplantation assay (Figure 3) and are summarized below:

a) The earliest phenotypic alterations as consequence of tumor-stroma interactions were always observed in the stromal compartment by the induction of granulation tissue formation and of angiogenesis.
b) The onset of this stromal activation and its intensity was correlated to the degree of transformation of transplanted cells, being delayed and weaker

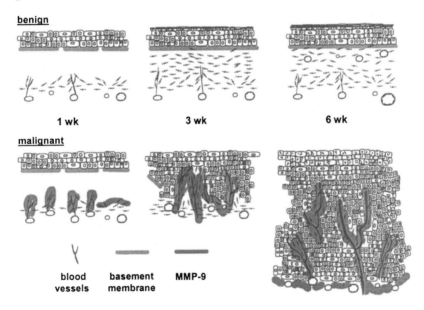

Figure 3. Dynamics of stroma activation and angiogenesis in benign and malignant transplants. With downregulation of angiogenesis the benign epithelium consolidates to a slightly dysplastic stratified epithelium lined by a continuous basement membrane. Concomitantly with ongoing angiogenesis, vascular infiltration and tumor invasion proceed. This was paralleled by the sequential expression of MMP-13, -9 and -3 by perivascular stromal cells.

with benign, while fastest and strongest with the most progressed (metastatic) carcinoma cells (Fusenig and Boukamp, 1998).

c) Whereas stromal activation and angiogenesis persisted in malignant (invasive) transplants, both phenomena were downregulated in benign transplants. This occurred as soon as the granulation tissue had fully replaced the collagen gel, concomitant with the consolidation of a differentiating benign epithelium (Skobe et al, 1997).

d) Moreover, the characteristics of the granulation tissue induced by benign versus malignant epithelial transplants differed markedly in their cellular composition, extracellular matrix components and protease expression (unpublished results).

e) The differential dynamics of angiogenesis induction and persistence in benign and malignant transplants was controlled by the regulation of the VEGF receptor 2 which was downregulated in the stroma of benign but not malignant transplants. Remarkably, VEGF expression persisted in both types of tumor cell transplants (Skobe et al, 1997).

f) Concomitantly, with stromal activation and blood vessel penetration towards tumor cells, interesting dynamics of stromal matrix metalloprotease (MMP) expression was observed in malignant transplants. This started with MMP-13 localized in cells exhibiting earliest infiltration into the collagen gel located in front of the penetrating blood vessels, followed by MMP-9 and MMP-3 when stromal elements had approached the tumor cells (Airola et al, submitted). Remarkably, in transplants of benign cells, none of these stromal proteases were expressed. Moreover, expression of MMP-1 and -9 observed in cultured benign tumor cells was completely switched off in transplants *in vivo*, whereas it was maintained and even upregulated in transplanted malignant cells (Airola and Fusenig, unpublished data).

Collectively, these data strongly suggest that the activated state of the newly formed stroma and blood vessels and its close vicinity to the tumor cells play an essential role in determining the tumor phenotype: sustained activation of stromal cells and blood vessels seems to be prerequisite for tumor invasion. The early onset of stromal activation, the rapid penetration of vessels and perivascular cells through the collagen gel (towards the tumor cells on the surface) and their eventual infiltration into the malignant tumor tissue usually preceeds recognizable tumor cell invasion.

According to these data, the infiltration of stromal strands, together with blood vessels into the expanding tumor mass is the leading event and prerequisite for the onset of tumor invasion. Whether the activated stromal elements, in particular the newly formed blood vessels, create a permissive environment for tumor infiltration by modulation of the extracellular matrix (ECM) and expression of ECM-degrading proteases or both, is a subject of ongoing research. The crucial role of tumor stroma for the malignant phenotype is also supported by observations that many matrix-degrading proteases are expressed in stromal, mostly perivascular cells, often in close vicinity to the tumor border (for review see Noël et al, 1997). Their activity may also be responsible for the disappearance of basement membrane structures in malignant transplants at the time when stromal elements get in close vicinity to the tumor cells (Tomakidi et al, 1999). Although many details of the complex interaction of malignant tumor cells with their specific stroma still need to be unravelled, the causal correlation between activated stromal components and tumor invasion is becoming more and more obvious and shall be examplified in the following in four different experimental settings aimed to inhibit or activate granulation tissue and angiogenesis.

5. STROMAL INTERACTIONS DETERMINE THE TUMOR PHENOTYPE

5.1. Inhibition of angiogenesis blocks tumor vascularization and invasion

Inhibition of angiogenesis blocks tumor vascularization and invasion in malignant transplants of skin squamous carcinoma cells and delays tumor expansion. Based on the observation that tumor invasion was associated with ongoing angiogenesis and that the latter correlated to persistent expression of VEGFR-2 by endothelial cells we hypothesized that inactivation of VEGFR-2-mediated signaling would not only block angiogenesis but also affect tumor invasion. This assumption has been proven to be correct. By blocking VEGFR-2 with a specific monoclonal antibody (DC101, ImClone, New York) applied systemically (i.p.) into animals carrying transplants of malignant keratinocytes, both angiogenesis and invasion could be abrogated. Although this treatment did not exhibit marked effects on granulation tissue formation and blood vessel development within the first two weeks (after transplantation and start of treatment), significant effects and striking alterations were observed after three and four weeks, respectively (Skobe et al, 1997). Whereas transplants treated with control antibodies exhibited the typical phenotype of a heavily vascularized squamous cell carcinoma with many proliferating tumor and stromal cells, this phenotype was dramatically changed in animals treated with the DC101 antibody. Morphologically, the DC101-treated transplants resembled those formed by benign cells displaying moderately dysplastic epithelia covered by a thick parakeratotic stratum corneum. One major difference, however, to benign transplants

215

was the maintained high proliferative activity (comparable to the invasive control transplants), and the localization of proliferating cells throughout all epithelial layers (Skobe et al, 1997). On the other hand, the underlying stroma exhibited a drastic reduction in vessel density and number of proliferating stromal cells.

Strikingly, the benign-looking malignant epithelia were completely free of penetrating stromal strands and blood vessels. Thus, a blockade of endothelial-cell activation abrogated new blood vessel formation in the adjacent tumor stroma and, moreover, prevented their penetration into the tumor tissue. The difference in tumor vascularization upon DC101-treatment was even more pronounced in transplants of the more aggressive and heavily vascularized HaCaT line A5-RT3. The effect was similarly observed when the start of DC101 treatment was delayed for two weeks, a time when vessel infiltration into the tumor mass had already started. The initial tumor vascularization was drastically reduced or had disappeared completely in animals treated for six weeks so that transplants consisted of a small rim of vital but avascular tumor area adjacent to a poorly vascularized stroma, whereas most parts of the tumor were necrotic (Vosseler and Fusenig, in preparation). When DC101-treatment was discontinued, tumor vascularization was rapidly restored to a level seen in the heavily vascularized control tumors.

Similar correlations between inhibition of angiogenesis, tumor vascularization and blockade of invasion and tumor expansion were observed in tumors formed by subcutaneously injected A5-RT3 carcinoma cells in DC101-treated animals. Tumor expansion and vascularization were drastically inhibited in a dose- and application frequency-dependent manner. In turn, both tumor growth and vascularization were rapidly restored when treatment was discontinued (Vosseler and Fusenig, in preparation).

Whether this remarkable interdependence of tumor vascularization and invasion is mechanistically based on the modulation of ECM components and/or protease expression and activation is a matter of ongoing studies. A close correlation between onset of angiogenesis and tumor vascularization with tumor invasion has also been observed in clinical and experimental systems where the angiogenic switch usually preceeds the invasive stage of a developing tumor (Hanahan and Folkman, 1996; Smith-McCune and Weidner, 1994). In skin carcinoma patients, however, increased vascular density was only seen in later stage carcinomas which had a higher metastatic probability, whereas premalignant and early malignant lesions did not exhibit higher vascularization (Strieth et al, 2000). This may relate to a generally slower growth rate in these authochthonous tumors.

5.2. Dysbalance of matrix components and stromal protease activity

Dysbalance of matrix components and stromal protease activity prevents tumor vascularization, invasion and expansion in two different model systems.

Comparable striking consequences of stromal alterations and tumor expansion have been noticed following overexpression of the ECM component thrombospondin-1 (TSP-1) usually found in the provisional wound matrix and in tumor stroma. Upon transfection and overexpression of TSP-1 in a human skin squamous carcinoma cell line (SCC), these cells had for the most part lost their tumorigenic potential upon s.c. injection, whereas their proliferative potential *in vitro* was unaltered (Bleuel et al, 1999). Comparable to DC101-mediated blockade of VEGF-R2, the TSP-1 transfectants exhibited a transient block in tumor invasion in transplants, and the TSP-1 overexpressing tumor masses were free of penetrating vessels and stromal strands. Again, initial angiogenesis was not inhibited and blood vessels accumulated in the surrounding stroma. Remarkably, the overexpressed TSP-1 had accumulated preferentially at the tumor-stroma border, detectable as an intensely stained deposit which presumably functioned as a barrier preventing the infiltration of stromal strands and blood vessels into the tumor. The causal role of this TSP-1 deposition and its inhibitory function of vessel penetration for the observed blockade of tumor invasion and expansion was confirmed by downregulation of TSP-1 expression using antisense oligonucleotides. Coincident with abrogation of TSP-1 expression and deposition at the tumor-stroma boundary, the tumors became heavily vascularized and expanded much alike to the untransfected control carcinoma cells (Bleuel et al, 1999). Whether the TSP-1 deposits acted as a physical barrier for endothelial or fibroblast migration or functioned through modulation of growth factor or protease activity is not known at present. In any case, the data demonstrate, however, that an imbalance in one single ECM component may have a dramatic impact on tumor vascularization and subsequently on the process of tumor invasion and expansion.

Corresponding, while initially surprising results were obtained when the balance of the serine protease plasminogen activator (uPA) and its endogenous inhibitor (PAI-1) was deranged in the stromal tissue. For this study, malignant mouse keratinocytes were transplanted onto PAI-1 knockout. Contrary to the presumption that a deficiency in protease inhibitor would enhance tumor growth and invasion, the grafted mouse skin carcinoma cells completely failed to invade the stroma of the PAI-1 deficient host (Bajou et al, 1998). Although, in PAI-1 knockout animals tumor cells induced angiogenesis and granulation tissue formation beneath the collagen gel, but the vessels were unable to penetrate further into the vicinity of the tumor tissue. Thus, in contrast to the well vascularized invasive transplants in wild-type animals, the absence of PAI-1 in the host stroma prevented tumor vascularization and, as seen in the other models, tumor invasion. The causal role of the absence of PAI-1 for this vascular deficiency was confirmed by adenovirus-mediated restoration of PAI-1 in the knockout animals. This lead to both tumor vascularization and invasion in only those animals with elevated PAI-1 serum levels (Bajou et al, 1998). Targeted mutations of the PAI-1 gene demonstrated that the binding site for uPA was essential for this restoration, while mutations in the binding site for vitronectin (important for endothelial migration) did not affect the restoring efficacy of PAI-1 (Bajou et al, submitted).

Thus, also the imbalance of a single stromal protease due to interference with its inhibitor causing enhanced protease activity (in this case of plasmin) can disturb vessel formation, tumor vascularization finally prevents tumor invasion and expansion. This is in accordance with earlier observations that increased plasmin activity prevents vessel morphogenesis in an *in vitro* angiogenesis assay (Monteasano et al, 1990), although the underlying mechanism may be diffi- cult.

5.3. Modulation of the tumor phenotype by stromal cell activation

Modulation of the tumor phenotype by stromal cell activationhas also been observed in several experimental systems.

While the importance of the appropriate microenvironment for the develop- ment of transplanted carcinomas is well recognized (for review see Fidler, 1992), much less is known about the nature of the tumor cell-induced stroma and its role in the transformation process. Studies on fibroblasts isolated from stroma of carcinomas demonstrated a stable potential to enhance progression of pre- malignant cells to tumorigenicity when coinoculated into nude mice (Olumi et al, 1999). Although several phenotypic changes have been documented in carcinoma-associated fibroblasts (Schor et al, 1988; Nakamura et al, 1987), their contribution to tumor development and progression is still poorly understood.

We have recently shown that constant activation of stromal cells by the potent stromal activator platelet-derived growth factor (PDGF) modulates immortal, but non tumorigenic, HaCaT cells to tumorigenicity, although to the benign phenotype only (Skobe and Fusenig, 1998). Previously, we had observed that in transplants of malignant HaCaT-*ras* cells expression of PDGF was activated, but only transiently, during the early phase of stroma induction. Furthermore, PDGF itself, when applied in the transplantation assay onto collagen gels, was a strong inducer of granulation tissue and angiogenesis (Skobe, 1996). In order to study the further role of PDGF in stroma formation and tumor development, we have stably transfected PDGF-B into HaCaT cells, causing enhanced expression and secretion of active PDGF-BB. Although the transfected HaCaT cells (they do not express PDGF receptors) exhibited unaltered growth *in vitro*, they formed tumors after subcutaneous injection into nude mice (Skobe and Fusenig, 1998). These tumors were histologically benign encapsulated cysts with a rim of hyperproliferative cells, lining the slowly enlarging and keratinizing non-invasive tumors. In their early growth phase a strong angiogenic response and stromal activation was noticed, but this was lost at later tumor stages, although PDGF overexpression was maintained in the transplanted epithelia.

In surface transplants on collagen gels the distinct kinetics of stromal activation by the PDGF transfectants became more evident underlining once more the advantages of this model. Following an initial strong induction of granulation tissue and angiogenesis, this activation declined after four to six weeks with a drastic reduction in vessel density and stromal cell numbers. This decline was comparable to that seen in transplants of benign HaCaT-*ras* cells. Concomitant with this downregulation of the stromal elements a hyperplastic, but noninvasive, stratified epithelium had established ressembling the phenotype of transplants of benign HaCaT-ras cells (Lederle et al, in preparation). Thus, PDGFB was able to induce stromal activation and angiogenesis but was less efficient in maintaining angiogenesis and promoting tumor vascularization. Nevertheless, ongoing PDGF secretion modulated the stroma to induce keratinocyte hyperproliferation and by this promoted benign tumor formation. As seen in wound healing and *in vitro* studies, PDGF induces keratinocyte growth factor (KGF) expression in fibroblasts, which in turn stimulates keratinocyte proliferation (Brauchle et al, 1994). Thus, although the detailed mechanism of this biphasic effect of PDGF on stromal activation is still a matter of ongoing research, the data add to the emerging picture that tumor and stromal cells interact via a complex network of diffusible factors resulting in reciprocal modulation of cell growth and function, which may eventually lead to tumor formation in a permissive stromal environment.

6. CONCLUSIONS

The above summarized findings of this laboratory on tumor-stroma interactions, together with a growing number of other reports contribute to the accumulating evidence that the stromal part of epithelial tumors plays a more active role in epithelial tumor development and progression than until recently recognized. The transplantation assay developed by us represents in *in vivo* system particularly suited to highlight early tumor-stroma interactions and to discriminate tumor stage-dependent characteristics in this interplay. Furthermore, by the unique assembly and geometry of this model the essential role of tumor-stroma interactions for tumor invasion has been documented unimbigously for the first time. Thus, the significance of extracellular matrix composition, stromal protease activity and growth factor interactions for modulating the tumor phenotype has been evidenced in different experimental settings. In addition to the transplantation assay comparable culture systems *in vitro* provide relevant models to study the mechanistic details of the complex interplay between tumor and stroma cells. These investigations will not only increase our knowledge on the important role of stromal cells in tumor biology, but may yield additional targets for novel therapeutic strategies aiming at genetically normal cells according to the principle of antiangiogenic therapy.

ACKNOWLEDGMENTS

We would like to thank our colleagues W. Peter and M. Mappes who have contributed to these studies. Work has been supported by grants of the EU (EURAM/AIR/BIOMED), the German Granting Organization (DFG FU 91-4, FU 91-5; NF, DB BR 530/8-1) and from FAB, Abano Therme. Mihaela Skobe had a grant from Boehringer Ingelheim Foundation and Nicolae Mirancea was as guest scientist grant holder of the DKFZ. We also appreciate the stylistic improvements and the expert typing by Martina Kegel.

REFERENCES

Bajou K, Noël, A, Gerard RD, Masson V, Brunner N, Holst-Hansen C, Skobe M, Fusenig NE, Carmeliet P, Collen D, Foidart JM. Absence of host plasminogen activator inhibitor 1 prevents cancer invasion and vascularization. Nature Med 1998; 4: 923–928.

Bajou K, Masson V, Gerard RD, Schmitt PM, Albert, V, Lund, L.R, Frandsen, TL, Brunner N, Dano, K, Fusenig, NE, Loskutoff, D, Collen, D, Carmeliet P, Foidart JM, Noël A. The plasminogen activator inhibitor PAI-1 controls in vivo tumor vascularization by interaction with proteases, not vitronectin: implications for anti-angiogenic strategies. J Cell Biol 2000; in press.

Bleuel K, Popp S, Fusenig NE, Stanbridge EJ, Boukamp P. Tumor suppression in human skin carcinoma cells by chromosome 15 transfer or thrombospondin-1 overexpression through halted tumor vascularization. Proc Natl Acad Sci (USA) 1999; 96: 2065–2070.

Borchers AH, Powell MB, Fusenig NE, Bowden T. Paracrine factor and cell-cell contact-mediated induction of protease and c-ets gene expression in malignant keratinocyte/dermal fibroblast cocultures. Exp Cell Res 1994; 213: 143–147.

Borchers AH, Steinbauer H, Schafer BS, Kramer M, Bowden T. Fibroblast-directed expression and localization of 92-kDa type IV vollagenase along the tumor-stroma interface in an in vitro three-dimensional model of human squamous cell carcinoma. Molec Carcinog 1997; 19: 258–266.

Boukamp P, Dzarlieva-Petrusevska RT, Breitkreutz D, Hornung J, Markham A, Fusenig NE.

220

Normal keratinization in a spontaneously immortalized aneuploid human keratinocyte cell line. J Cell Biol 1988; 106: 761–771.

Boukamp P, Stanbridge EJ, Foo DY, Cerutti PA, Fusenig NE. c-Ha-ras oncogene expression in immortalized human keratinocytes (HaCaT) alters growth potential in vivo but lacks correlation with malignancy. Cancer Res 1990; 50: 2840–2847.

Boukamp P, Popp S, Altmeyer S, Hülsen A, Fasching C, Cremer T, Fusenig NE. Sustained non-tumorigenic phenotype correlates with a largely stable chromosome content during long-term culture of the human keratinocyte line HaCaT. Genes, Chromsomes & Cancer 1997; 19: 201–214.

Brauchle M, Angermeyer K, Hübner G, Werner S. Large induction of keratinocyte growth factor expression by serum growth factors and pro-inflammatory cytokines in cultured fibroblasts. Oncogene 1994; 9: 3199–3204.

Breitkreutz D, Boukamp P, Ryle CM, Stark HJ, Roop DR, Fusenig NE. Epidermal morphogenesis and keratin expression in c-Ha-ras-transfected tumorigenic clonesof the human HaCaT cell line. Cancer Res 1991; 51: 4402–4409.

Breitkreutz D, Stark HJ, Plein P, Baur M, Fusenig NE. Differential modulation of epidermal keratinization in immortalized (HaCaT) and tumorigenic human skin keratinocytes (HaCaT-ras) by retinoic acid and extracellular Ca2+. Differentiation 1993; 5: 201–217.

Breitkreutz D, Stark HJ, Mirancea N, Tomakidi P, Steinbauer H, Fusenig NE. Integrin and basement membrane normalization in mouse grafts of human keratinocytes – implications for epidermal homeostasis. Differentiation 1997; 61: 195–209.

Breitkreutz D, Schoop VM, Mirancea N, Baur M, Stark HJ, Fusenig NE. Epidermal differentiation and basment membrane formation by HaCaT cells in surface transplants. Eur J Cell Biol 1998; 75: 273–286.

Cornil J, Theodorescu D, Man S, Herlin J, Jambrosic J, Kerbel RS. Fibroblast cell interactions with human melanoma cells affect tumor cell growth as a function of tumor progression. Proc Natl Acad Sci (USA) 1991; 88: 6028–6032.

Dingemans KP, Zeeman-Boeschoten IM, Keep RF, Pranab K. Transplantation of colon carcinoma into granulation tissue induces an invasive morphotype. Int J Cancer 1993; 54: 1010–1016.

Dvorak HF. Tumors: wounds that do not heal. Similarities between tumor stroma generation and wound healing. New Engl Med 1986; 315: 1650–1659.

Fidler IJ. Critical factors in the biology of human cancer metastasis: twenty-eight GHA Clowes memorial lecture. Cancer Res 1990; 50: 6130–6138.

Fusenig NE, Valentine EA, Worst PKM. Growth behaviour of normal and transformed mouse epidermal cells after reimplantation in vivo. In: Richards RJ, Rajan KT (eds), *Tissue Culture in Medical Research (II)*. Pergamon Press, 1980, pp. 87–95.

Fusenig NE, Breitkreutz D, Dzarlieva RT, Boukamp P, Bohnert A, Tilgen W. Growth and differentiation characteristics of transformed keratinocytes from mouse and human skin in vitro and in vivo. J Invest Dermatol 1983; 81: 168–175.

Fusenig NE. Cell interaction and epithelial differentiation. In: Freshney RI (ed), *Culture of Epithelial Cells*. Wiley-Liss Inc, New York, 1992, pp. 25–57.

Fusenig NE. Epithelial-mesenchymal interactions regulate keratinocyte growth and differentiation in vitro. In: Leigh I, Lane B, Watt F (eds), *The Keratinocyte Handbook*. Cambridge University Press, 1994, pp. 71–94.

Fusenig NE, Boukamp P. Multiple stages and genetic alterations in immortalization, malignant transformation, and tumor progression of human skin keratinocytes. Molecular Carcinogenesis 1998; 23: 144–158.

Gregoire M, Lieubeau B. The role of fibroblasts in tumor behavior. Cancer Metastasis Rev 1995; 14: 339–350.

221

Hanahan D, Folkman J. Patterns and emerging mechanisms of the angiogenic switch during tumorigenesis. Cell 1996; 86: 353–364.

Hornung J, Bohnert A, Phan-Than L, Krieg T, Fusenig NE. Basement membrane formation by malignant mouse keratinocyte cell lines in organotypic culture and transplants: correlation with degree of morphologic differentiation. J Cancer Res Clin Oncol 1987; 113: 325–341.

Maas-Szabowski N, Shimotoyodome A, Fusenig NE. Keratinocyte growth regulation in fibroblast cocultures via a double paracrine mechanism. J Cell Sci 1999; 112: 1843–1853.

Maas-Szabowski N, Stark HJ, Fusenig NE. Keratinocyte growth regulation in defined organotypic cultures through IL-1-induced keratinocyte growth factor expression in resting fibroblasts. J Invest Dermatol 2000; 114: 1075, 1084.

Montesano R, Pepper MS, Möhle-Steinlein U, Risau W, Wagner EF, Orci L. Increased proteolytic activity is responsible for the aberrant morphogenetic behavior of endothelial cells expressing the middle T oncogene. Cell 1990; 62: 435–445.

Morikawa K, Walker SM, Nakajima M, Pathak S, Jessup JM, Fidler IJ. Influence of organ environment on the growth, selection, and metastasis of human colon carcinoma cells in nude mice. Cancer Res 1988; 48: 6863–6871.

Mueller MM, Peter W, Mappes M, Huelsen A, Steinbauer H, Boukamp P, Vaccariello M, Garlick J, Fusenig. In vivo microenvironment promotes tumor progression of skin carcinomas by clonal selection and mutagenesis. Submitted.

Nakamura T, Matsumoto K, Kiritoshi A, Tano Y, Nakamura T. Induction of hepatocyte growth factor in fibroblasts by tumor-derived factors affects invasive growth of tumor cells: in vitro analysis of tumor-stromal interactions. Cancer Res 1997; 57: 3305–3313.

Noël A, Gilles C, Bajou K, Devy L, Kebers F, Lewalle JM, Maquoi E, Munaut C, Remacle A,, Foidart JM. Emerging roles for proteinases in cancer. Invasion Metastasis 1997; 17: 221–239.

Noser FK, Limat A. Organotypic culture of outer root sheath cells from human hair follicles using a new culture device. In Vitro Cell Develop Biol 1987; 23: 541–545.

Olumi AF, Grossfeld GD, Hayward SW, Carroll PR, Tisty TD, Cunha GR. Carcinoma-associated fibroblasts direct tumor progression of initiated human prostatic epithelium. Cancer Res 1999; 59: 5002–5011.

Pauli BU, Knudson W. Tumor invasion: a consequence of destructive and compositional matrix alterations. Hum Pathol 1988; 19: 628–639.

Ryle CM, Breitkreutz P, Stark HJ, Leigh IM, Steinert PM, Roop D, Fusenig NE. Density-dependent modulation of synthesis of keratins 1 and 10 in the human keratinocyte line HaCaT and in ras-transfected tumorigenic clones. Differentiation 1989; 40: 42–54.

Schoop V, Mirancea N, Fusenig NE. Epidermal organization and differentiation of HaCaT keratinocytes in organotypic coculture with human dermal fibroblasts. J Invest Dermatol 1999; 112: 343–353.

Schor SL, Schor AM, Grey AM, Rushton G. Foetal and cancer patient fibroblasts produce an autocrine migration-stimulating factor not made by normal adult cells. J Cell Sci 1988; 90: 391–399.

Skobe M. Mechanisms of tumor-stroma interactions with emphasis on angiogenesis and its significance for tumor growth and invasion, Doctoral Thesis, Technische Hochschule Darmstadt, Fachbereich Biologie, 1996.

Skobe M, Rockwell P, Goldstein N, Vosseler S, Fusenig NE. Halting angiogenesis suppresses carcinoma cell invasion. Nature Med 1997; 11: 1222–1227.

Skobe M, Fusenig NE. Tumorigenic conversion of immortal human keratinocytes through stromal cell activation. Proc Natl Acad Sci (USA) 1998; 95: 1050–1055.

Smith-McCune KK, Weidner N. Demonstration and characterization of the angiogenic properties of cervical dysplasia. Cancer Res 1994; 54: 800–809.

222

Bernfield et al, 1999; David, 1993; Wight et al, 1992; Repraeger, 1993). HS chains generally consist of clusters of sulfated disaccharide units (predominantly N-sulfated glucosamine linked to α-L-iduronic acid residues) separated by low or non-sulfated regions (predominantly disaccharide units of N-acetylated glucosamine linked to β-D-glucuronic acid) (Kjellen and Lindahl, 1991; Bernfield et al, 1999; David, 1993).

Studies of the involvement of ECM molecules in cell attachment, growth and differentiation revealed a central role of HSPGs in embryonic morphogenesis, angiogenesis, metastasis, neurite outgrowth, and tissue repair (Kjellen and Lindahl, 1991; Bernfield et al, 1999; David, 1993; Wight et al, 1992; Repraeger, 1993). Transmembrane HSPGs (syndecans) are emerging as molecules that mediate cell interactions with components of the microenvironment that control cell shape, adhesion, proliferation and differentiation (Bernfield et al, 1999; David, 1993; Wight and Kinsella, 1992). The HS chains, unique in their ability to bind a multitude of proteins, ensure that a wide variety of effector molecules cling to the cell surface (Repraeger, 1993). For example, HSPGs are responsible for lipoprotein lipase cycling and herpes simplex virus infection (Vlodavsky et al, 1993). Moreover, transmembrane and membrane anchored HSPGs have a co-receptor role in which the proteoglycan in concert with the other cell surface molecules, comprises a functional receptor complex that binds the ligand and mediates its action (Rapraeger, 1993; Vlodavsky et al, 1992, 1997). Syndecans and possibly other species of HSPGs are also involved in early embryogenesis, epithelial-mesenchymal interactions, morphogenesis and differentiation (Bernfield et al, 1999; Wight et al, 1992). The ability of HS side chains to interact with enzymes (e.g. coagulation factors, mast cell proteases, lipoprotein lipase), cytokines (GM-CSF, IFN, IL-3, IL-7) and various members of the heparin binding growth factor family (e.g., bFGF, VEGF, hepatocyte growth factor) (Rapraeger, 1993; Vlodavsky et al, 1993, 1997; Iozzo, 1998) suggests an involvement in the control of normal and pathologic processes such as wound, healing tumor growth and vessel formation. HSPGs are also prominent components of blood vessels (Wight, 1989). In large vessels, they are concentrated mostly in the intima and inner media, whereas in capillaries, they are found mainly in the subendothelial basement membrane where they support proliferating and migrating endothelial cells and stabilize the structure of the capillary wall. Enzymatic degradation of HS in ECM and BMs appears, therefore, to be involved in fundamental biological phenomena ranging from pregnancy and development to inflammation, angiogenesis, and cancer metastasis.

3. MAMMALIAN HEPARANASE: GENE CLONING AND MOLECULAR PROPERTIES

Mammalian enzymes degrading HS, commonly referred to as heparanases, have been studied during the last three decades. These enzymes cleave the glycosidic bond with a hydrolase mechanism and are thus distinct from bacterial eliminases called heparinases and heparitinase (Erns et al, 1995). HS polysaccharide chains ($M_r \sim 30,000-100,000$) are cleaved by heparanase at only a few sites resulting in HS fragments of still appreciable size ($M_r \sim 5,000-10,000$). This suggests substrate specificity of the enzyme recognizing a particular and quite rare HS structure (Vlodavsky et al, 1983; Nakajima et al, 1988; Pikas et al, 1998). Heparanase enzymatic activity was first described in human placenta (Klein and Von Figura, 1976). Since then the enzyme has been identified in a variety of normal and malignant cells and tissues among which are skin fibroblasts, cytotrophoblasts, hepatocytes, endothelial cells, platelets, mast cells, neutrophils, macrophages, T and B lymphocytes, lymphoma, melanoma and carcinoma cells (Nakajima et al, 1988; Vlodavsky et al, 1992, 1994; Parish et al, 1987; Goshen et al, 1996; Freeman and Parish, 1998; Oosta et al, 1992). Normally, extracellularly acting heparanase is thought to participate in embryonic development, tissue repair, angiogenesis and inflammation, permitting BM degradation and cellular invasion into the ECM. Heparanase activity has also been described in hematopoietic cell types, correlating with the capacity of these cells to traverse the subendothelial BM and enter sites of inflammation in response to antigen expression (Vlodavsky et al, 1992).

Research on heparanases has for too long remained descriptive because of difficulties in purifying the protein and cloning the gene. A major impediment to studying the enzyme has been the lack of a simple assay for detecting heparanase activity. Heparanase assays were cumbersome and time consuming in both preparation of the labeled substrate and the methods required for the separation of degradative products from the uncleaved substrate. Also, the enzyme is unstable during purification and is found in low abundance in cells and tissues (for example 1 mg of purified heparanase protein is obtained from one unit of human platelets, 1×10^9 highly metastatic tumor cells, or 10 g of rat liver) (Freeman and Parish, 1998). A unique rapid quantitative assay for the detection of mammalian heparanase activity took advantage of an observation that the HS-binding plasma protein, histidine-rich glycoprotein (HRG) masks heparanase cleavage sites on HS chains. Following heparanase digestion, radio-labelled HS fragments are not bound by HRG-coupled Sepharose beads, unlike the remaining intact and partially degraded substrate, allowing a rapid separation of the cleaved product from the substrate (Freeman and Parish, 1998).

There have been several attempts to purify heparanase; for example, various species of heparanase were purified from human platelets with molecular weights of 137 kDa (Oosta et al, 1982), 50 kDa (Freeman and Parish, 1998) and 32–40 kDa (Hoogewerf et al, 1995). The latter was proposed to be an endoglucosaminidase consisting of four subunits, each closely related to the CXC chemokines CTAP-III and NAP-2 (Hoogewerf et al, 1995). A 98 kDa heparanase was purified from mouse melanoma and partially sequenced (Jin et al, 1990). This sequence was later attributed to an endoplasmin-like contaminant (De Vouge et al, 1994). No direct evidence for the biological function of any of these isolated enzymes was reported.

The cloning of a single human heparanase cDNA sequence (HPSE) and its expression in mammalian cells was independently reported by several groups, using amino acid sequences derived from heparanase enzymes purified from human platelets, placenta, hepatoma cells, and transformed embryonic fibroblasts (Vlodavsky et al, 1999; Helett et al, 1999; Kussie et al, 1999; Toyoshima and Nakajima, 1999; Fairbanks et al, 1999, Dempsey et al, 2000). An identical cDNA sequence was also derived from a human T-cell lymphoma cell line (Hulett et al, 1999). HPSE contains an open reading frame of 1,629 bp, which encodes for a unique 61.2 kDa polypeptide of 543 amino acids (Figure 1). The mature 50 kDa enzyme isolated from tissues has its N-terminus 157 amino acids downstream from the initiation codon (Vlodavsk et al, 1999; Hulett et al, 1999; Kussie et al, 1999) (Figure 1), suggesting post-translational processing of the heparanase polypeptide. The active enzyme has recently been claimed to be a heterodimer of the 50 kDa subunit (Ly^{s158} to Ile^{543}), non-covalently associated with an 8.2 kDa peptide (Gln^{36} to Glu^{109}), which arises from proteolytic processing of the pre-proheparanase protein (Fairbanks et al, 1999). It is not known whether the association of the 50 kDa polypeptide with the 8.2 kDa fragment is essential for expression of heparanase activity. The protease activities responsible for processing of heparanase have not been identified. The predicted amino acid sequence encodes for six putative N-glycosylation sites, five of which cluster in the first 80 amino acids of the 50 kDa mature protein. De-N-glycosylation decreased the Mr to 58 kDa, but did not reduce the enzyme activity (Vlodavsky et al, 1999; Hulett et al, 1999). The sequence also contains a putative N-terminal signal peptide sequence (Met^1 to Ala^{35}) and a candidate transmembrane region (Pro^{515} to Ile^{534}) (Figure 1), consistent with the requirement for detergent to completely solubilize the enzyme (Freeman and Parish, 1998; Hulett et al, 1999).

Alignment of the human, mouse and rat heparanase amino acid sequences corresponding to the 50 kDa human mature enzyme (Lys^{158} to Ile^{543}) demonstrated 80.0%, 79.7% and 92.7% identity between the human and mouse, human, and rat, and mouse and rat heparanases, respectively (Hulett et al, 1999). A 58–61% homology was found between the recently cloned chicken heparanase

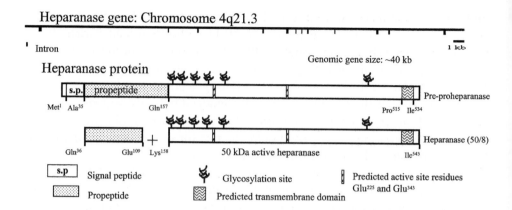

Figure 1. Scheme of the human heparanase gene and protein.

(Goldshmidt et al, 2001) and the human, mouse and rat enzymes (Figure 1). Both the rat and mouse heparanase amino acid sequences have a highly conserved putative transmembrane region at their C-termini and only 4 potential N-glycosylation sites, all of which are conserved in human heparanase. This accounts for the size differences between the isolated human, rat and mouse enzymes (Freeman and Parish, 1998; Hulett et al, 1999). No significant similarity or homology to any other reported protein including CTAP-III, other heparin-binding proteins or any of the bacterial heparin lyases was found, consistent with the different substrate specificities of the bacterial and mammalian enzymes (Ernst et al, 1995). The fact that highly homologous cDNA sequences were derived from human platelets, placenta, metastatic human rat and mouse tumor cells, and activated mouse splenic T-cells is consistent with the notion that one dominant endoglucuronidase is expressed by all mammalian cells (Vlodavsky et al, 1999; Hulett et al, 1999; Kussie et al, 1999; Toyoshima and Nakajima, 1999; Fairbanks et al, 1999; Dempsey et al, 2000). Unlike the large number of proteases that can solubilize polypeptides in the ECM (Kleiner and Stetler-Stevenson, 1993; Liotta et al, 1983), the present data suggest that only one heparanase is used by cells to degrade ECM heparan sulfate. Heparanase may, therefore, represent an attractive target for the development of new anti-metastatic drugs (Finkel, 1999).

3.1. Active site

Human heparanase contains two regions of clustered basic amino acid regions (272–278 and 157–162), which conform to previously proposed heparin and HS-binding protein consensus motifs (Cardin et al, 1991), as well as a highly basic cluster ranging from amino acid 426 to 432 (Dempsey et al, 2000). Search of PSI-blast databases using the amino acid sequences of the human, rat, mouse and chicken heparanases revealed weak similarities to members of the glycosyl hydrolase family. Furthermore, secondary structure predictions suggested that the enzyme contained a (α/β) 8 TIM barrel fold, which is conserved in several of the glycosyl hydrolase families. The identification of significant identity between regions containing active-site proton donor and nucleophile residues of specific TIM-barrel glycosyl hydrolases (e.g., xylanases, iduronidase and endo-glucanases) and heparanase suggests that heparanase exhibits a similar catalytic mechanism. Substitution of the putative proton donor (Glu[225]), or nucleophile (Glu[343]) residues, with alanine, followed by expression of these mutant heparanases in COS-7 cells, abolished the HS-degrading capacity of the enzyme. Substitution of two other glutamic acid residues predicted to reside outside the active site, did not affect the expressed heparanase activity (Hulett et al, 2000).

3.2. Genomic locus

The genomic locus which encodes heparanase spans ~40 kb. It is composed of 12 exons separated by 11 introns, is localized on human chromosome 4q21.3, and is linked to the genetic marker D4S400 (Vlodavsky et al, 1999; Hulett et al, 1999; Dempsey et al, 2000) (Figure 1). Southern blot analysis of human genomic DNA digested with a range of restriction enzymes demonstrated a simple hybridization pattern, consistent with the human heparanase gene being a single-copy gene (Hulett et al, 1999). However, the possible existence of tissue-specific isoforms derived by alternate splicing, or distantly related heparanases can not be excluded. The mouse heparanase gene has been localized to the E3-E5 region of mouse chromosome 5, which is syntenic to the centromere-proximal arm of human chromosome 4 (Dempsey, 2000).

231

3.3. Processing and activation

Expression of the cloned HPSE cDNA in mammalian cells yielded 65 kDa and 50 kDa recombinant proteins. The 50 kDa enzyme represents an N-terminal processed enzyme which is at least 200-fold more active than the full length 65 kDa form (Vlodavsky et al, 1999). Processing was readily demonstrated during incubation of the full length recombinant enzyme with intact tumor cells (Vlodavsky et al, 1999). The nature of the cellular, possibly membrane bound enzyme(s) involved in activation of the latent heparanase has not been characterized. Attempts to express the truncated 50 kDa protein Lys[158] to Ile[543] failed to yield active enzyme, suggesting that the region N-terminal to Lys[158] may play a functional role in mediating expression and/or function of the protein. Attempts to express full length heparanase cDNA lacking the C-terminal hydrophobic region also failed to yield active enzyme (Hulett et al, unpublished results).

Conversion of a proenzyme into an active enzyme provides an attractive means by which heparanase mediated cleavage of HS is regulated at the protein level, under physiological and pathological conditions. A proteolytic activation of a pro-enzyme is a common feature of enzymes (e.g., MMPs, plasminogen activators) involved in degradation of ECM proteins and in cell invasion (Kleiner and Stetler-Stevenson, 1993). The same principle appears to hold for endoglycosidic enzymes that degrade HS glycosaminoglycans. Proteases may thus regulate degradation of HS through activation of latent heparanase (Vlodavsky et al, 1999) and through a better exposure of HS side chains embedded in the ECM to heparanase activity (Vlodavsky et al, 1983, 1992).

3.4. Regulation

HS plays important roles in a wide range of biological processes. Since heparanase may play a regulatory role in many of these processes, it is likely that the enzyme activity would be tightly regulated because of the potential tissue damage that could result from inadvertent cleavage of HS. Heparanase activity may be regulated at the nucleotide level by transcription factors and post-transcriptionally through cytokine induction cell-cell interaction, activation of an inactive precursor, removal of endogenous inhibitors, control of local pH, cellular localization, and, at the substrate level, by directly masking the heparanase-cleavage site in the HS substrate.

Malignant melanoma which is neuroendocrine in origin, has a high frequency of metastasis to the brain. Treatment of murine and human melanoma cells with nerve growth factor or neurotrophin-3 stimulated both heparanase activity and invasion through a reconstituted BM (Walch et al, 1999). Both parameters were not stimulated in non-metastatic cell variants, nor in cell variants which were metastatic to other tissue sites. Heparanase activity may be inhibited by competing HS-binding proteins. Heparin/HS-interacting protein (HIP) which is expressed on the surface of epithelial and endothelial cells, binds to HS, thereby preventing heparanase digestion of the subendothelial ECM (Marchetti et al, 1997). Similarly, the plasma protein histidine-rich glycoprotein (HRG) was shown to bind along the heparanase cleavage site, thus inhibiting HS degradation (Freeman and Parish, 1998) and protecting the vascular cell surface HS.

Factors affecting the cellular localization of the enzyme may also play a role in its regulation. For example, the subcellular localization of cathepsin B in breast cancer cells was shown to change from within lysosomes to the plasma membrane with increasing metastatic potential. Similarly, while catheprsin B is localized on the surface of invasive bladder cancer cells, it is confined to lysosomes in the respective non-invasive cell line variant or normal bladder epithelium (Weiss et al, 1990). Interestingly, mannose-6-phosphate was reported to inhibit T-lymphocyte heparanase degradation of ECM due to displacement of the enzyme from the cell surface (Bartlett et al, 1995). Although lacking cell surface 300 kDa mannose-6-phosphate receptor (MPR-300) while in the circulation and within lymphoid organs, T lymphocytes gain cell surface expression of MPR-300 when they enter inflammatory sites.

3.5. Cellular localization of heparanase

While it is likely that degradative enzymes expressed on the cell surface would be more effective than intracellular enzymes in solubilizing the ECM during cell migration, the cellular location of heparanase has not been fully characterized. Heparanase immunoreactivity was observed both on the cell surface and cytoplasm of human colon adenocarcinoma (Friedmann et al, 2000) and meyloid leukemia cells (Bitan et al, 2002). Complete solubilization of heparanase activity from human platelets, rat and human tumor cells and from rat liver, required the presence of a detergent during homogenization, suggesting that up to 25% of the heparanase activity in cells and platelets was membrane associated (Freeman and parish, 1998; Hulett et al, 1999). The relatively low pH optimum for heparanase activity (Vlodavsky et al, 1992, 1994, 1999; Hulett et al, 1999) suggests that the enzyme has a lysosomal localization. Heparanase activity was isolated from rat liver lysosomes (Kjellen et al, 1985) and has been demonstrated to be present in both chloroquine-sensitive (lysosomal) and insensitive (endosomal) compartments in rat ovarian cancer cells and human colon carcinoma cells (Yanagishita, 1985). It has been localized in the tertiary granules of human neutrophils, co-localizing with gelatinase activity (Matzner et al, 1992; Mollinedo et al, 1997).

Studies with intact cells revealed a decreased, but still significant heparanase activity at pH 7.2 (Freeman and Parish, 1998; Hulett et al, 1999; Graham and Underwood, 1996). It was also suggested that physiological pH, heparanase binds to and associates with HS chains within the ECM rather than degrading them, thereby anchoring human T-lymphocytes (Gilat et al, 1995). HSPGs may thus tether inactive heparanase in the ECM, thereby serving as a reservoir for heparanase activity to facilitate leukocyte extravasation into the tissues in response to inflammatory conditions, or stimulate neovascularization during tumor growth (Gilat et al, 1995).

3.6. Substrate specificity

Although HS consists of long stretches of glucuronic acid (GlcA)-rich domains, it appears that only a small number of specific linkages are cleaved by the heparanase endoglucuronidase activity. The actual sequence within HS, which is cleaved by the enzyme, has not been fully characterized. Studies have been contradictory regarding the influence of 2-O-sulfate groups, iduronic acid residues, and whether N-substituted glucosamine residues are necessary for cleavage. It is agreed that decarboxylated heparin and HS are not cleaved (Freeman and Parish, 1998; Hulett et al, 1999; Freeman et al, 1999). Freeman and Parish (Freeman and Parish, 1998) demonstrated that neither the presence of N- nor O-sulfation was an absolute requirement for substrate cleavage. Whereas totally de-sulfated lung heparin was not a substrate, platelet heparanase cleaved both the re-N-acetylated and re-N-sulfated analogs of desulfated heparin. These and other results suggest that the enzyme may, in fact, cleave a non-sulfated substrate, providing that IdoA residues are also present and the glucosamine residues are substituted. In fact, the platelet and melanoma heparanases cleaved both de-N-sulfated heparin and its re-N-acetylated analog (Nakajima et al, 1998; Freeman and Parish, 1998). In contrast, other studies proposed that 2-O-sulfation is required for cleavage by human platelet (Pikas et al, 1998) and CHO cell (Bame et al, 1998) heparanases. The CHO cells appear to contain at least four heparanase activities, differing in their sizes (30–45 kDa) and pIs, and possessing different substrate specificity (Bame et al, 1998).

Sequential enzymatic and chemical modification of the capsular polysaccharide produced by E. coli K5 strain, revealed that human platelet and hepatoma heparanases require the presence of O-sulfation with no essential requirement for N-sulfation or IdoA residues (Pikas et al, 1998). Heparanase cleavage of the AT-III heparin-derived octasaccharide was unaffected by selective 6-O-desulfation, but was inhibited by selective 2-O-desulfation, implying that a 2-O sulfate group on a hexuronic acid residue located two monosaccharide units away from the cleavage site is essential for substrate recognition by heparanase (Pikas et al, 1998). On the basis of these studies, the minimal HS sequence cleaved by heparanase is within the sequence [HexA-GlcNS/Ac(6S)-GlcA-GlcNS/Ac-HexA2S-GlcNS/Ac-HexA (Pikas et al, 1998)]. It should be noted that the above studies demonstrated only the absolute structural requirements for substrate cleavage, occurring during a prolonged incubation. A comparison of the effect of various substrate structural features on the rate of cleavage, and at the optimal pH for each structurally defined substrate, needs to be performed in order to identify important physiological structural features which will prove useful for characterization of the enzyme's active site and subsequent development of highly specific heparanase inhibitors.

4. PREFERENTIAL EXPRESSION OF THE HEPARANASE GENE AND PROTEIN IN HUMAN TUMORS

4.1. Normal tissues

Expression of the human heparanase mRNA in normal tissues is restricted primarily to the placenta and lymphoid organs. Northern blot analysis of human non-immune tissues using the full length human nucleotide sequence demonstrated a high expression of a 2 kb heparanase mRNA in placenta, low levels in colon, stomach and testis, and none in heart, brain, lung, liver, skeletal muscle, kidney, or pancreas (Hulett et al, 1999; Kussie et al, 1999). A 1.4 kb mRNA was also detected in testis. A 4.4 kb mRNA derived by alternate polyadenylation was detected strongly in placenta, and weakly in all other tissues (Dempsey et al, 2000). Immunohistochemistry of normal tissues revealed staining of the human heparanase protein in neutrophils, macrophages, platelets, cytotrophoblasts, proximal convoluted tubules and mesangial cells capillary endothelial cells ganglion cells, and nerves. Fibroblasts and most connective tissue cells, endothelial cells of medium and large vessels, and normal epithelial cells of the colon, breast and liver, showed little or no staining.

4.2. Breast carcinoma

Heparanase activity is significantly higher (4–10-fold higher) in highly metastatic rat and human mammary adenocarcinoma cell lines compared to their non-metastatic variants (Vlodavsky et al, 1999; Freeman et al, 1999). Northern blot analysis of human and rat breast cancer cell lines demonstrated high levels of a 2 kb heparanase mRNA in highly metastatic rat mammary adenocarcinoma cell lines, compared to their non-metastatic variants, demonstrating a good correlation between heparanase mRNA enzyme activity and the cell's metastatic potential (Vlodavsky et al, 1999; Hulett et al, 1999).

Semi-quantitative RT-PCR was applied to evaluate the expression of the *hpa* gene by human breast carcinoma cell lines. While the expected 585 bp PCR product of the *hpa* cDNA was not detected in non-metastatic MCF-7 breast carcinoma cells (Figure 2a; inset: lane 1), moderate (MDA 231 lane 2) and highly (MDA 435 lane 3) metastatic breast carcinoma cell lines exhibited a marked increase in *hpa* gene expression. The differential pattern of the *hpa* gene expression correlated with the pattern of heparanase activity (Figure 2a) (Vlodavsky et al, 1999, 2000). An increased expression of both the heparanase gene and enzymatic activity was also seen when nearly normal breast epithelial cells (MCF 10A) derived from a patient with fibrocystic breast disease were compared to cells transfected with prooncogenic (MCF 10AneoN) and oncogenic (MCF 10AneoT) forms of C-H ras.

We applied sense and antisense deoxigenin-labeled *hpa* RNA probes to screen archival paraffin embedded human breast tissue for expression of the *hpa* gene transcripts. Hybridization of the heparanase antisense riboprobe to invasive duct carcinoma tissue sections resulted in a massive positive staining localized specifically to the carcinoma cells (Figure 2b right). The *hpa* gene was also expressed in areas adjacent to the carcinoma, showing fibrocystic changes (not shown). Normal breast tissue derived from reduction mammoplasty failed to express the *hpa* transcript, yielding the same staining both with the antisense (Figure 2b left) and sense probes (Vlodavsky et al, 1999). Similarly, immune staining of normal looking breast epithelial cells revealed weak staining (Figure 2c left) as compared to breast carcinoma cells present in the same specimen (Figure 2c right). Interestingly, myoepithelial cells of fibroadenomas expressed the heparanase protein as compared to little or no expression of the enzyme in the myoepithelium of normal breast tissue (not shown).

4.3. Colon carcinoma

Expression of the heparanase gene and protein was detected at early stages of colon carcinoma progression, already at the stage of adenoma, while the adjacent normal-looking colonic tissue showed no expression of the enzyme (Friedmann et al, 2000). Gradually increasing expression of heparanase was evident as the cells progressed from severe dysplasia through well differentiated to poorly differentiated colon carcinoma. Deeply invading colon carcinoma cells and adjacent desmoplastic stromal fibroblasts showed the highest levels of the heparanase mRNA and protein (Friedmann et al, 2000). Both the heparanase gene and protein were also highly expressed in colon carcinoma metastasizing to the lung, liver and lymph nodes, as well as in the accompanying stromal fibroblasts (Figure 3) (Friedmann et al, 2000). A similar pattern of expression was observed both at the mRNA (*in situ* hybridization) and protein (immuno-

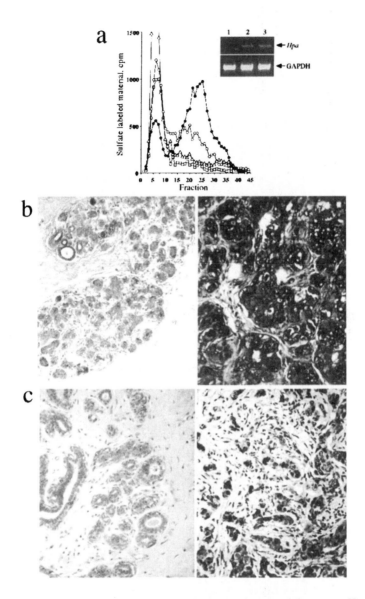

Figure 2. Preferential expression of heparanase in human breast carcinoma. **a.** Human breast carcinoma cell lines exhibiting different degrees of metastasis were tested for expression of the hpa gene (inset) and heparanase activity. MCF-7 ($\triangle$) MDA-231 ($\circ$) MDA-435 ($\bullet$) cells, or control medium alone ($\square$) were incubated in contact with sulfate labeled ECM. Labeled degradation products were analyzed by gel filtration on Sepharose 6B. **Inset.** Total RNA was subjected to RT-PCR using heparanase (top) and GAPDH (bottom) specific primers. Lane 1: non-metastatic MCF-7 cells; Lane 2: moderately metastatic MDA-231 cells; Lane 3: highly metastatic MDA-435 cells. **b.** and **c.** Paraffin embedded specimens derived from normal breast (left) and invasive ductal carcinoma of breast (right) were subjected to *in situ* hybridization (**b**) and immunohisto-chemistry (**c**).

237

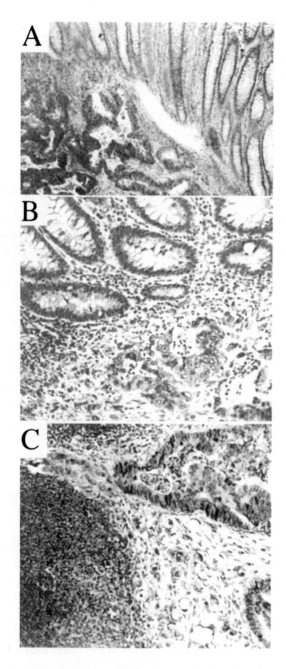

Figure 3. Preferential expression of the heparanase mRNA and protein in human colon adeno-carcinoma cells vs. 'normal looking' colonic gland epithelium adjacent to the tumor. **A.** *In situ* hybridization; **B.** immunohistochemistry. **C.** High expression of the heparanase protein in colon carcinoma cells metastatic to a lymph node.

238

histochemistry) levels, indicating that both the heparanase gene and protein are expressed already at early stages of carcinogenesis, continuing through later stages. The heparanase protein was detected both in the cytoplasm and on the cell surface, suggesting that some of the enzyme is membrane associated and/or secreted.

Our results strongly suggest that heparanase expression is related to the presumed stages in colon carcinoma progression. These results were supported by the finding that both the heparanase protein, detected by Western blot analysis, and enzymatic activity, measured by release of HS degradation fragments from intact ECM, were found in much higher levels in the colon tumor tissue than in the adjacent normal appearing tissue (Friedmann et al, 2000). Heparanase expression was inversely related to tumor grade, being the strongest in poorly differentiated tumor areas, suggesting that heparanase may reflect the differentiation status and metastatic nature of the cells. Heparanase may thus play a role in colon tumor progression, most probably through its effect on the tumor microenvironment, resulting in an enhanced tumor cell invasiveness and vascularization (Friedmann et al, 2000).

4.4. Other tumors

Tissue specimens derived from adenocarcinoma of the ovary, metastatic melanoma, squamous cell carcinoma of the cervix, prostate, bladder and hepatocellular carcinomas exhibited strong staining with the anti-sense *hpa* RNA probe and with the anti-heparanase antibodies, as compared to the surrounding connective tissue and the respective normal-looking control tissues (Vlodavsky et al, 2000 and our unpublished results).

5. INVOLVEMENT OF HEPARANASE IN TUMOR METASTASIS AND ANGIOGENESIS

5.1. Tumor metastasis

A critical event in the process of cancer invasion and metastasis is degradation of various ECM constituents including collagen, laminin, fibronectin and HSPGs (Liotta et al, 1983). The malignant cell is able to accomplish this task through the concerted sequential action of enzymes such as metalloproteinases, serine proteases and endoglycosidases. The ability of HSPGs to interact with various ECM macromolecules, and with different attachment sites on plasma membranes, suggests a key role for this proteoglycan in the self-assembly and insolubility of ECM components, as well as in cell adhesion and locomotion (Kjellen and Lindahl, 1991; Bernfield et al, 1999; David, 1993; Wight et al, 1992; Rapraeger, 1993; Vlodavsky et al, 1993). Cleavage of HS may, therefore, result in disassembly of the subendothelial ECM, and hence may play a decisive role in extravasation of blood-borne cells (Nakajima et al, 1988; Vlodavsky et al, 1992, 1994). Expression of HS degrading heparanase correlates with the metastatic potential of mouse lymphoma, fibrosarcoma, breast carcinoma, and melanoma (Nakajima et al, 1988; Vlodavsky et al, 1994, 1999; Parish et al, 1987) cells. Moreover, elevated levels of heparanase were detected in sera of metastatic tumor bearing animals and cancer patients (Nakajima et al, 1988), and in tumor specimens (Friedmann et al, 2000). Interestingly, heparanase activity was detected in the urine of some metastatic cancer patients, as opposed to no detectable levels in normal donors (Vlodavsky et al, 1997 and our unpublished observations). It is likely that heparanase can preferentially and readily cross the glomerular BM barrier by virtue of its ability to degrade HS and hence destroy its permselectivity properties.

We and others have previously demonstrated that heparanase inhibiting molecules (e.g., non-anticoagulant species of heparin, polysulfated polysaccharides, polyanionic molecules) markedly reduced (> 90%) the incidence of lung metastases induced by B16 melanoma, Lewis lung carcinoma, and mammary adenocarcinoma cells (Nakajima et al, 1988, 1998; Vlodavsky et al, 1994; Parish et al, 1997; Coombe et al, 1987; Miao et al, 1999). Although the anti-metastatic activity of these molecules correlated with their anti-heparanase activity, other explanations (i.e. effect on cell adhesion) can not be ruled out (Koenig et al, 1998). More convincing evidence for a direct role of heparanase in tumor metastasis was provided by the conversion of Eb T-lymphoma cells from a non-metastatic to metastatic behavior, following stable transfection and over-expression of the heparanase gene (Vlodavsky et al, 1999). For this purpose, heparanase transfected and mock transfected Eb cells were injected subcutaneously into DBA/2 mice followed by measurements of survival time and liver metastases. All mice injected with cells transfected with control pcDNA3 plasmid alone survived during the first 4 weeks of the experiment vs. a 75% mortality observed in mice inoculated with Eb cells transfected with the *hpa* containing expression plasmid (Figure 4c). Macroscopic and microscopic examination revealed that the liver of mice inoculated with *hpa* transfected cells was infiltrated with numerous Eb lymphoma cells (Figure 4d, bottom-right), while metastatic lesions could not be detected in the liver of mice inoculated with mock transfected control Eb cells (Figure 4d, bottom-left) (Vlodavsky et al, 1999). Similarly, transient transfection of the heparanase gene into low metastatic B16-F1 mouse melanoma cells, followed by intravenous inoculation, resulted in a 3- to 5-fold increase in lung colonization, versus that of mock transfected cells.

240

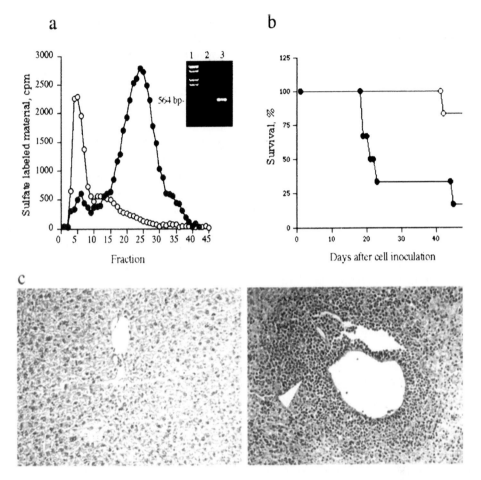

Figure 4. Overexpression of heparanase in non-metastatic Eb T-lymphoma cells leads to liver metastasis and accelerated mortality. **a:** Heparanase gene expression and activity. Eb cells transfected with control plasmid alone (○ inset: lane 2) or with *hpa* containing plasmid (● inset: lane 3) were incubated with sulfate labeled ECM. Labeled degradation fragments were analyzed by gel filtration. **b** and **c:** Mortality and liver metastasis. DBA/2 mice were inoculated (s.c; 2×10^5 cells/mouse) with Eb cells transfected with control vector alone (○) or *hpa* containing plasmid (●) (20 mice per group). Mice were evaluated for mortality (**b**) and infiltration of the liver tissue by lymphoma cells (**c**). Liver tissue specimens were taken (day 28) from mice inoculated with mock transfected (left) and *hpa* transfected (right) Eb cells.

5.2. Tumor angiogenesis

Heparin, HS and related polysaccharides have long been implicated in the angiogenic process. The earliest indication that heparin may be involved in the regulation of angiogenesis was the finding that mast cells accumulate at the site of tumor angiogenesis before capillary ingrowth. Mast cells or the medium in which they were incubated significantly, stimulated the locomotion of capillary endothelial cells *in vitro*. This activity was attributed to heparin since it was abolished by protamine and heparinase (Folkman and Shing, 1992). Heparin also played a key role in the purification of the first tumor derived angiogenic factor which was found to be bFGF (Folkman and Shing, 1992). Subsequently, several other growth promoting factors were purified based on their affinity to heparin, constituting a growing family of heparin-binding growth factors of which many (e.g., VEGF; bFGF) are highly angiogenic (Folkman and Shing, 1992). It soon became apparent that the heparin-affinity of these growth factors was more than just a useful technique for purification. Both heparin and HS were found to i) potentiate the mitogenic effect of FGFs on vascular endothelial cells *in vitro*; ii) stabilize and protect FGFs from inactivation; and iii) function as low affinity receptors that sequester bFGF and facilitate its interaction with high affinity signaling receptors on the cell surface (Vlodavsky et al, 1991, 1993, 1996, 1997; Aviezer et al, 1994). The heparin affinity of FGFs also appears to be the basis for their storage in BMs and ECM of cells and tissues, where they are bound to HS, and can be released in an active form by species of heparin and heparin-like molecules and by heparin/HS degrading enzymes (Vlodavsky et al, 1991, 1993, 1996, 1997; Aviezer et al, 1994). The released FGFs and other heparin-binding growth factors may then stimulate cell proliferation and migration associated with neovascularization. Angiogenesis represents a coordinated multicellular process that requires the functional activity of a wide variety of molecules, including growth factors, ECM components, adhesion receptors and matrix-degrading enzymes (Folkman and Shing, 1992). HSPGs and HSPG-degrading enzymes are therefore implicated in a number of angiogenesis-related cellular events, including cell invasion, migration, adhesion, differentiation and proliferation (Kjellen and Lindahl, 1991; Bernfield et al, 1999; David, 1993; Wight et al, 1992; Rapraeger, 1993; Vlodavsky et al, 1993, 1997).

A most important early step in the angiogenic cascade is degradation of the subendothelial capillary BM by proliferating endothelial cells and formation of vascular sprouts (Stetler-Stevenson, 1999). Heparanase, degrading the polysaccharide scaffold (HSPGs) of BM is presumed to markedly contribute to the invasive ability of endothelial cells and their migration through the ECM toward the angiogenic stimulus (e.g., growing tumor). It has been previously suggested that stimulated endothelial cells secrete heparanase-like activity (Sivaram et al, 1995). In recent experiments, we have demonstrated the presence of heparanase mRNA transcripts in proliferating human umbilical vein endothelial cells (HUVEC). Immunohistochemical staining of paraffin-embedded sections of human, colon and breast carcinomas with anti-heparanase mono-clonal antibodies revealed preferential expression of the heparanase protein by endothelial cells of sprouting capillaries in the vicinity of the tumor vs. little or no staining of mature vessels (Elkin et al, 2001).

In addition to direct involvement in BM invasion by endothelial cells, degra-dation of HS may elicit an indirect angiogenic response by releasing HS-bound angiogenic growth factors (i.e., bFGF, VEGF) from ECM and BMs and gener-ating HS degradation fragments that promote angiogenic growth factor activity (Vlodavsky et al, 1991, 1993, 1996, 1997; Aviezer et al, 1994). Of particular significance is the interaction of HS side chains with heparin-binding growth factors (e.g., HB-EGF, bFGF, VEGF, hepatocyte growth factor) (Rapraeger, 1993; Vlodavsky et al, 1993, 1996, 1997; Iozzo, 1998). Interactions of HS with bFGF were studied extensively. Basic FGF requires HSPG as cofactor for sig-naling. Cell surface HSPGs bearing specific binding sequences function as accessory co-receptors for bFGF, facilitating binding of bFGF to high affinity cell surface tyrosine kinase receptors, inducing bFGF-receptor dimerization and signaling (Vlodavsky et al, 1991, 1996; Aviezer et al, 1994). ECM and BM resident HSPGs appear to be less active than cell surface HS in mediating bFGF/FGF-receptor complex assembly and function (Vlodavsky et al, 1997; Green et al, 1992). Rather, they bind specifically bFGF and therefore serve as its extracellular reservoir. ECM sequestration of bFGF by HSPGs is well doc-umented. Basic FGF was extracted from the subendothelial ECM *in vitro* and from both endothelial and epithelial basement membranes of the cornea (Vlodavsky et al, 1991, 1993, 1996, 1997). Similarly, bFGF is distributed ubiq-uitously in BMs of all sizes of blood vessels (Vlodavsky et al, 1991). Despite the ubiquitous presence of bFGF in normal tissues, EC proliferation in these tissues is usually very low, suggesting that bFGF is sequestered from its site of action (Vlodavsky et al, 1991, 1993, 1996, 1997).

It appears that HS moieties are specific for binding and sequestration of bFGF in BMs; other glycosaminoglycans such as chondroitin sulfate, dermatan sulfate, or keratan sulfate do not bind bFGF. In support of specific binding of bFGF to HS is the observation that up to 90% of the bound growth factor was displaced by heparin or HS (Vlodavsky et al, 1991, 1996). Similarly, heparanase that specifically degrades HS was found to be a most efficient specific releaser of active bFGF from ECM and cell surfaces (Vlodavsky et al, 1991, 1993, 1996, 1997). Our studies indicate that both recombinant mammalian heparanase and heparanase secreted by platelets, tumor and inflammatory cells (Vlodavsky et al, 1991) releases bFGF as a complex with HS fragment, yielding a highly active form of bFGF, which may readily interact with high affinity receptors on the surface of endothelial cells and thus elicit an angiogenic response. The size of HS required for optimal stimulation of bFGF receptor binding and dimerization was similar to that of HS fragments released by heparanase (Vlodavsky et al, 1996). A role of heparanase in angiogenesis was demonstrated in our recent experiments applying the matrigel plug angiogenesis assay *in vivo*. Using this assay, we observed an increased angiogenic response to heparanase transfected Eb lymphoma cells vs. a small or no response to the parental mock transfected cells (Elkin et al, 2001) (Figure 5). Thus, cooperative interactions between heparanases from tumor, inflammation and endothelial sources appear to play an important role in the angiogenic cascade. The anticancerous potential of heparanase inhibitors is therefore not restricted solely to suppression of the invasive metastatic phenotype, but may also be due to suppression of tumor neovascularization. In fact, as detailed below, the heparanase inhibiting pentasaccharide phosphomannopentaose sulfate (PI-88) was found to reduce the vascularity, primary tumor growth and metastasis of rat mammary adenocarcinoma tumor (Parish et al, 1999).

6. SULFATED OLIGOSACCHARIDE INHIBITORS OF HEPARANASE ACTIVITY AND TUMOR PROGRESSION

A number of studies had shown that sulfated polysaccharides such as heparin, dextran sulfate and xylose sulfate were potent inhibitors of tumor metastasis. This inhibition was largely attributed to the anti-coagulant activity of these compounds. However, heparin which was drastically depleted of its anticoagulant activity by AT-III fractionation or by chemical modification was shown to retain its antimetastatic and heparanase inhibitory properties (Nakajima et al, 1988, 1998; Vlodavsky et al, 1994; Parish et al, 1987; Coombe et al, 1987). It was

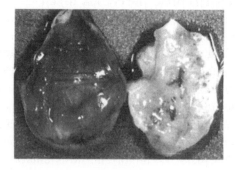

Figure 5. Heparanase mediated angiogenesis. Murine lymphoma Eb cells transfected with control vector alone (right) or *hpa* containing plasmid (left) were mixed with Matrigel and injected s.c. into mice. The Matrigel pellets were removed on day 6 and examined for extent of vascularization.

demonstrated that the sulfated polysaccharides heparin, fucoidin, pentosan sulfate, dextran sulfate and carrageena-lambda inhibited tumor cell heparanase activity and tumor metastasis, while chondroitin sulfate, carrageena-kappa and hyaluronic acid had a small or no effect (Parish et al, 1987; Coombe et al, 1987). Interestingly, Green et al (1992) reported a lower mortality in cancer patients treated with low Mr heparin compared to heparin therapy.

Using purified platelet heparanase and a novel quantitative heparanase assay, Freeman et al (Freeman and Parish, 1998) determined the IC50 for a variety of heparin analogs. Platelet heparanase was inhibited by 50% in the presence of 1.2 µg/ml of highly sulfated lung heparin. De-N-sulfated heparin and its N-acetylated derivative were 12- and 4-fold poorer inhibitors than heparin itself. De-N-sulfation would effectively reduce the overall negative charge of the inhibitor and this effect was partially relieved by N-acetylation of the inhibitor. In an earlier study, Vlodavsky et al (1994) reported that inhibition of both heparanase activity and melanoma lung colonization depended on the size and degree of sulfation of the heparin molecule, the position of sulfate groups and the occupancy of the N-position of the hexosamines. Inhibition of heparanase was best achieved by heparin species containing 16 sugar units or more and having sulfate groups at both the N and O positions. Low sulfate oligosaccharides were less effective heparanase inhibitors than medium and high sulfate fractions of the same size saccharide (Vlodavsky et al, 1994). While O-desulfation abolished the heparanase inhibiting effect of heparin, O-sulfated, N-substituted (e.g., N-acetyl or N-hexanoyl) species of heparin retained a high inhibitory activity, provided that the N-substituted molecules had a molecular size of about 4000 daltons or more. Likewise, 6-O-sulfation and N-acetylation rather than N-sulfation was required for inhibition of heparanase and tumor metastasis by chemically modified chitins (Saiki et al, 1990). Potent inhibition of heparanase activity, and tumor metastasis in animal models has also been demonstrated with calcium spirulin (Mishima et al, 1998), laminaran sulfate (Miao et al, 1999), sulfated chitin derivatives (Saiki et al, 1992), phosphorothioate DNA oligonucleotides (Miao et al, 1999), and suramin (Nakajima et al, 1991). An effect of these heparin-like polyanionic molecules on selectin mediated cell adhesion could not be excluded (Koenig et al, 1998). Structural requirements for inhibition of heparanase activity and lung colonization of melanoma cells by species of heparin were different from those identified for release of ECM-bound bFGF, and for stimulation of bFGF receptor binding and mitogenic activity (Vlodavsky et al, 1994). These results indicate that various non-anticoagulant species of heparin and other polyanionic molecules differing in size, sulfation and substituted groups can be designed to elicit specific effects on tumor metastasis and angiogenesis.

While many of the sulfated polysaccharides described above are as potent as heparin in inhibiting heparanase activity and tumor metastasis in animal models, none of these compounds apart from low M_r heparins have been used clinically. In fact, they are unlikely to be of general clinical use for a number of reasons. Firstly, the molecules are structurally heterogeneous and of relatively high molecular weight, which may preclude oral delivery of the compounds. Secondly, the high anticoagulant activity of many of the polysaccharides which often cannot be easily eliminated by chemical modification, possess a major toxicity problem. Thirdly, some of the polysaccharides exhibit macrophage toxicity as they cannot be degraded by lysosomal glycosidases. Therefore, sulfated oligosaccharides have been examined as potential heparanase inhibitors. Such molecules are structurally better defined, are of a sufficiently low molecular weight that oral delivery is feasible, are relatively easy to manufacture and should have minimal toxicity due to reduced anti-coagulant activity and ease of excretion.

A comprehensive screening program was undertaken by Parish et al (Parish et al, 1999) to identify sulfated oligosaccharides which inhibit tumor metastasis by inhibiting heparanase activity and which also cause tumor regression by blocking angiogenic growth factor action. A large number of oligosaccharides varying in sizem type of sugar units and linkage were synthesized or isolated following chemical or enzymatic degradation of natural products and were chemically O-sulfated. The sulfated oligosacccharides were examined for their ability to inhibit heparanase activity and angiogenesis *in vitro*, as well as hematogenous metastasis using the highly metastatic rat mammary adenocarcinoma 13,762 MAT cells (Parish et al, 1999). The oligosaccharide chain length and degree of sulfation were more important parameters than the sugar composition and type of linkage. With increasing sulfation, there was a steady increase in the ability of maltohexaose to inhibit heparanase activity and experimental metastasis which plateaued when sulfation was 85% or greater (Parish et al, 1999). Optimum heparanase inhibitory activity was achieved with highly sulfated oligosaccharides of five or more monosaccharides in length. Whereas maltose sulfate was ineffective, the tetrasaccharides stachyose sulfate and maltotetraose sulfate exhibited modest inhibitory activity, while phosphomannopentaose sulfate (PI-88) and maltohexaose sulfate were comparable to heparin in their inhibitory activity with IC_{50}'s of 2 1.5 and 1 µg/ml respectively. There was a good correlation between heparanase inhibition *in vitro* and the ability of a compound to inhibit metastasis *in vivo*. PI-88 continuously administered to rats by mini-osmotic pumps at 20 µg/kg/day, starting 3 days prior to i.v. injection of the tumor cells, gave approximately 90% inhibition of lung metastasis (Parish et al, 1999). The effect of continuously administered PI-88 on primary tumor growth was assessed following injection of 13762 MAT cells into the hind footpads of rats. Primary tumor growth was reduced by about

50%, tumor vascularity by approximately 30%, and the presence of metasta-sizing tumor cells in the draining popliteal lymph nodes was reduced by nearly 40% (Parish et al, 1999).

PI-88 could be conveniently prepared in large quantities following chemical sulfation of the starting oligosaccharide phosphomannopentaose which is easily prepared from the polysaccharide secreted by the yeast *Pichia holstii*. PI-88 has successfully undergone exhaustive animal toxicity tests and a phase I clinical trial in healthy humans has demonstrated its low toxicity. An international multi-center phase II trial is underway.

NOTE ADDED IN PROOFS

Articles published since the submission of this chapter have demonstrated that cancer patients exhibiting high levels of heparanase in the tumor tissue had a significantly shorter postoperative survival time than patients whose tumors contained relatively low levels of heparanase (Koliopanos et al, 2001; Gohji et al, 2001). High levels of heparanase also correlate with a high density of angio-genic blood vessels in the tumor (Gohji et al, 2001), further corroborating the significance of heparanase in the most critical aspects of human cancer pro-gression (Vlodavsky and Friedmann, 2001; Parish et al, 2001).

Given the potential tissue damage that could result from inadvertent cleavage of HS, tight regulation and balance are essential. An attractive regulatory target is the apparently membrane bound protease, converting the heparanase from a latent 65 kDa protein into an active 50 kDa form. Regulation of heparanase promoter activity (e.g., methylation and identification of regulatory response elements and effective modulators) is being investigated. Applying *in vivo* models of cancer metastasis and non-invasive MRI analysis of vascular density, functionality and maturation, we have demonstrated that the potent pro-angio-genic and pro-metastatic properties of heparanase are tightly regulated by its cellular localization and secretion (Goldshmidt et al, 2002). Cell surface binding, activation, and uptake of extracellular heparanase into late endosomes appear to control its activation, clearance, and storage within the cells (Nadav et al, 2002; Goldshmidt et al, 2002). Our results (Goldshmidt et al., submitted for publication) indicate that cell surface expression of the enzyme also elicits a firm cell adhesion, independent of its enzymatic activity, suggesting a possible involvement of heparanase in signal transduction and non-enzymatic functions. Mammary glands of transgenic mice over-expressing the heparanase enzyme exhibit precocious branching and widening of ducts, associated with vascular-ization, BM disruption and early signs of hyperplasia. This, together with its preferential early expression in the developing vascular and nervous systems

(Goldshmidt et al, 2001) suggest a role for heparanase in normal embryogenesis and tissue morphogenesis and regeneration. Development of mice with target disruption of the heparanase gene is needed to elucidate its normal roles in embryonic development, tissue remodeling and the mature individual.

ACKNOWLEDGMENTS

This work was supported by grants from the Center for the Study of Emerging Diseases (CSED); the Israel Science Foundation founded by the Israel Academy of Sciences and Humanities; the Israel Cancer Research Fund; the Association for International Cancer Research UK; the Breast Cancer Research Program of the US Army; and Progen Industries Brisbane Australia.

REFERENCES

Aviezer D, Hecht D, Safran M, Eisinger M, David G, Yayon A. Perlecan basal lamina proteoglycan promotes basic fibroblast growth factor-receptor binding, mitogenesis and angiogenesis. Cell 1994; 79: 1005–1013.

Bame KJ, Hassall A, Sanderson C, Venkatesan I, Sun C. Partial purification of heparanase activities in Chinese hamster ovary cells: evidence for multiple intracellular heparanases. Biochem J 1998; 336: 191–200.

Bartlett MR, Cowden WB, Parish CR. Differential effects of the anti-inflammatory compounds heparin, mannose-6-phosphate and castanospermine on degradation of the vascular basement membrane by leukocytes, endothelial cells and platelets. J Leukoc Biol 1995; 57: 207–213.

Bernfield, M Gotte, M Park, PW Reizes, O Fitzgerald ML, Lincecum J, Zako M. Functions of cell surface heparan sulfate proteoglycans. Annu Rev Biochem 1999; 68: 729–777.

Bitan M, Polliack A, Zecchina G, Nagler A, Friedmann Y, Nadav L, Deutsch V, Pecker I, Eldor A, Vlodavsky I, Katz B-Z. Heparanase expression in human leukemias is restricted to acute myeloid leukemias. Exp Hematol 2002; 30: 34–41.

Cardin AD, Demeter DA, Weintraub HJ, Jackson RL. Molecular design and modeling of protein-heparin interactions. Methods Enzymol 1991; 203: 556–583.

Chang Z, Meyer K, Rapraeger AC, Friedl A. Differential ability of heparan sulfate proteoglycans to assemble the fibroblast growth factor receptor complex in situ. FASEB J 2000; 14: 137–144.

Coombe DR, Parish CR, Ramshaw IA, Snowden JM. Analysis of the inhibition of tumour metastasis by sulphated polysaccharides. Int J Cancer 1987; 39: 82–88.

David G. Integral membrane heparan sulfate proteoglycans. FASEB J 1993; 7: 1023–1030.

Dempsey LA, Plummer TB, Coombes SL, Platt JL. Heparanase expression in invasive trophoblasts and acute vascular damage. Glycobiology 2000; 10: 467–475

De Vouge MW, Yamazaki A, Bennett SA, Chen JH, Shwed PS, Couture C, Birnboim HC. Immunoselection of GRP94/endoplasmin from a KNRK cell-specific lambda gt11 library using antibodies directed against a putative heparanase amino-terminal peptide. Int J Cancer 1994; 56: 286–294.

Elkin M, Ishai-Michaeli R, Friedmann Y, Papo O, Pecker I, Vlodavsky I. Heparanase as mediator of angiogenesis: mode of action. FASEB J 2001; 15: 1661–1663.

248

Ernst S, Langer R, Cooney CL, Sasisekharan R. Enzymatic degradation of glycosaminoglycans. Crit Rev Biochem Mol Biol 1995; 30: 387–444.

Fairbanks MB, Mildner AM, Leone JW, Cavey GS, Mathews WR, Drong RF, Slightom JL, Bienkowski MJ, Smith CW, Bannow CA, Heinrikson RL. Processing of the human heparanase precursor and evidence that the active enzyme is a heterodimer. J Biol Chem 1999; 274: 29587–29590.

Finkel E. Potential target found for anti-metastasis drugs. Science 1999; 285: 33–34.

Folkman J, Shing Y. Control of angiogenesis by heparin and other sulfated polysaccharides. Adv Exp Med Biol 1992; 313: 355–364.

Freeman C, Parish CR. Human platelet heparanase: purification characterization and catalytic activity. Biochem J 1998; 330: 1341–1350.

Freeman C, Browne AM, Parish CR. Evidence that platelet and tumour heparanases are similar enzymes. Biochem J 1999; 342: 361–368.

Friedmann Y, Vlodavsky I, Aingorn H, Aviv A, Peretz T, Pecker I, Pappo O. Expression of heparanase in normal dysplastic and Neoplastic human colon mucosa and stroma. Am J Pathol 2000; 108: 341–347.

Gilat D, Hershkoviz R, Goldkorn I, Cahalon L, Korner G, Vlodavsky I, Lider O. Molecular behavior adapts to context: heparanase functions as an extracellular matrix-degrading enzyme or as a T cell adhesion molecule depending on the local pH. J Exp Med 1995; 181, 1929–1934.

Gohji K, Hirano H, Okamoto M, Kitazawa S, Toyoshima M, Dong J, Katsuoka Y, Nakajima M. Expression of three extracellular matrix degradative enzymes in bladder cancer. Int J Cancer 2001; 95: 295–301.

Goldshmidt O, Nadav L, Aingorn H, Irit C, Feinstein N, Ilan N, Zamir E, Geiger B, Vlodavsky I, Katz BZ. Human heparanase is localized within lysosomes in a stable form. Exptl Cell Res 2002; 281: 50–62.

Goldshmidt O, Zcharia E, Abramovitch R, Metzger S, Aingorn H, Friedmann Y, Mitrani E, Vlodavsky I. Cell surface expression and secretion of heparanase markedly promote tumor angiogenesis and metastasis. Proc Natl Acad Sci USA 2002; 99: 10031–10036.

Goldshmidt O, Zcharia E, Aingorn H, Guatta-Rangini Z, Atzmon R, Michal I, Pecker I, Mitrani E, Vlodavsky I. Secretion and expression pattern of human and chicken heparanase are determined by their signal peptide sequences. J Biol Chem 2001; 276: 29178–29187.

Goshen R, Hochberg AA, Korner G, Levy E, Ishai-Michaeli R, Elkin M, de Groot N, Vlodavsky I. Purification and characterization of placental heparanase and its expression by cultured cytotrophoblasts. Mol Hum Reprod 1996; 2: 679–684.

Graham LD, Underwood PA. Comparison of the heparanase enzymes from mouse melanoma cells, mouse macrophages and human platelets. Biochem Mol Biol Int 1996; 39: 563–571.

Green D, Hull RD, Brant R, Pineo GF. Lower mortality in cancer patients treated with low-molecular-weight versus standard heparin [letter]. Lancet 1992; 339: 1476.

Hoogewerf AJ, Leone JW, Reardon IM, Howe WJ, Asa D, Heinrikson RL, Ledbetter SR. CXC chemokines connective tissue activating peptide-III and neutrophil activating peptide-2 are heparin/heparan sulfate-degrading enzymes. J Biol Chem 1995; 270: 3268–3277.

Hulett MD, Freeman C, Hamdorf BJ, Baker RT, Harris MJ, Parish CR. Cloning of mammalian heparanase, an important enzyme in tumor invasion and metastasis. Nat Med 1999; 5: 803–809.

Hulett MD, Hornbu JR, Ohms SJ, Zuegg J, Freeman C, Gready JE, Parish CR. Identification of active-site of the pro-metastatic endoglycisidase heparanase. Biochemistry 2000; 39: 15659–15667.

Iozzo RV. Matrix proteoglycans: from molecular design to cellular function. Annu Rev Biochem 1998; 67: 609–652.

249

Jin L, Nakajima M, Nicolson GL. Immunochemical localization of heparanase in mouse and human melanomas. Int J Cancer 1990; 45: 1088–1095.

Kjellen L, Lindahl U. Proteoglycans: structures and interactions. Annu Rev Biochem 1991; 60: 443–475.

Kjellen L, Pertoft H, Oldberg A, Hook M. Oligosaccharides generated by an endoglucuronidase are intermediates in the intracellular degradation of heparan sulfate proteoglycans. J Biol Chem 1985; 260: 8416–8422.

Klein U, Von Figura K. Partial purification and characterization of heparan sulfate specific endoglucuronidase. Biochem Biophys Res Commun 1976; 73: 569–576.

Kleiner DE Jr, Stetler-Stevenson WG. Structural biochemistry and activation of matrix metallo-proteases. Curr Opin Cell Biol 1993; 5: 891–897.

Koenig A, Norgard-Sumnicht K, Linhardt R, Varki A. Differential interactions of heparin and heparan sulfate glycosaminoglycans with the selectins. Implications for the use of unfraction-ated and low molecular weight heparins as therapeutic agents. J Clin Invest 1998; 101: 877–889.

Koliopanos A, Friess H, Kleeff J, Shi X, Liao Q, Pecker I, Vlodavsky I, Zimmermann A, Büchler MW. Heparanase expression in primary and metastatic pancreatic cancer. Cancer Res 2001; 61: 4655–4659.

Kussie PH, Hulmes JD, Ludwig DL, Patel S, Navarro EC, Seddon AP, Giorgio NA, Bohlen P. Cloning and functional expression of a human heparanase gene. Biochem Biophys Res Commun 1999; 261: 183–187.

Liotta LA, Rao CN, Barsky SH. Tumor invasion and the extracellular matrix. Lab Invest 1983; 49: 636–649.

Marchetti D, Liu S, Spohn WC, Carson DD. Heparanase and a synthetic peptide of heparan sulfate-interacting protein recognize common sites on cell surface and extracellular matrix heparan sulfate. J Biol Chem 1997; 272: 15891–15897.

Matzner Y, Vlodavsky I, Bar-Ner M, Ishai-Michaeli R, Tauber AI. Subcellular localization of heparanase in human neutrophils. J Leukoc Biol 1992; 51: 519–524.

Miao HQ, Elkin M Aingorn E, Ishai-Michaeli R, Stein CA, Vlodavsky I. Inhibition of heparanase activity and tumor metastasis by laminarin sulfate and synthetic phosphorothioate oligo-deoxynucleotides. Int J Cancer 1999; 83: 424–431.

Mishima T, Murata J, Toyoshima M, Fujii H, Nakajima M, Hayashi T, Kato T, Saiki I. Inhibition of tumor invasion and metastasis by calcium spirulan (Ca-SP), a novel sulfated polysaccha-ride derived from a blue-green alga Spirulina platensis. Clin Exp Metastasis 1998; 16: 541–550.

Mollinedo F, Nakajima M, Llorens A, Barbosa E, Callejo S, Gajate C, Fabra A. Major co-local-ization of the extracellular-matrix degradative enzymes heparanase and gelatinase in tertiary granules of human neutrophils. Biochem J 1997; 327: 917–923.

Nadav L, Yacoby-Zeevi O, Zamir E, Pecker I, Ilan N, Geiger B, Eldor A, Vlodavsky I, Katz BZ. Activation, processing and trafficking of extracellular heparanase by primary human fibroblasts. J Cell Sci 2002; 115: 2179–2187.

Nakajima M, DeChavigny, A Johnson CE, Hamada J, Stein CA, Nicolson GL. Suramin. A potent inhibitor of melanoma, heparanase and invasion. J Biol Chem 1991; 266: 9661–9666.

Nakajima M, Irimura T, Nicolson GL. Heparanases and tumor metastasis. J Cell Biochem 1988; 36: 157–167.

Oosta GM, Favreau LV, Beeler DL, Rosenberg RD. Purification and properties of human platelet heparitinase. J Biol Chem 1982; 257: 11249–11255.

Parish CR, Coombe DR, Jakobsen KB, Bennett FA, Underwood PA. Evidence that sulphated polysaccharides inhibit tumour metastasis by blocking tumour-cell-derived heparanases. Int J Cancer 1987; 40: 511–518.

Parish CR, Freeman C, Brown KJ, Francis DJ, Cowden WB. Identification of sulfated oligosac-

250

charide-based inhibitors of tumor growth and metastasis using novel in vitro assays for angiogenesis and heparanase activity. Cancer Res 1999; 59: 3433–3441.

Parish CR, Freeman C, Hulett MD. Heparanase: a key enzyme involved in cell invasion. Biochem Biophys Acta 2001; 1471: M99–M108.

Pikas DS, Li JP, Vlodavsky I, Lindahl U. Substrate specificity of heparanases from human hepatoma and platelets. J Biol Chem 1998; 273: 18770–18777.

Rapraeger AC. The coordinated regulation of heparan sulfate syndecans and cell behavior. Curr Opin Cell Biol 1993; 5: 844–853.

Saiki I, Murata J, Nakajima M, Tokura S, Azuma I. Inhibition by sulfated chitin derivatives of invasion through extracellular matrix and enzymatic degradation by metastatic melanoma cells. Cancer Res 1990; 50: 3631–3637.

Sivaram P, Obunike JC, Goldberg IJ. Lysolecithin-induced alteration of subendothelial heparan sulfate proteoglycans increases monocyte binding to matrix. J Biol Chem 1995; 270: 29760–29765.

Stetler-Stevenson WG. Matrix metalloproteinases in angiogenesis: a moving target for therapeutic intervention. J Clin Invest 1999; 103: 1237–1241.

Toyoshima M, Nakajima M. Human heparanase. Purification characterization cloning and expression. J Biol Chem 1999; 274: 24153–24160.

Vlodavsky I, Bar-Shavit R, Ishai-Michaeli R, Bashkin P, Fuks Z. Extracellular sequestration and release of fibroblast growth factor: a regulatory mechanism? Trends Biochem Sci 1991; 16: 268–271.

Vlodavsky I, Bar-Shavit R, Korner G, Fuks Z. Extracellular matix-bound growth factors enzymes and plasma proteins. In: Rohrbach DH, Timpl R (eds), *Basement Membranes: Cellular and Molecular Aspects*. Academic Press Inc, Orlando, FL, 1993, pp. 327–343.

Vlodavsky I, Eldor A, Haimovitz-Friedman A, Matzner Y, Ishai-Michaeli R, Lider O, Naparstek Y, Cohen IR, Fuks Z. Expression of heparanase by platelets and circulating cells of the immune system: possible involvement in diapedesis and extravasation. Invasion Metastasis 1992; 12: 112–127.

Vlodavsky I, Elkin M, Pappo O, Aingorn H, Atzmon R, Ishai-Michaeli R, Aviv A, Pecker I, Friedmann Y. Mammalian heparanase as mediator of tumor metastasis and angiogenesis. Is Med Assoc J 2000; 2: 37–45.

Vlodavsky I, Friedmann Y. Molecular properties and function of heparanase in cancer metastasis and angiogenesis. J Clin Invest 2001; 108; 341–347.

Vlodavsky I, Friedmann Y, Elkin M, Aingorn H, Atzmon R, Ishai-Michaeli Bitan M, Pappo, O, Peretz T, Michal I, Spector L, Pecker I. Mammalian heparanase: gene cloning expression and function in tumor progression and metastasis. Nat Med 1999; 5: 793–802.

Vlodavsky I, Fuks Z, Bar-Ner M, Ariav Y, Schirrmacher V. Lymphoma cell-mediated degradation of sulfated proteoglycans in the subendothelial extracellular matrix: relationship to tumor cell metastasis. Cancer Res 1983; 43: 2704–2711.

Vlodavsky I, Miao H-Q, Benezra M, Lidaer O, Bar-Shavit R, Schmidt A, Peretz T. Involvement of the extracellular matrix heparan sulfate proteoglycans and heparan sulfate degrading enzymes in angiogenesis and metastasis. In: Lewis CE, Bicknell R, Ferrara N (eds), *Tumor Angiogenesis*. Oxford University Press, Oxford, UK, 1997, pp. 125–140.

Vlodavsky I, Miao HQ, Medalion B, Danagher P, Ron D. Involvement of heparan sulfate and related molecules in sequestration and growth promoting activity of fibroblast growth factor. Cancer Metastasis Rev 1996; 15: 177–186.

Vlodavsky I, Mohsen M, Lider O, Svahn CM, Ekre HP, Vigoda M, Ishai-Michaeli R, Peretz T. Inhibition of tumor metastasis by heparanase inhibiting species of heparin. Invasion Metastasis 1994; 14: 290–302.

Walch ET, Albino AP, Marchetti D. Correlation of overexpression of the low-affinity p75 neurotrophin receptor with augmented invasion and heparanase production in human malignant melanoma cells. Int J Cancer 1999; 82: 112–120.

Weiss RE, Liu BC, Ahlering T, Dubeau L, Droller MJ. Mechanisms of human bladder tumor invasion: role of protease cathepsin B. J Urol 1990; 144: 798–804.

Wight TN. Cell biology of arterial proteoglycans. Arteriosclerosis 1989; 9: 1–20.

Wight TN, Kinsella MG, Qwarnstrom EE. The role of proteoglycans in cell adhesion migration and proliferation. Curr Opin Cell Biol 1992; 4: 793–801.

Yanagishita M. Inhibition of intracellular degradation of proteoglycans by leupeptin in rat ovarian granulosa cells. J Biol Chem 1985; 260: 11075–11082.

INDEX